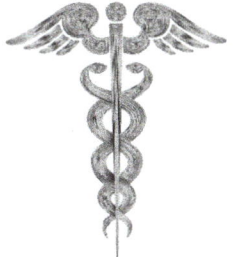

# Medical School Bound

## The ESSENTIAL Guide to BS/MD, BS/DO, BS/DDS, & Pre-Med Programs

### For High School Students

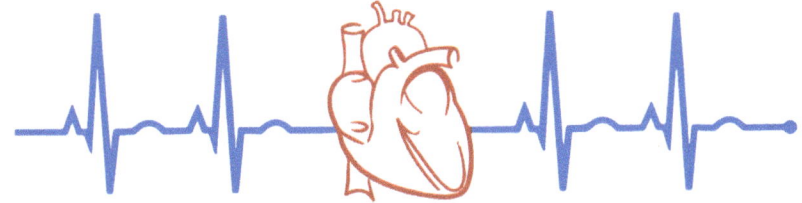

## Rachel A. Winston, Ph.D.

*Researcher, Professor, Admissions Expert, Motivational Speaker*

Lizard Publishing is not sponsored by any college. While data was derived from school, state, or nationally published sources, some statistics may be out of date, since published sources vary widely based upon the date of submission and currency of numbers. Attempts were made to obtain the best information during the writing of this book from NCES, U.S. Census Bureau, U.S. Department of Education, Common Data Set, College Board, *U.S. News & World Report*, college, and organizational sites. Descriptions of colleges are a compilation of college website information as well as interviews with student, faculty, and staff interviews providing their unique experiences and impressions. Attempts were made to triangulate multiple points of light. If you would like to share program information, data, or an impression of a specific college, please write to Lizard Publishing at the address below or at the e-mail address: *collegeguide@yahoo.com*

ISBN (hardback); 978-1-958558-51-5 (paperback); 978-1-958558-52-2 (e-book); 978-1-958558-53-9

LCCN: 2025904874

Lizard Publishing, 7700 Irvine Center Drive, Suite 800, Irvine, CA 92618 *www.lizard-publishing.com*

Lizard Publishing creates, designs, produces, and distributes books and resources to provide academic, admissions, and career information. Our mental process is fueled by three tenets:

- Ignite the hunger to learn and the passion to make a difference
- Illuminate the expanse of knowledge by sharing cutting edge thinking
- Innovate to create a world that makes the transition from dreams to reality

We work with academic leaders who transform the educational landscape to publish relevant content and advise students of their educational and professional options, with the aim of developing 21st-century learners and leaders. We also work with students to publish their books and present widely diverse ideas to the college/graduate school-bound community. With headquarters in Irvine, California, Lizard Publishing works virtually with authors to edit, publish, and distribute digital, paperback, and hard copy books.

This book was published in the U.S.A. Lizard Publishing is a premium quality provider of educational reference, career guidance, and motivational publications/merchandise for global learners, educators, and stakeholders in education.

Book design by Michelle Tahan *www.michelletahan.com*

Book formatting by Obinna Chinemerem Ozuo *(ozuobinna@gmail.com)*

Book website: *www.bsmdguide.com*

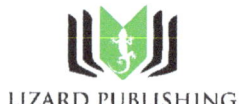

LIZARD PUBLISHING

# ACKNOWLEDGEMENTS

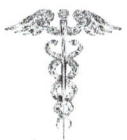

There is never enough room to acknowledge every person who contributed to an individual's perspective, assisted in the development of a person's knowledge base, or taught indelible lessons that last a lifetime. In this book, I gratefully acknowledge David Waugh, Malka Mirvis, Robert Helmer, Zenobia Murray, Michelle Tahan, Jasmine Jhunjhnuwala, and Obinna Ozuo as well as my family, friends, colleagues, and professors.

I would also like to thank the thousands of students I have taught, counseled, or tutored in my more than forty years of service in education.

Isaac Newton once said, "If I see so far, it is because I stand on the shoulders of giants." A few of those giants whose broad shoulders lifted me higher and taught me invaluable lessons include: Lauren/Patrick Bayeh, Jill Board, Dan Burke, Ria/Pria Chawla, Anabella/Andersen Cheong, Lana/Rita Debbaneh, Arya/Farangis Ebrahimi, Joey/Ricky Hanzich, Annette Hartenstein, Chase/Chad Heger, Joel Horwich, Raymond Hunter, Skipper John, Arpi/Ashray Kapuria, Kim Kelly, Riki Kucheck, Linda Lebile, Chelsea Lee, Caley Lynch, Jim Manion, Samantha Mann, JaNice Marshall, John Mearsheimer, Leigh Moore, Zenobia Murray, Tamar Nicherie, Michael Ortell, Sornya/Skorn Ponrartana, Eesa/Maryam Quraishi, Mary Retterer, Steve Robinson, Martha Rogers, John E. Roueche, Maya/Taya Salman, Sandra Savage, John Smart, James Sullivan, Michelle Temby, Natalie Tran, Harrison White, and Jacqueline Xu.

*"If I see so far, it is because I stand on the shoulders of giants."*
*— Isaac Newton*

Lizard Publishing creates, designs, produces, and distributes books and resources to provide academic, admissions, and career information.

As a faculty member in the UCLA College Counseling Certificate Program, I met many dedicated counselors who devote their lives to serving and supporting students. Meaningful contributions to this book have also been made indirectly by admissions representatives, college counselors, and faculty members who took a special interest in its success.

Finally, there would be no book covering university BS/MD, BS/DO, BS/DDS, BS/DVM, and medical programs and no career in college admissions counseling without the support of Robert Helmer, whose tireless efforts support me every single day.

# ABOUT THE AUTHOR

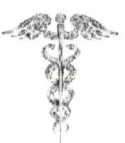

D r. Rachel A. Winston is a tireless student-advocate. She has served the educational community as a university professor, college advisor, statistician, cryptanalyst, motivational speaker, medical scientist, lifelong student, Faculty Member of the Year, Academic Senate President, and elected statewide college leader. As one of the leading experts in college counseling, Dr. Winston has spent her lifetime learning, teaching and mentoring students on their pathway from high school to medical school and residency.

She started college at thirteen and graduated from college programs in such widely ranging disciplines as chemistry, mathematics, educational computing, liberal arts, international relations, business administration, higher education leadership, interpreting, college counseling, and publishing. Throughout her education, she attended Harvard, UChicago, NYU, GWU, Syracuse, Maryland, UCLA, UCI, CSUF, CSUDH, Cal Poly, ASU, Claremont Graduate University, Pepperdine, and USC among other colleges.

Her position working in Washington, D.C. on Capitol Hill and with the White House in the 1980s took her to approximately a hundred universities training campaign managers at colleges from Colorado to California, thoroughly dotting the western states. Later, she led college tours with students and their families on road trips throughout the United States. She has taught or counseled thousands of students over her career and speaks at conferences and academic programs throughout the world.

As a professor and avid writer for numerous publications, she won the 2012 McFarland Literary Achievement Award and numerous other awards, including National Science Foundation grants, Leadership Tomorrow Leader of the Year, and college service and leadership awards. Studying Human Capital at Claremont Graduate University, she was a scholarship recipient at the Drucker School of Management. She was also elected to positions in national science organizations and the Board of Directors of the Newport Chamber of Commerce.

She served as a faculty member for the UCLA College Counselor Certificate Program, the Director of Mathematics at Brandman University, and a professor at Embry Riddle Aeronautical University, Chapman University, Cal State Fullerton, and a few California Community Colleges, including Cerro Coso College where she also served as the Academic Senate President and retired in 2016. Over her career, she taught mathematics online, on television, live interactive satellite, telecourses, and in large and small lecture halls.

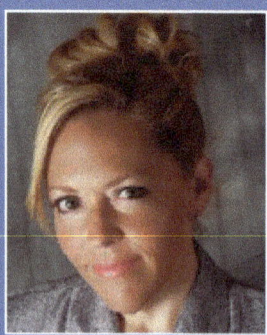

## Rachel A. Winston, Ph.D.
### Researcher, Professor, Admissions Expert, Motivational Speaker

*"Knowledge has to be improved, challenged, and increased constantly; or it vanishes."*

# AUTHOR'S NOTE

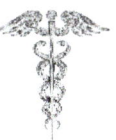

You are reading this book because you are considering a medical school education. Whether you choose to pursue the BS/MD, BS/DO, BS.DDS, or premedical route, or apply to programs with the goal of deciding later, you are in the right place. Right now, you need to gather information to make informed decisions. While many people offer advice, suggestions differ. Friends will tell you the 'right' way or the way their neighbor was accepted.

Graciously accept this anecdotal information while you commit to learning more. This is your future. Dig deeper to consider both expert and current information from counselors who have worked with hundreds of BS/MD students. Changes in programs, curricula, requirements, and links happen each year. Double-check each program's specifics yourself. This guide has valuable information with each school's school's website. However, new programs come and go. A few programs have been discontinued. Be diligent and persistent in reviewing current information for changes, updates, and opportunities. Medical professionals will continue to be in high demand. You are on your way!

There are a few good books on BS/MD programs written by talented and experienced counselors. I admire and cheer on their efforts. This colorful guide is different in that a resource full of lists, timelines, and unique ways of organizing information. I hope you find this book a valuable resource.

> "We are what we think. All that we are arises with our thoughts. With our thoughts, we make the world."
> Buddha

Your job is to begin early by assembling information for the schools you are considering, creating a road map, and setting yourself on a clear path. If you see an error in this book or even a suggestion for a future edition, please write to me and let me know at collegeguide@yahoo.com. I will fix the entry with the next version I print.

All of that said, this book was written for you in mind. There is a wealth of information on the Internet with free downloads, FAQs, testimonials, and offers to help you with your applications. Some of these advisors are knowledgeable and could help you. Some are all hype with fancy marketing and inexperienced neophytes. Yet, students and parents hunt around the web searching for a tremendous number of hours seeking the information they need. This book was designed to make your search easier.

For now, though, I will assume that you are reasonably confident that you want to attend medical school and are exploring this avenue as a possible way to take advantage of a program that will get you on your way toward your goal. I will also assume that you are a highly academic candidate who is willing to work very hard. You should also have a curiosity about or fascination with the human body, passion for medicine, or a commitment to serve others selflessly. These are virtually prerequisites for BS/MD, BS/DO, or BS/DDS programs.

As you investigate colleges, you might find differences in the names of these programs - BS/MD, BA/MD, BS/DO, BA/DO, BS/DDS, BS.DMD, direct med, early acceptance, or early assurance programs. Applying to and writing essays for each application requires research. While you might have in your mind that direct med programs are relatively similar, each program's nuances make them very different. While these changes may seem confusing, my goal with this book is to demystify the process.

# CONTENTS

## Part One

### The Road to Medical School

There Is No Royal Road
1

The Right & Wrong Reasons
5

Preparing For The Journey
9

Is The Direct Route or The Traditional Premed Path Right For You?
13

Medicine & Affiliated Medical Careers
19

Covid-19 & The Medical School Pipeline
25

## Part Two

### Preparation for BS/MD & BS/DDS Programs

Coursework and GPA
33

Testing
37

Volunteer & Service Activities
43

Research & Healthcare Experiences
47

Academic Preparation & Competitions
53

Athletics, Clubs, Involvement
73

Summer Programs
77

Study Skills & Tutoring
121

Desired Qualities
125

# Part Three

## Timelines, Calendars, and Checklists

Planning Ahead 8th – 10th Grade
131

Junior Year Ramp Up
135

Senior Year Seriousness
139

College Prep Calendar
143

College Admission Checklist
147

Words of Advice
151

Note to Parents
155

# Part 4

## Which Programs Are Best for You?

Researching Schools
161

Allopathic Vs. Osteopathic Medicine
165

BS/MD, BS/DO, Direct Med, Early Acceptance
171

Curriculum, Catalog, & Requirements
177

Support Services
183

College Visits
189

College Events, Fairs, & Representatives
193

Narrowing Your List
197

Where to Apply?
201

International Student Pathway
205

Reconsidering the Traditional Pathway
209

Dental School, PA, PharmD, Vet School
213

Looking Ahead - MCAT, Med School
217

# Part Five

## Application & Admissions Process

The College Admissions Process
223

ED, EA, REA, RD, & Rolling
227

Your College Counselor
231

Choosing a Major
235

Recommendations
239

Essays, Supplement Essays, and AI
243

Resume
247

Portfolios, Abstracts, Talent
251

Interviews
257

Portals, Verification, Validity
261

Financial Aid & Scholarships
267

Deferrals, Waitlists, & Decisions & Waitlists
279

Next Steps: Transitioning to College
285

# Part six

## Profiles of BS/MD, BA/MD, BS/DO Programs

List of BS/MD and BS/DO Programs
293

Northeast
294

Midwest
312

South
320

West
332

# Part 7

## Lists of College Programs

List of B/MD, B/DO, EAP, and Direct Med by State/City
340

BS/MD State Residency Required List
342

D.O. Schools List
347

Dental Schools List
349

PharmD. Schools List
351

Vet Schools List
355

BS/MD Timeline
357

Index
359

# GLOSSARY AND ACRONYMS

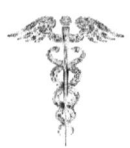

## ACADEMIC FIELDS OF STUDY

**Biological Sciences:** biochemistry, biomedicine, cell biology, conservation, ecology, genetics, human biology, immunology, microbiology, pathobiology, and physiology

**Humanities:** ancient culture, art, dance, English, film, foreign languages, history, law, literature, music, philosophy, politics, religion, and theater

**Math and Statistics:** actuarial science, artificial intelligence, bioinformatics, biostatistics, computational neuroscience, cryptology, data science, demographics, econometrics, epidemiological modeling, operations research, optimization, population genetics, predictive analysis, reliability analysis, and statistics

**Physical Sciences/Engineering:** astronomy, chemistry, computer science, engineering, geology, meteorology, physical geography, physics

**Social Sciences:** anthropology, criminal justice, economics, geography, history, international relations, political science, sociology, and psychology

**Specialized Health Sciences:** dietetics, gerontology, kinesiology, nursing, nutrition, occupational therapy, public health

## APPLICATION TERMS

**AMCAS Work & Activities Section** - This area allows you to present and describe more than a dozen activities you have pursued.

**Clinical Hours** - These experiential hours include work in a hospital/clinic, shadowing physicians, or working directly with patients.

**Research Hours** - This includes time spent in laboratory or clinical research experiences.

**Rolling Admission** - This is when schools review applications as they arrive. Typically, when the spots are filled, there are no additional spaces. So, apply early.

**Shadowing** - Students observe doctors in hospitals or clinics to better understand the practice of a physician.

# ACRONYMS

**AAMC** - American Association of Medical Colleges
**AACOM** - American Association of Colleges of Osteopathic Medicine
**AMCAS** - American Medical College Application Service
**BCPM** - Biology, Chemistry, Physics, and Math
**CSS** - College Scholarship Service
**DAT** - Dental Admissions Test
**DDS** - Doctor of Dental Surgery
**DMD** - Doctor of Medicine in Dentistry or Doctor of Dental Medicine
**DO** - Doctor of Osteopathic Medicine
**EA** - Early Action
**EAP** - Early Admission Program, Early Acceptance Program, or Early Assurance
        Program depending upon the school
**ED** - Early Decision
**FAFSA** - Free Application for Federal Student Aid
**GAP** - Guaranteed Admissions Program
**GPPA** – Guaranteed Professional Programs Admissions
**HOBY** - Hugh O'Brian Youth (Leadership Program)
**HPM** – Health Professions Mentoring
**HPME** –  Honors Program in Medical Education
**JAMP** – Joint Admissions Medical Program
**JAS** – Joint Admissions Scholars
**LECOM** - Lake Erie College of Osteopathic Medicine
**MCAT** - Medical College Admission Test
**MD** – Medical Doctor or Doctor of Medicine
**MITES** - Minority Introduction to Engineering and Science
**MPH** – Master of Public Health
**MSAR** - Medical School Admission Requirements
**MSP** –  Medical Scholars Program
**NEOMED** – Northeast Ohio Medical University
**Ph.D.** – Doctor of Philosophy
**PLME** – Program in Liberal Medical Education
**Post-Bacc** – Post Baccalaureate (programs after earning a BA or BS)
**PPSP** – Pre-Professional Scholars Program
**RD** - Regular Decision
**REA** - Restricted Early Action
**REMS** – Rochester Early Medical Scholars
**RHOP** – Rural Health Opportunities Program
**SLOs** – Student Learning Objectives
**SPiM** – Special Program in Medicine
**STEM** - Science, Technology, Engineering, and Mathematics
**TMDSAS** - Texas Medical & Dental Schools Application Service
**UMKC** - University of Missouri, Kansas City
**USMLE** - United States Medical Licensing Examination

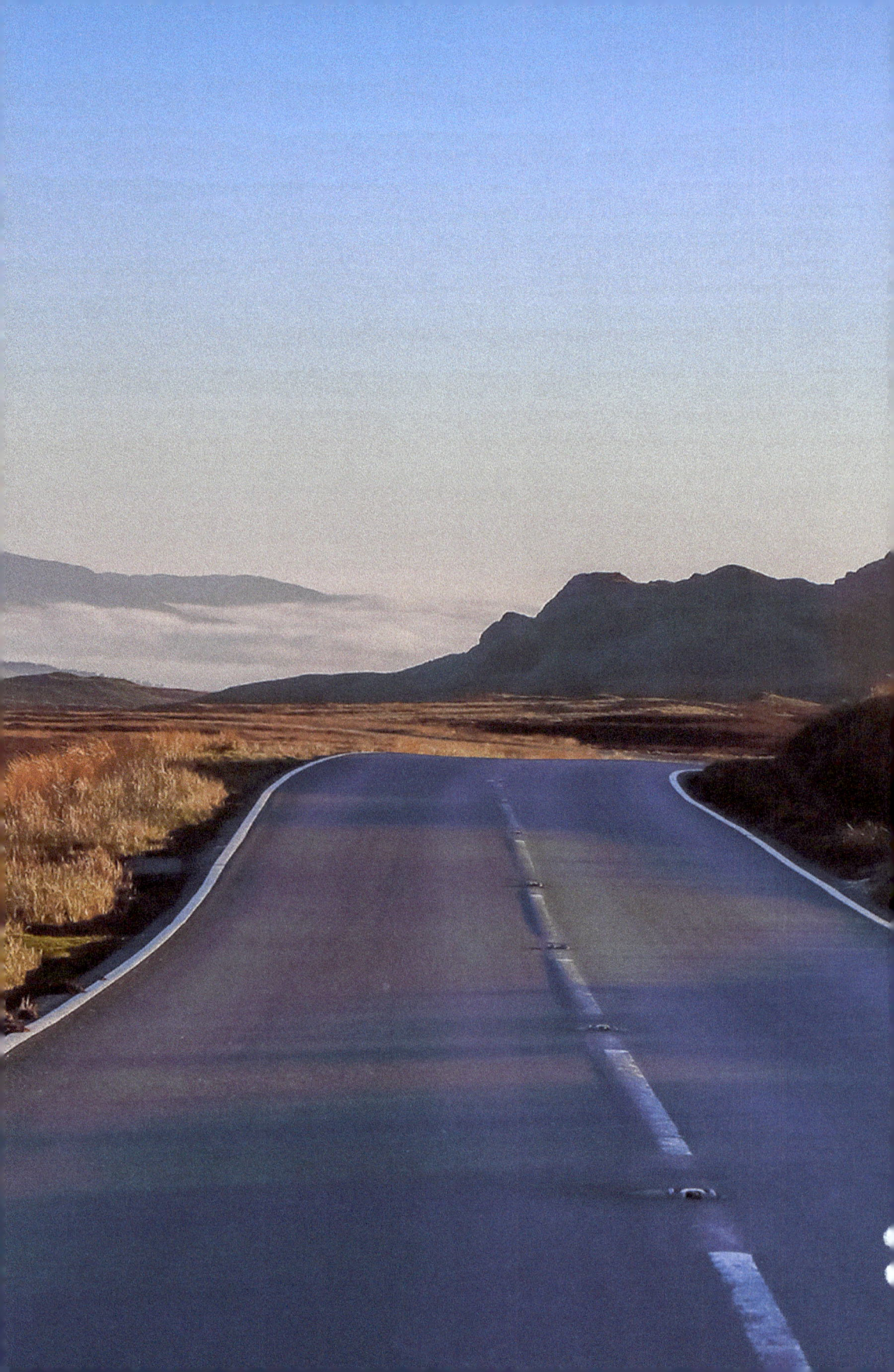

# PART ONE

# THE ROAD TO MEDICAL SCHOOL

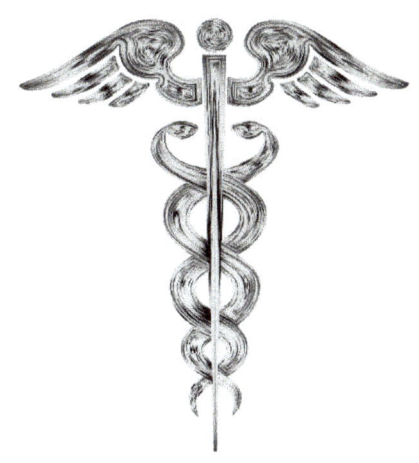

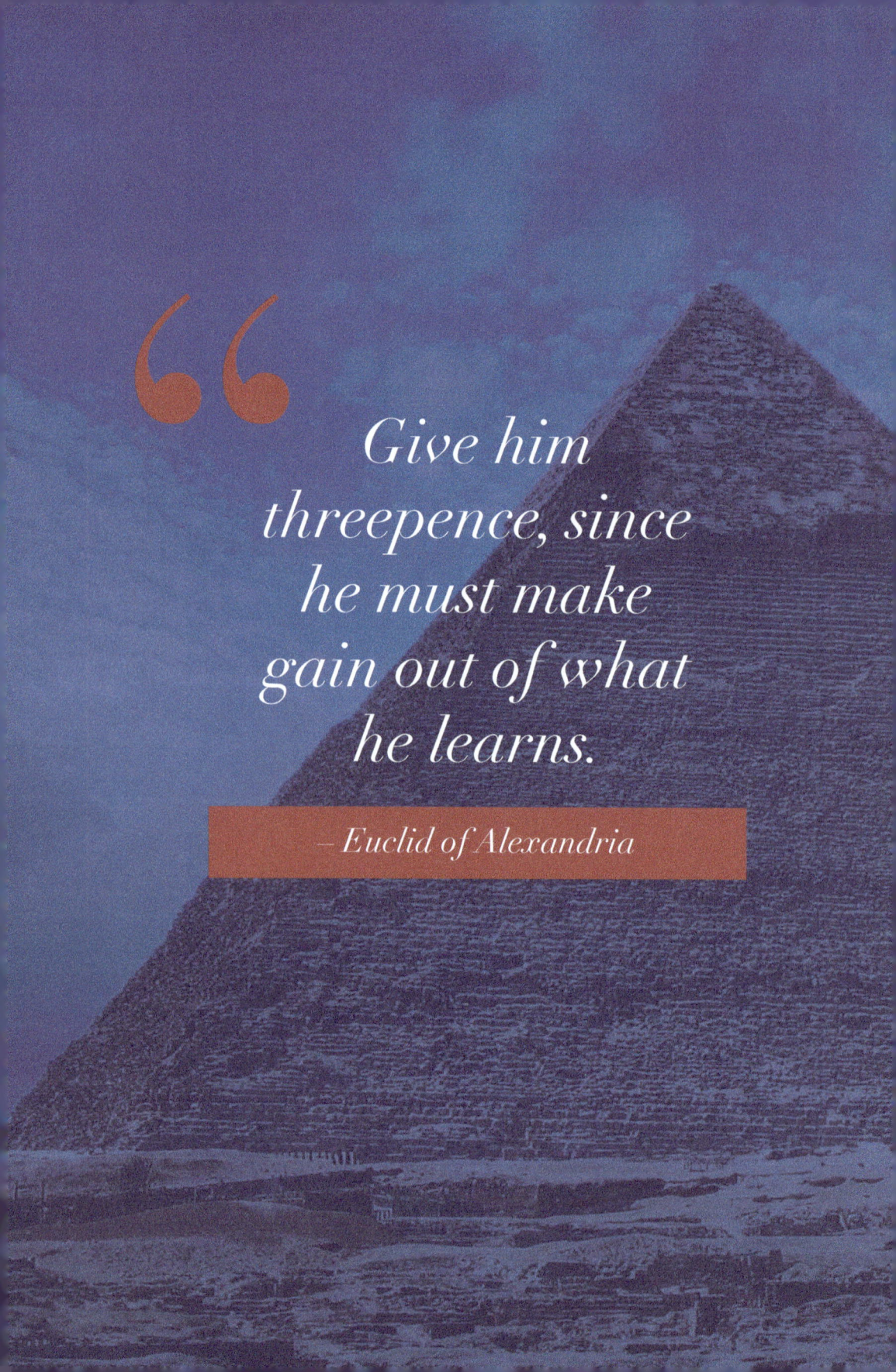

"

*Give him
threepence, since
he must make
gain out of what
he learns.*

*— Euclid of Alexandria*

## CHAPTER ONE

# THERE IS NO ROYAL ROAD

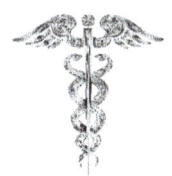

Euclid of Alexandria (~365 BCE – ~300 BCE), a mathematician who was thought to be a student of Plato, wrote one of the most widely read collection of books in all of history called *Elements*. This series of thirteen texts rigorously lays the foundation for mathematics, proofs, and spatial representations. The books emphasize deduction, logically constructed from explicitly stated assumptions. Although much of the contents were known long beforehand, Euclid systematically organized the definitions, abstractions, and proofs in a comprehensive set of texts.

Proclus Lycaeus (412 AD – 485 AD) wrote that when Ptolemy 1 was studying *Elements*, he struggled with the concepts. Ptolemy 1 asked if there was an easier way to learn the material. Euclid responded to the future ruler of Egypt (323 BCE – 283 BCE), "There is no royal road to geometry."

Similarly, there is no royal road to BS/MD, BS/DO, or BS/DDS programs. The road is long, difficult, and not designed for those who want an easy path. Students must take the hardest courses and earn the top scores on the SAT or ACT, while also participating in service, leadership, clinical, and/or research.

Fortunately, the MCAT or DAT is not required in a few direct medical/dental school programs. In these, students are guaranteed admission if they keep up their grades. The saving grace is the peace of mind that if they learn the required material, they will not have to sweat another grueling and very competitive admissions process with no assurance of admission. After all, Harvard Medical School has a 3.8% chance of acceptance.

In another anecdote, a frustrated student asked what he would get out of studying geometry. Euclid, in a sarcastic reply, told his servant, "Give him threepence, since he must make gain out of what he learns." Admissions representatives are keenly aware of students who complete only the minimum community service, clinical, and research requirements to 'look good'. Euclid might say, "Must you get credit or 'make gain out of what you learn' or are you so passionate about your chosen activities that you would do them anyway?"

There is another saying that goes, "Do what you love, and the money will come." Relating this to your current pursuit might translate to, "Do what you love, and you will enjoy your life no matter what happens in the future." Undoubtedly, both attitudes are recognizable during interviews. Trained interviewers look for passion and commitment.

STEM teachers and athletic coaches remind students that disciplined learning is often not easy. Effort and practice are required for mastery. This is particularly true for coursework in pursuit of medical school since 'failure is not an option'. Students must be persistent in mastering the required subject matter. Organic chemistry notoriously challenges students to their limits. Note: Study more chemistry in high school!

You may not realize the reasons for studying theoretical concepts that may seem too abstruse or abstract to be necessary or relevant. Nevertheless, there are many reasons for learning and mastering difficult concepts, not the least of which are logical reasoning and rigorous analysis of assumptions. There are no short cuts to medicine or 'royal road' that will smooth out your path. However, with persistence, diligence, and serious study, you will find that the result is worth the effort.

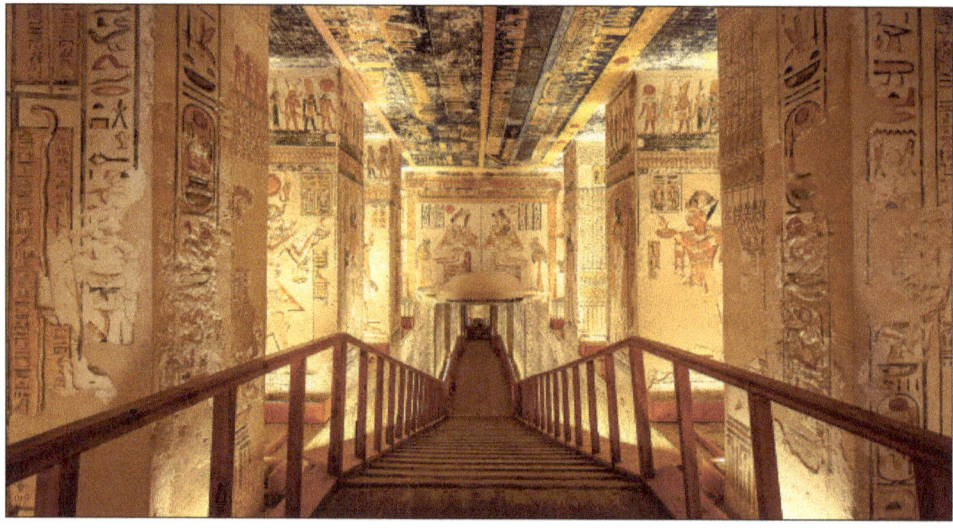

There is truly no royal road to medical school no matter what people say. Direct medical programs are just one path. You can reach the same destination via four-year college programs. However, you also should know that recently more than half of medical school applicants who did not pursue a direct medical program have taken one or more gap years.

Many students take the extra time to gain clinical and research experiences. The average age of medical school matriculants is between 24 and 25 (variability noted). At this moment, consider your options. You can choose the 6, 7, or 8 year road if accepted to a BS/MD, BS/DO, BS/DDS or the 9, 10, or 11 year traditional path.

Most physicians and dentists who pursued a direct medical/dental program do not regret their decision, particularly as they watch the scribes and medical assistants who work for them struggle for years to gain admission. Yet, the most important part of this road to medical school is coupling discipline, integrity, and work ethic. Go above and beyond your high school curriculum while gaining enough familiarity with medical/dental science and practice to be certain of your goal.

No matter how good you were in high school, remember, everyone admitted to one of these programs was near the top of their class, earned high test scores, and had character-defining attributes. Beware, though. Overconfidence can lead to blind spots and a sense of entitlement or supremacy. Dispel that notion immediately. BS/MD, BS/DO, BS/DDS, BD/DMD programs are typically not win-lose games where competition reigns supreme. Support your classmates. In these programs, you are all headed in the same direction and will be colleagues for life.

Ultimately, there is no one road and certainly not a royal road. *U.S. News & World Report* presented an article in June 2025 entitled, "Why a Capstone Is No Longer Optional for Top College Admissions". Magnet program coordinators call them capstones, Boy Scouts call them Eagle Awards, Girl Scouts call them Gold Awards, and students call these passion projects. Either way, they are now common to showcase leadership, organization, financial management, and vision. Consider a capstone.

Nevertheless, if you have taken the most challenging courses and possibly some in college, you also need to stand out as an athlete, dancer, filmmaker, sail maker or farmhand. Whether you are a virtuoso violinist, soccer star, computer geek, robotics team leader, or Chemistry Olympiad champion, your persistence, and dedication will show through on your application, recommendations, and interviews.

So, go boldly on this journey to serve others. The medical/dental profession awaits your selflessness, kindness, and empathy. Work hard and diligently carve your own unique path and discover your passions at the same time.

*Allow your passion to become your purpose, and it will one day become your profession.*

— Gabrielle Bernstein

CHAPTER TWO

# THE RIGHT AND WRONG REASONS

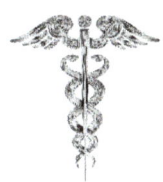

The journey to and through medical/dental school is long, but the reward is worth the effort. "No pain–no gain," as the saying goes, is the appropriate mantra. No matter how smart you are or how little you had to study to excel in the toughest classes in high school or college, the medical/dental field will demand much of you mentally and physically – more than you expected. You must be disciplined in your study habits and organized in your thinking to prepare for medical or dental school, even in a direct or accelerated program.

There are dozens of reasons why you might believe that the medical field is inspiring, rewarding, and/or appealing. A few that come to mind include:

| | |
|---|---|
| » *To serve.* | » *To extend compassion.* |
| » *To support.* | » *To work with a team of professionals.* |
| » *To care.* | » *To improve other people's lives.* |
| » *To save lives.* | » *To immerse yourself in patient care.* |
| » *To diagnose.* | » *To fix a broken system.* |
| » *To treat.* | » *To provide healthcare for the underserved.* |
| » *To resolve.* | » *To follow a rewarding path.* |
| » *To learn.* | » *To make a difference.* |
| » *To collaborate.* | » *To understand the human body.* |
| » *To research.* | » *To always be fascinated.* |
| » *To empathize.* | » *To connect to your curiosity.* |
| » *To reassure.* | » *To be intellectually stimulated.* |
| » *To help families cope with death.* | » *To get paid to do what you love.* |
| » *To persistently seek cures.* | » *To resolve issues of access and disparity.* |

These are all good reasons. The medical or dental school journey, though, is arduous. Many change their path during college. The time you invest to read and study will be long. However, the hours working day and night as a medical school intern will be even longer. Real-life medicine is not like television medical shows like *The Pitt, Doctor Odyssey, Pulse, Hyper Knife, The Trauma Code, Chicago Med, ER, House, Grey's Anatomy, The Good Doctor, Scrubs,* or *Code Black.* Even if you have the stamina, the practice of medicine demands keen attentiveness and responsive caring for fellow humans who have families, loved ones, and people who count on them.

Pursue medicine for the right reasons. Otherwise, you are likely to hit a massive roadblock. There will be times when you do not understand a concept, you hunkered down on a chemistry assignment for too long, or are simply exhausted. You might be deliriously ill, or your computer may crash after you have completed the twentieth page of a twenty-five-page paper due the next day. An internal engine with a booster shot of adrenaline can kick in at the last minute if you are certain where you are headed. Let passion fuel your heart and mind.

Patients count on you. They put their bodies and lives in your hands. Medicine and dentistry are not for people who want to be a hero, show off their intelligence, or merely gain a prestigious reputation. Many students feel the pressure to pursue medicine because their parents were doctors, or their family is urging them to go into a field where they can make a lot of money. Others simply feel that becoming a doctor will make their parents happy or proud. One or more of these wrong reasons may resonate with you, but do not let the wrong reasons be your driving force.

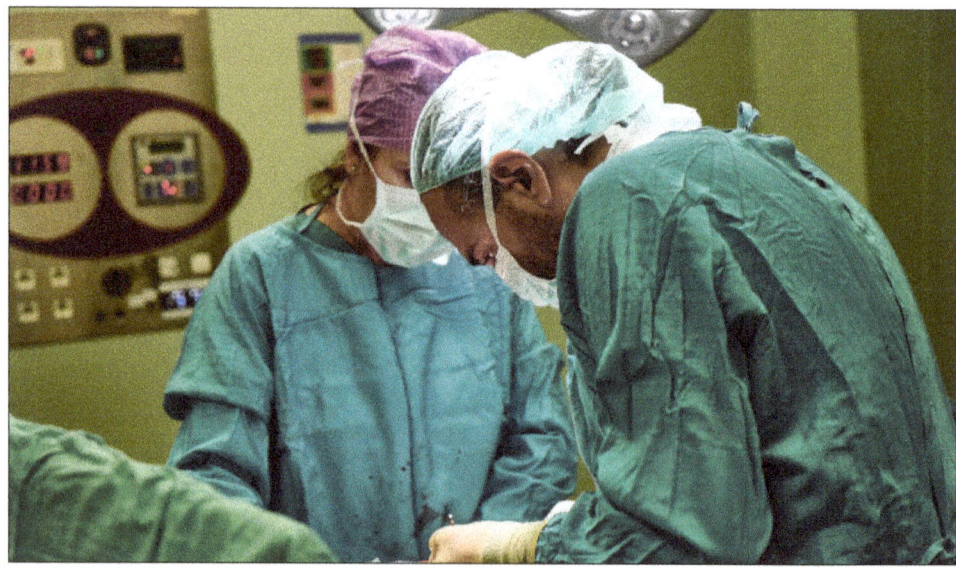

Choosing to pursue a BS/MD, BS/DO, or BS/DDS program as a high school student is one of the boldest, most life-shaping decisions you can make. Done for the right reasons, this pursuit represents a fierce commitment to service, a passion for science, and a vision for a life spent healing and innovating. Students who dream of being doctors must also envision themselves as leaders, advocates, and explorers at the frontiers of medicine. These specialized programs help you earn your degree faster as you enter a lifelong career of compassion, resilience, and transformation.

The right reason to pursue a BS/MD, BS/DO, or BS/DDS is an unwavering passion for medicine or dentistry. Applicants volunteered in clinics, served in hospitals, shadowed dentists, and feel empathy for other's suffering. They must understand human biology, stay up late reading about breakthroughs in cancer therapies, tissue regeneration, and brain-body connections. Medicine or dentistry must be a calling, not a shortcut.

There are wrong reasons to pursue a BS/MD, BS/DO, or BS/DDS program too. Choosing a direct medical/dentistry program solely for job security, parental approval, or being "set for life" will erode motivation when inevitable difficulties arise. Medical training demands more than intelligence; it demands emotional stamina, humility, and sacrifice. If your foundation is not based on genuine passion, the long years of study and confrontations with human suffering will feel hollow.

The right student embraces academic and emotional rigor with an awareness of the sacrifices, knowing that a commitment to medicine means delayed gratification, continuous growth, and tireless learning. They see setbacks not as signs they are unworthy, but as invitations to deepen their character. They approach the journey with the knowledge that their future patients deserve nothing less than their full-hearted effort. BS/MD, BS/DO, BS/DDS and, frankly, serious pre-med/pre-dent students do not ask, "What will I get out of this?" but rather, "Who can I become?" and, "Who can I serve with my knowledge?"

Ultimately, pursuing a BS/MD, BS/DO, or BS/DDS program is about believing in something bigger than oneself. It is a declaration that despite the obstacles, despite the years of hard work, you will persist because you know that in someone's most vulnerable moment, your hands, your mind, and your heart can make the difference. That is the kind of passion that carries students through sleepless nights and into operating rooms, research labs, and communities in need. This kind of passion deserves a place in a BS/MD, BS/DO, or BS.DDS program.

If you feel the commitment in your heart, you are pursuing this course toward a BS/MD, BS/DO, or BS/DDS for the right reasons.

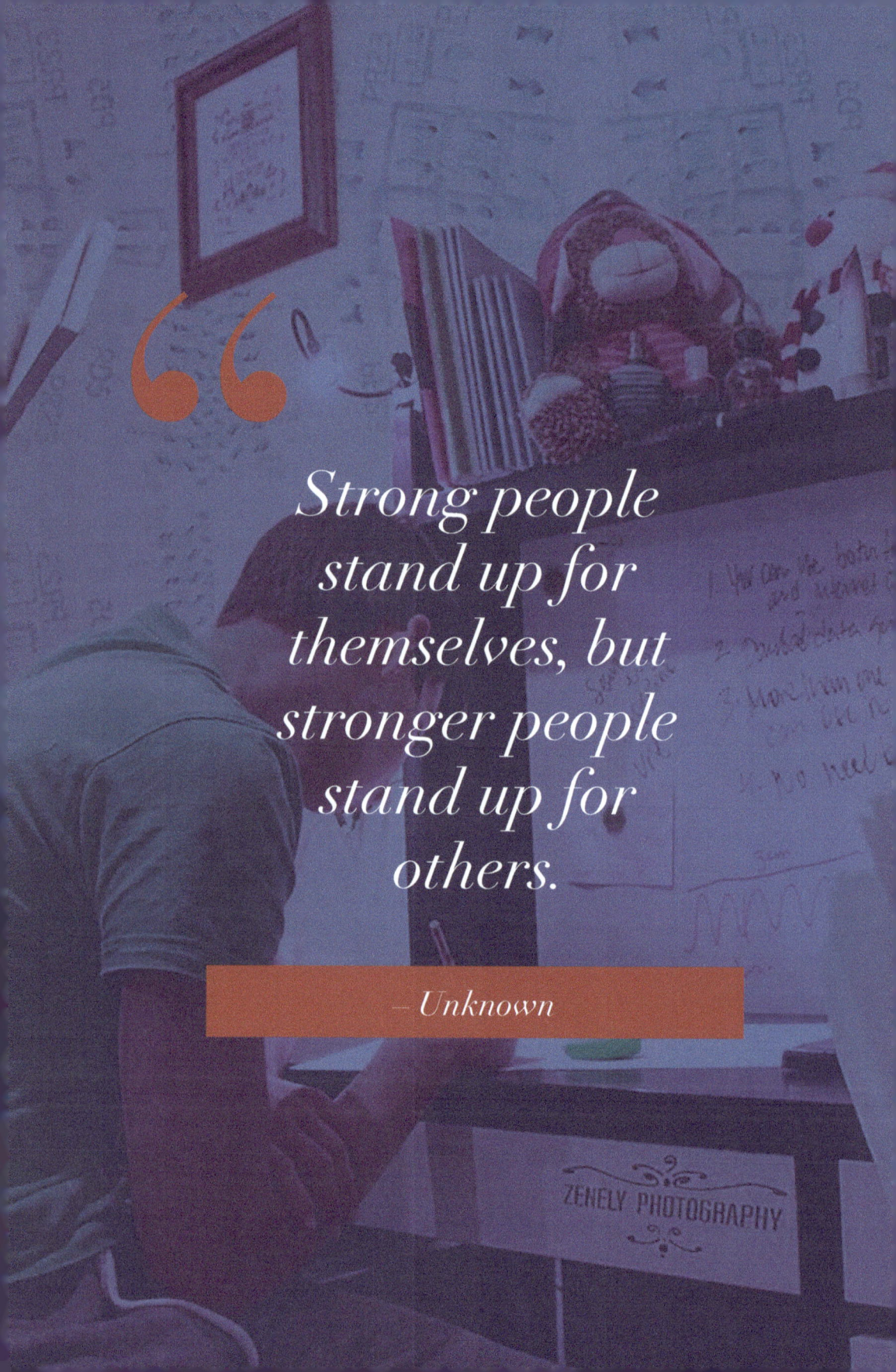

CHAPTER THREE

# PREPARING FOR THE JOURNEY

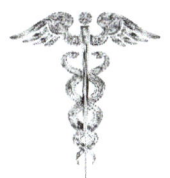

cademic choices in middle school and high school determine your trajectory. Although you can often catch up with additional math and science courses later, starting early is helpful. Depending upon the high school you attend, you may not be able to take AP or honors science classes due to restrictions or without taking prerequisites. Also, a solid math foundation is a necessity. In some cases, you need a teacher recommendation or a certain grade to proceed to higher levels. Determine the requirements and procedures for the school you attend at the outset. Most community colleges allow students to take courses to get ahead, build skills, and gain knowledge.

Academics are important, but they are not everything. Many students who seemingly study 24/7, have high grades. Yet, they do not participate in school activities, clubs, athletics, or leadership. Some have never served in the community or shadowed a doctor. These academic powerhouses are unlikely to be accepted into a BS/MD, BS/DO, or BS/DDS program.

Get involved! First, to understand the world around you and the diverse people you will serve, interact with your community. Tutor underprivileged kids. Cut vegetables at a soup kitchen. Volunteer at a retirement home. Help at a homeless shelter. Take a leadership role in Girl Scouts, Boy Scouts, National Charity League, Assistance League, or the National League of Young Men. Coach soccer, assist domestic violence victims, work with the disabled, or volunteer with refugee organizations. Ultimately, you will treat the old and young, rich and poor, and people from every ethnicity and background.

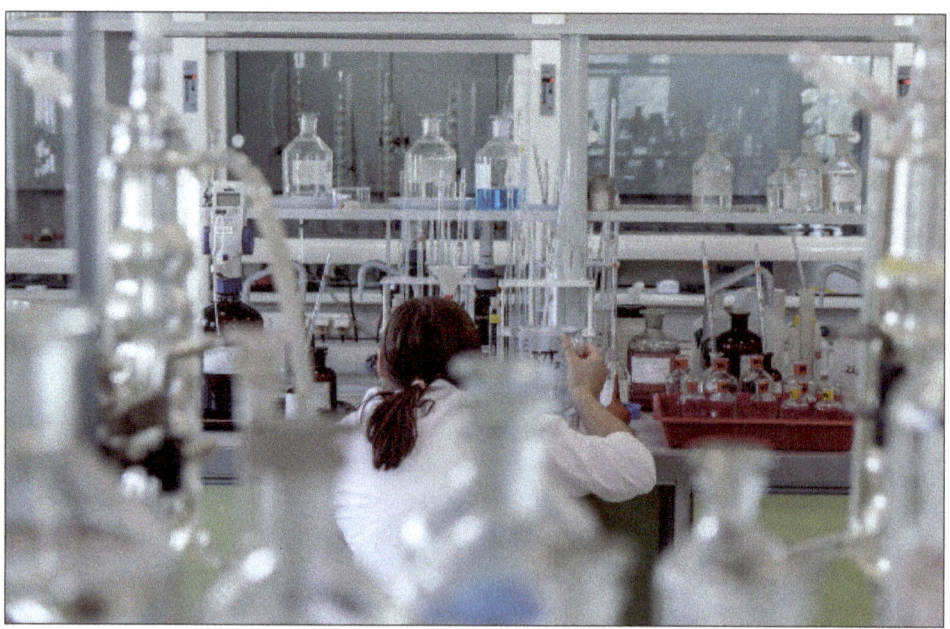

Discover activities you can do to support groups of people in your community.

| | | | |
|---|---|---|---|
| » | *Old* | » | *Gang Members* |
| » | *Young* | » | *Rural Community Members* |
| » | *Homeless* | » | *Farmers* |
| » | *Disadvantaged* | » | *Disabled* |
| » | *Rape Victims* | » | *Hospitalized* |
| » | *Refugees* | » | *Veterans* |
| » | *Immigrants* | » | *Addicts or those in Rehabilitation* |
| » | *Athletes* | » | *Victims of Domestic Violence, etc.* |

If you cannot drive, take a bus or Uber. Otherwise, you could take phone orders for food deliveries or collect donations from people in your neighborhood. You might create and donate art or write thank you letters/e-mails to the people who are important in your life; send care packages to veteran's homes; sponsor a drive to provide necessities to older or disabled people who cannot leave their residences.

Due to the pandemic, society has a heightened consciousness of the challenges and opportunities of doctors, nurses, and other health professionals. We knew, heard, or watched stories of the many vulnerable people who lived on the streets with chronic conditions and limited access to healthcare. Those who lived from paycheck to paycheck chose between paying their rent or buying food. Some did not have the money for medical appointments, medicines, or necessary procedures.

What can you do to make people's lives better? How can you improve the health of others? Do not wait until you attend medical/dental school to make a difference in the mental or physical health of people in your community. Epitomize selfless service now. Help people in your community. Figure it out. Find a unique way to serve. Do not wait for a program to ask you to join them. Start one. People within a few miles of wherever you live have lifesaving needs. Your proactive steps can make a difference.

Preparing for the journey is as much about being part of your school and regional society as it is about your education. Getting involved in high school is a good indicator of whether or not you will get involved in college and take an active role in the BS/MD, BS/DO, BS/DDS community.

Even if you cannot stay after school for sports, debate, theatre, MUN, Mock Trial, robotics, rocketry, Science Olympiad, or clubs, find other ways to participate in student government, musicals, artistic groups, or volunteer service. Get involved in weekend events, homeless shelters, community events, research, or hospital activities.

By taking part in your school and community, you gain a better understanding of the critical state of people, old and young. You will hear stories from those you will eventually serve while collaborating on projects and achieving success together.

Of course, this is not to say that academics is unimportant, but many students focus solely on academics and believe they are worthy just because of their high school and college transcripts. BS/MD, BS/DO, or BS/DDS programs seek well-rounded students who care about others rather than isolate and review their books.

Summer is your chance to shine in a basic science or clinical research program or hospital or shadowing opportunity. You might do a medical mission trip overseas in Fiji, Laos, Peru, or Senegal. Numerous groups take students like Refugee Health Alliance, Volunteers Around the World, Vida Volunteer, International Medical Relief, and Global Medical Brigades. Some even serve with their families. Another option is Maranatha Volunteers International which organizes the "Ultimate Workout," a two-week mission trip specifically designed for high school students aged 14–18. This cultural and service program engages students in construction projects, community outreach, and basic health education in various countries, primarily in Latin America.

Keep looking for what fits your interests, experiences, and passion. Remember, you do not have to do everything, but you must do something.

Here is a quote to live by.

*I am only one, but I am one.*
*I cannot do everything, but I can do something.*
*And I will not let what I cannot do interfere with what I can do.*

**- Edward Everett Hale**

> # "
> ## *Life is a matter of choices, and every choice you make makes you.*

– John C. Maxwell

CHAPTER FOUR

# IS THE DIRECT ROUTE OR THE TRADITIONAL PREMED PATH RIGHT FOR YOU?

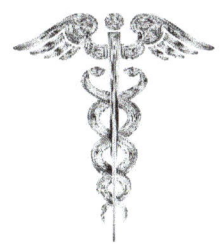

You probably already know that BS/MD, BS/DO, and BS/DDS programs are highly competitive. The most popular programs like Brown's PLME (Program in Liberal Medical Education), the University of Rochester's REMS (Rochester Early Medical Scholars), Case Western Reserve's PPSP (Pre-Professional Scholars Program), and George Washington's Seven-Year Dual BA/MD Program have low acceptance rates and are highly selective. You will need more than the minimum requirements.

The most competitive schools only accept the very best math and science students. Many valedictorians are rejected. Students with perfect test scores are set aside for more well-rounded students or those who fit the school's state residency or diversity requirements. Now is the time for you to gain medical, leadership, service, and research experiences.

You have probably 'received the memo' that says you should take four years of the highest level of AP/IB science classes and mathematics at your school (through AP Calculus BC and AP Physics C, if offered). Many students also take college classes that go above the high school curriculum. You will need to take the SAT or ACT. These testing requirements are essential indicators of aptitude in problem solving, critical thinking, language fluency, reading comprehension, and quantitative ability.

Of course, you need high grades and high test scores. A listed minimum GPA is the lowest possible score the school will even consider. Admitted students to BS/MD, BS/DO, and BS/DDS programs have significantly higher average scores. Additionally, requirements listed on the college website simply get you to the starting plate to swing the bat. The goal is for you to hit a home run. Lots of students begin their journey to medical school and arrive at first, second, or third base with decent successes along the way. Yet, they miss the home run, which in your case is medical school, whether you go the long way or shorter route.

## IS THE PRE-MED/PRE-DENT TRACK BETTER FOR YOU?

If you are a highly academic student who is certain medical/dental school is in your future, you should consider is the BS/MD, BS/DO, or BS/DDS track. Frankly, the direct med programs are a lot shorter since few students gain admission to medical or dental  school right out of college. Furthermore, your college classmates will be equally focused on medicine and driven to achieve their goals. If you are not absolutely sure you want to pursue medicine or dentistry, the BS/MD,  BS/DO, BS/DDS avenue is the wrong road. You have other options. Attend college, choose an interesting major, take the required courses, and apply to medical school after your four years of study.

If you head toward the four year college route, you should know that a degree in biology is not required to enter medical school. You can major in any field provided you take the required science coursework and the  MCAT. I provided a chart on the next page with alternative majors having higher acceptance rates.

By following the pathway to medical school, while gaining medical training, scientific research, and community service, you will learn more about yourself and your specific career interests. There are many roads to choose that can translate your interest in medicine into a related field. You might consider dental school, vet school, or pharmacy school. Maybe you would prefer to be a physician's assistant, nurse practitioner, or medical researcher. You might find psychology, public health, or community medicine more appealing. By choosing to pursue the premedical pathway, you will navigate college while continuing to discover what subjects and activities you enjoy the most. Maybe you will find that medicine is not right for you.

Most students take the longer road to medical or dental school through undergraduate universities because this avenue is more flexible. You can explore majors, while considering alternative career paths. For many students who want to attend medical or dental school, this is the most appropriate. Students can choose any major while taking their premedical requirements.

# LOOKING AT THE DATA

The following is a table from the AAMC website that offers 2024 statistical data of GPA, MCAT, and majors for students who applied and those who matriculated. The AAMC website provides tons of valuable information. Check it out. While you may not yet be applying to medical school, keep your eye on the prize. Look at where you are headed to make good decisions now as to how to get to your future as an MD or DO.

## AAMC TABLE A-17 APPLICANTS AND MATRICULANTS TO U.S. MEDICAL SCHOOLS 2024

| Applicants | Total MCAT | | GPA Science | | GPA Non-Science | | GPA Total | | Total Applicants |
|---|---|---|---|---|---|---|---|---|---|
| | Mean | SD | Mean | SD | Mean | SD | Mean | SD | |
| Biological Sciences | 506.3 | 9.8 | 3.56 | 0.41 | 3.80 | 0.25 | 3.65 | 0.33 | 30,054 |
| Humanities | 509.0 | 9.1 | 3.52 | 0.44 | 3.77 | 0.28 | 3.65 | 0.32 | 1,661 |
| Math & Statistics | 511.9 | 9.6 | 3.66 | 0.37 | 3.76 | 0.28 | 3.69 | 0.32 | 344 |
| Other | 505.1 | 10.3 | 3.52 | 0.44 | 3.76 | 0.29 | 3.64 | 0.34 | 9,064 |
| Physical Sciences | 509.1 | 9.6 | 3.61 | 0.39 | 3.75 | 0.28 | 3.67 | 0.32 | 4,228 |
| Social Sciences | 505.8 | 10.1 | 3.45 | 0.48 | 3.71 | 0.33 | 3.59 | 0.36 | 4,844 |
| Specialized Health Sciences | 503.3 | 10.5 | 3.49 | 0.45 | 3.75 | 0.28 | 3.62 | 0.33 | 2,382 |
| All Applicants | 506.3 | 10.0 | 3.54 | 0.42 | 3.78 | 0.27 | 3.64 | 0.33 | 52,577 |

| Matriculants | Total MCAT | | GPA Science | | GPA Non-Science | | GPA Total | | Total Matriculants |
|---|---|---|---|---|---|---|---|---|---|
| | Mean | SD | Mean | SD | Mean | SD | Mean | SD | |
| Biological Science | 511.5 | 6.9 | 3.72 | 0.29 | 3.87 | 0.18 | 3.78 | 0.23 | 13,050 |
| Humanities | 513.1 | 6.3 | 3.67 | 0.32 | 3.84 | 0.21 | 3.76 | 0.23 | 861 |
| Math & Statistics | 516.1 | 6.1 | 3.77 | 0.24 | 3.83 | 0.19 | 3.79 | 0.21 | 180 |
| Other | 511.2 | 6.9 | 3.69 | 0.30 | 3.85 | 0.19 | 3.78 | 0.22 | 3,767 |
| Physical Sciences | 513.8 | 6.6 | 3.73 | 0.28 | 3.82 | 0.23 | 3.77 | 0.24 | 2,094 |
| Social Sciences | 511.6 | 6.7 | 3.64 | 0.34 | 3.80 | 0.25 | 3.73 | 0.26 | 2,065 |
| Specialized Health Sciences | 510.2 | 6.8 | 3.69 | 0.30 | 3.84 | 0.20 | 3.77 | 0.22 | 964 |
| All Applicants | 511.7 | 6.9 | 3.71 | 0.30 | 3.85 | 0.20 | 3.77 | 0.23 | 22,981 |

To get a clearer picture of the applicant's majors, MCAT scores, GPAs, and their matriculation to medical school, here is a condensed version of that chart along with percentages of applicants who became medical school matriculants. You can view data for the current year by looking this up on the AAMC website.

| ACADEMIC FIELD | MATRICULANTS | APPLICANTS | PERCENTAGE |
|---|---|---|---|
| Biological Sciences | 12,050 | 30,054 | 40.09% |
| Humanities (Phil., Rel., Lit., etc.) | 861 | 1,661 | 51.83% |
| Math & Statistics | 180 | 344 | 52.33% |
| Other | 3,767 | 9,064 | 41.56% |
| Physical Sciences | 2,094 | 4,228 | 49.53% |
| Social Sciences (Psych., Soc., Anthro.) | 2,065 | 4,844 | 42.63% |
| Specialized Health Sciences | 964 | 2,382 | 40.47% |

Notice on the chart that the academic major with the highest probability of matriculating to medical school is Math & Statistics, with Humanities (Philosophy, Religion, Ethnic Studies, Logic, and Languages) and Physical Sciences (Chemistry, Physics, and Engineering) close behind. Surprisingly, the lowest probability of acceptance is the Biological Sciences, though there are more applicants in that area than any other set of majors. Specialized Health Sciences (Public Health, Nutrition, Kinesiology, and Health Education) programs next with Other and the Social Sciences (Psychology, Sociology, Anthropology, History, and Political Science) close behind.

Most students believe that the chances are higher in the biological sciences, but this is not the case. The problem-solving skills of the physical and mathematical sciences are fundamental in medical school. People may wonder why the humanities is so high. This is possibly because of the logic, critical reasoning, and depth of introspection required of philosophy and religion students.

The most challenging related courses in college are typically those in chemistry, physics, and biomedical engineering. Students more often get stuck along the road in physics, chemistry, and mathematics classes and not in biology or social sciences. While that knowledge is valuable, medical schools want to be sure you can succeed in the most academically challenging problem-solving classes.

Another interesting consideration is that the MCAT scores are higher for students majoring in Mathematics & Statistics, Physical Sciences, and Humanities. The GPAs are relatively consistent, though slightly lower in the Social Sciences category for both applicants and matriculants. These inferences must be taken in light of the many other factors that determine admission since acceptance is not based solely on GPA and MCAT scores. Nevertheless, if you look carefully at the range of GPAs and MCAT scores, the number are relatively consistent.

So, choose a major you enjoy. Take classes that fulfill you. Note that your major does make a difference particularly regarding thinking vs. memorizing and analysis vs. multiple choice. You might consider dual majoring, a major/minor, or earning a graduate degree. Irrespective of your major, you must take the required and possibly even the recommended courses to better prepare you for medical or dental school.

In conclusion, major in a field that fascinates you. However, my take is that medicine will be more technical and technological in the future. Each day, you will use computers, biotechnologies, and machines to test physiological functioning, process lab results, and perform surgery. Critical thinking and analysis will be required to diagnose and treat patients given generated outputs using accumulated wisdom. With artificial intelligence and quantum computing, medicine is entering a new realm where humanity and empathy are essential, but so are problem-solving and technology.

# BS/MD VS. EARLY ASSURANCE PROGRAMS

Traditionally, BS/MD and BS/DO programs have a direct-to-medical-school pathway, although many colleges still require students to take the MCAT and/or apply with AMCAS (the medical school application service, much like the Common App). When the AMCAS application is required, (1) some schools offer an automatic admit upon achieving the requirements, (2) others require candidates to apply to the affiliated medical school using the AMCAS binding Early Decision option, (3) and still others allow students to complete the first four years and choose another medical school upon completion. There is little consistency between programs.

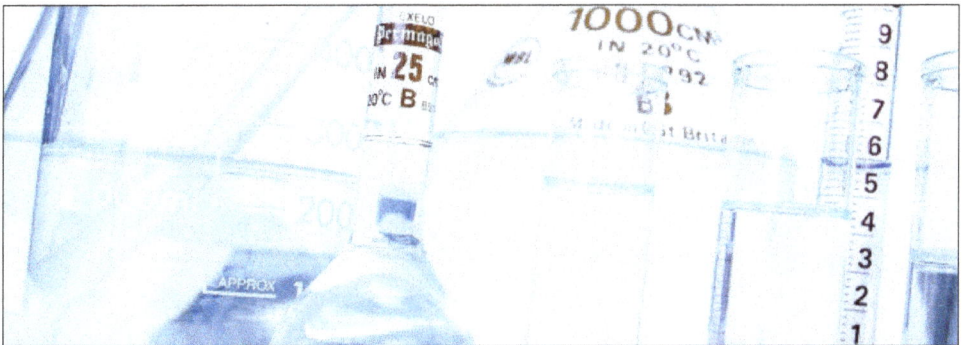

Outside of applying directly to BS/MD, BS/DO, and BS/DDS, other options include Early Assurance Programs or Early Acceptance Programs (EAPs). With EAPs, students are accepted to an undergraduate college. After completing a set of prerequisites they can apply to the university's direct med program. Programs like these include include Tufts MSP (Medical Scholars Program), BU's MMEDIC (Modular Medical Integrated Curriculum), and GWU's Early Selection Program.

This specialized premedical pathway guarantees admission provided the student achieves the requisite grades and MCAT scores or at least these students are prioritized the in the medical school admissions process. Some of these programs require students to take the MCAT and/or complete the AMCAS; some do not. This book includes a few of these programs even though you do not apply straight out of high school just so you can plan accordingly.

Finally, some college's BS/MD or BS/DO programs are surprisingly not connected to their medical college, but to a different medical school. Students complete four years and attend one of the affiliated schools. A pathway is made to take candidates who have successfully completed all of the requirements.

"

*There is no elevator to success. You have to take the stairs.*

—Zig Ziglar

# CHAPTER FIVE

# MEDICINE AND AFFILIATED MEDICAL CAREERS

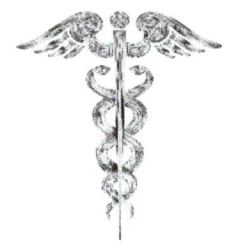

## MEETING THE NEED FOR HEALTHCARE WORKERS

According to the Bureau of Labor Statistics , the healthcare industry is expected to grow faster than the average for all other occupations. With a projected increase of 14 percent from 2026 to 2036, approximately 1.9 million new jobs will be available each year for those interested in medical related careers. The pandemic fueled demand for medical services. However, greater increases are anticipated due to the aging population in a demographic shift, sometimes referred to as the "gray tsunami." In 2030, twenty percent of the U.S. population will be over 65.

According to the U.S. Census Bureau, baby boomers, born between 1946 and 1964, are turning 65 at a rate of about 10,000 per day. By 2030, when the next census is taken, all baby boomers will have crossed that threshold. This information is critical to understanding all careers in healthcare and is the key reason why the healthcare profession will have a surge of jobs. Hospitals, emergency services, home healthcare, nursing homes, and mental health services will require professionals to meet the rising need. Wages in healthcare professions are likely to rise in the next decade.

## WHAT MEDICAL PROFESSION IS RIGHT FOR YOU?

When students ponder the pursuit of medicine, they tend to consider medical school as the quintessential career and life objective. No doubt medical school is the right pursuit for many students. Yet, there are many rewarding options and there is more than one road to get to your goal.

In the 1990s, a Harvard interviewer asked one of my very talented Hispanic students why she wanted to attend Harvard if she wanted to pursue nursing. My student answered the question without hesitation, explaining that her mom had a DNP but always wished she had started her road with a rigorous liberal arts education. However, I never stopped thinking about that question. Sure, a specialized undergraduate nursing education is a more direct pathway and her desired route would extend her timeline, but she was committed to expanding her knowledge base. After we talked, I came to understand her long-term objective. She did not get accepted to Harvard, but she did attend Columbia and she is now a nurse practitioner.

There are numerous possibilities for students who find medicine, healthcare, and human biology fascinating. Popular choices for those who complete graduate school include allopathic medicine (MD), osteopathic medicine (DO), dentist (DDS or DMD), podiatrist (DPM), veterinarian (DVM), pharmacist (PharmD), psychologist (M.A., Ph.D., Psy.D.), psychiatrist (MD), optometrist (OD), chiropractor (DC), physician's assistant (PA), physical therapist (PT), speech pathologist, nurse practitioner (MSN, DNP), occupational therapist (MSOT, DOT), and nurse anesthetist (MSN).

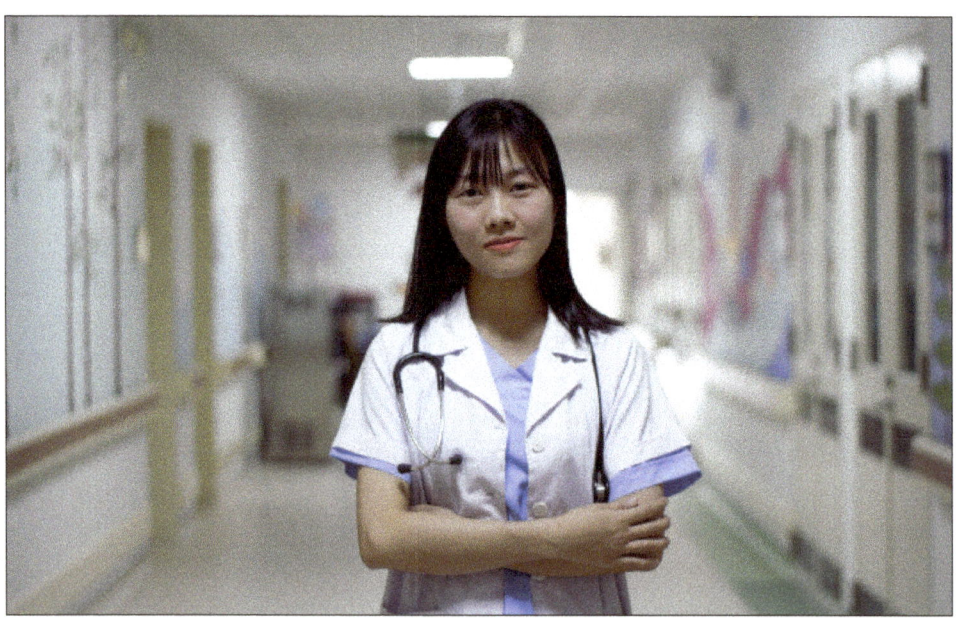

| OCCUPATION/DEGREE | ASSOCIATIONS, CERTIFICATION ORGANIZATIONS | BUREAU OF LABOR STATISTICS DATA (2024) |
|---|---|---|
| Medical Doctor (MD) Allopathic Medicine – AMCAS - 160 accredited colleges in the U.S.; 20 in Canada with 2 more opening by 2028 | *American Association of Medical Colleges (AAMC) *American Medical Association (MDs & DOs) | Median Annual Salary – $239,200 Number of Physicians & Surgeons (2025) – 667,189 Projected Job Change (2024 – 2034) – 8% increase |
| Physician (DO) Osteopathic Medicine – AACOMAS - 44 (2025) accredited colleges in the U.S. ; three new DO schools projected to open by 2027 | * American Association of Colleges of Osteopathic Medicine (AACOM) *American Osteopathic Association (AOA) *Bureau of Osteopathic Specialists (BOS) *Certifying Board Services (CBS) | Median Annual Salary – $239,200 Number of Physicians & Surgeons (2025) – 90,980 Projected Job Change (2024 – 2034) – 9% increase |
| Podiatrist (DPM) – CPME - 11 accredited colleges in the U.S.; there is 1 in Canada | *American Association of Colleges of Podiatry Medicine (AACPM) * Council on Podiatric Medical Education (CPME) | Median Annual Salary – $152,800 Number of Podiatrists (2025) – 18,000 Projected Job Change (2024 – 2034) – 3% increase |
| Dentistry (DDS or DMD) – ADEA AADSAS – 76 ADA accredited dental schools in the U.S.; 10 in Canada | *American Dental Education Association (ADEA) *American Dental Association (ADA) | Median Annual Salary – $179,200 Specialists - $239,200 Number of Dentists (2025) – 218,200 Projected Job Change (2024 – 2034) – 5% increase |
| Veterinary Medicine (DVM) – VMCAS - 35 accredited veterinary medical schools in the U.S.; 5 in Canada | *Association of American Veterinary Medical Colleges (AAVMC) *American Veterinary Medical Association (AVMA) | Median Annual Salary – $125,510 Specialists - $212,890 Number of Veterinarians (2025) – 130,415 Projected Job Change (2024 – 2034) – 19% inc. |
| Pharmacist (PharmD) – PharmCAS - 142 full or candidate accredited pharmacy schools in the U.S.; 11 pharmacy schools in Canada | *Accreditation Council for Pharmacy Education (ACPE) *American Pharmacists Association (APhA) | Median Annual Salary – $137,480 Number of Pharmacists (2025) – 350,000 Projected Job Change (2024 – 2034) – 5% inc. |
| Psychologist (MA, Ph.D., Psy.D) – numbers vary by type 223 Ph.D. Psychology programs and 80 APA-accredited for Psy.D. | *American Psychological Association (APA) | Median Annual Salary – $94,310 Number of Psychologists (2025) – 210,000 Projected Job Change (2024 – 2034) – 7% inc. |
| Psychiatrist (MD) | See MD | Median Annual Salary – $323,000 Number of Psychiatrists (2025) – 39,180 Projected Job Change (2024 – 2034) – 0% inc. |
| Optometrist (OD) - 27 accredited optometry schools in the U.S. and 2 in pre-accreditation; 2 in Canada | *Association of Schools and Colleges of Optometry (ASCO) *Association of Optometrists (AOP) | Median Annual Salary – $135,297 Number of Optometrists (2025) – 170,628 Projected Job Change (2024 – 2034) – 9% increase |

| OCCUPATION/DEGREE | ASSOCIATIONS, CERTIFICATION ORGANIZATIONS | BUREAU OF LABOR STATISTICS DATA (2018) |
|---|---|---|
| Chiropractor (DC)<br>- 21 chiropractic schools in the U.S.; 2 in Canada | *Association of Chiropractic Colleges (ACC)<br>*American Chiropractic Association (ACA)<br>*Council on Chiropractic Education | Median Annual Salary – $85,646<br>Number of Chiropractors (2025) – 70,000<br>Projected Job Change (2024 – 2034) – 9% increase |
| Physician's Assistant (PA)<br>- 314 ARC-PA accredited PA programs in the U.S.; 5 in Canada | *Accreditation Review Commission on Education for the Physician Assistant (ARC-PA)<br>*American Academy of Physician Assistants (AAPA) | Median Annual Salary – $133,260<br>Number of PAs (2018) – 178,700<br>Projected Job Change (2024 – 2034) – 28% increase |
| Physical Therapist (PT)<br>- Over 338 CAPTE accredited PT schools; 6 in Canada | *American Physical Therapy Association (APTA)<br>*Commission on Accreditation in Physical Therapy Education (CAPTE) | Median Annual Salary – $101,020<br>Number of PTs (2018) – 233,890<br>Projected Job Change (2024 – 2034) – 14% increase |
| Speech Pathologist<br>– 288 accredited programs; 38 programs awaiting accreditation; 12 in Canada | *<br>*American Speech–Language–Hearing Association (ASHA) | Median Annual Salary – $95,410<br>Number of Speech Pathologists (2025) – 172,100<br>Projected Job Change (2024 – 2034) – 18% increase |
| Nurse Practitioner ( NP)<br>MSN, DNP<br>- Approximately 400 NP programs ; 24 in Canada | *American Association of Colleges of Nursing (AACN)<br>*American Association of Nurse Practitioners (AANP) | Median Annual Salary – $129,210<br>Number of NPs (2025) – 267,000<br>Projected Job Change (2024 – 2034) – 45% increase |
| Occupational Therapist (MSOT, DOT)<br>- 471 fully accredited DOT programs; 36 in Canada | *American Occupational Therapy Association (AOTA)<br>* Accreditation Council for Occupational Therapy Education (ACOTE) | Median Annual Salary – $98,340<br>Number of Occupational Therapists (2025) – 150,500 Projected Job Change (2024 – 2034) – 11% increase |
| Nurse Anesthetist (MSN) - 163 accredited nurse anesthesia programs | See NP | Median Annual Salary – $223,210<br>Number of NPs (2025) – 49,900<br>Projected Job Change (2024 – 2034) – 10% increase |

# ALLIED HEALTH PROFESSIONS

The medical profession would not be able to serve the public without the talented and dedicated service of allied health professionals who support, assist, record, evaluate, and rehabilitate patients. From intake and testing to nutrition and maintenance, it 'takes a village'. Today, the village provides healthcare for patients who are multifaceted, multilingual, and multitalented. These careers often require interpersonal skills in communication and listening along with recordkeeping, problem solving, and critical thinking. In addition to healthcare administrators, managers, and insurance professionals, the following presents a list of some of the many professionals in the medical support community.

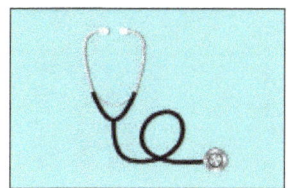

- » *Athletic Trainer*
- » *Audiologist*
- » *Cardiovascular Technologist*
- » *Clinical Laboratory Technician*
- » *Clinical Laboratory Technologist*
- » *Diagnostic Medical Sonographer*
- » *Emergency Medical Technician*
- » *Exercise Physiologists*
- » *Dental Assistant*
- » *Dietician (RD, RDN)*
- » *Dispensing Optician*
- » *Genetics Counselors*
- » *Health Information Technician*
- » *Home Health Aide*
- » *Kinesiologist*
- » *Massage Therapist*
- » *Medical Assistant*
- » *Medical Records Assistant*
- » *Medical Transcriptionist*
- » *Midwife*
- » *MRI Technologist*
- » *Nuclear Medicine Technologists*
- » *Nursing Assistant (CNA)*
- » *Nutritionist*
- » *Occupational Therapy Assistant*
- » *Orderly*
- » *Orthotists*
- » *Paramedics*
- » *Pharmacy Technician*
- » *Phlebotomist*
- » *Physical Therapy Assistant*
- » *Prosthetists*
- » *Psychiatric Aide*
- » *Recreational Therapist*
- » *Radiation Therapists*
- » *Radiologic Technologist*
- » *Registered Nurse (RN, BSN)*
- » *Respiratory Therapist*
- » *Ultrasound Technician*
- » *Veterinary Assistant*
- » *Veterinary Technologist*

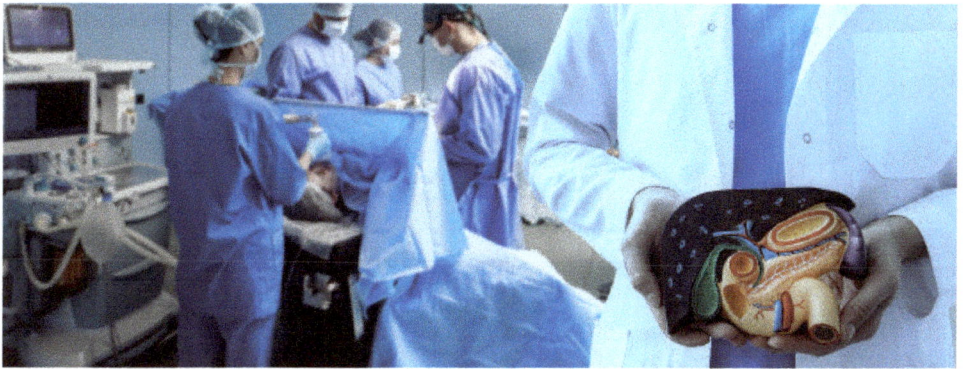

"

*A mind that is stretched by a new experience can never go back to its old dimensions.*

– *Oliver Wendell Holmes, Jr.*

## CHAPTER SIX

# COVID-19 & THE MEDICAL SCHOOL PIPELINE

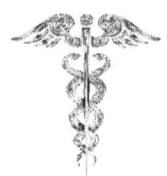

A tsunami transforming healthcare and educational practices was caused by a global quake of enormous magnitude. The rollout and repercussions could not have been predicted because society was not in the mindset of planning for an unprecedented medical catastrophe. Enhanced 'virtual clinical training' and 'ethics in telehealth procedures' were immediately conceptualized and established in some fields at the height of the pandemic to allow students to progress. Medical programs were adjusted to compensate for missed learning and experiences on all levels. Medical education adapted by enhancing patient relationships, ethical practices, and technical knowledge while emphasizing science foundation coursework, medical training, and board exams.

As pandemic surged, middle and high school kids entered the medical school pipeline seeking a fascinating and rewarding career with seemingly endless potential. Students needed additional support given the educational challenges of the quarantine, online education, and years spent while incorporating new ways of learning. A surge of medical school applicants flooded medical school admissions.

Medicine has come a long way since the Spanish Flu of 1918-1920 which terrified world for three years and killed nearly fifty million people. Yet, while the death toll was not as high, the fear was equally palpable. The consequences permeated people's lives as they came to grips with their mortality and sensed death around them. As soon as medical schools mitigated the pandemic's woes, technological progress added new twists to with artificial intelligence, 3-D printed organs, stem cell therapies, computerized implants, and quantum computing, Today, research centers, educational institutions, and pharmaceutical companies are adapting to changes while attempting to thwart future medical catastrophes.

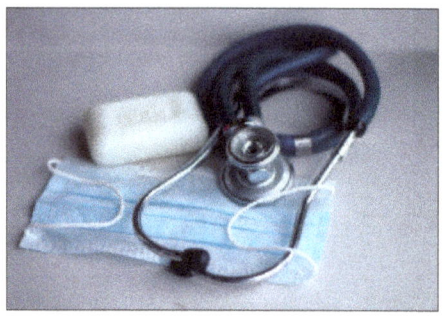

Global citizenry were awakened to the fact that the human body is not resilient to all new and virulent microbes. For lay people, this idea remained dormant in some undisturbed subterranean sector of our subconscious. Movies like *Contagion* left lingering reminders as they dramatized the possibility of global health emergencies. Yet, many did not want to believe a global pandemic was possible. Few in academia were prepared to manage this tumultuous ride. As the news shook cities and waves of the virus began to cross the Pacific Ocean, the threat seemed too far away in January and February of 2020 to contemplate that our lives would erupt and death would strike upon our doorposts.

Like the rippling effect of foreshocks to an earthquake that had not yet released its energy, most people in the academy did not plan for 'the big one' even as it began to rock Asia. Information from China had been cut off, so quantitative and qualitative data from the epicenter could not be accumulated. However, doctors in Italy were not silent. Deaths mounted. Hospitals and clinics were unprepared. Supplies were needed. Protection was limited. Nobody was immune - young, old, educated, skilled. From the garment worker to state leaders, COVID-19 passed through cities with its destructive force. Money could not stem the tide as people sang from their balconies and vehicles bearing coffins rolled down the streets. Accounts from nurses and physicians sent up flares, lighting the sky and warning all that this pernicious menace was headed their way.

Schools, heading the siren, acted quickly, though the consequences of stopping in-person school meant an abrupt change from classroom education to online chaos. Some schools were more prepared, but others languished with students who had no computers, tests that could not be proctored, and school lunches that would no longer be provided. The challenges did not just rest with K-12 education as colleges and medical schools struggled to determine how they would deliver lectures, hold labs, and support the thousands of students who were asked to leave their dormitory rooms. International students had nowhere to go, with flights grounded to their

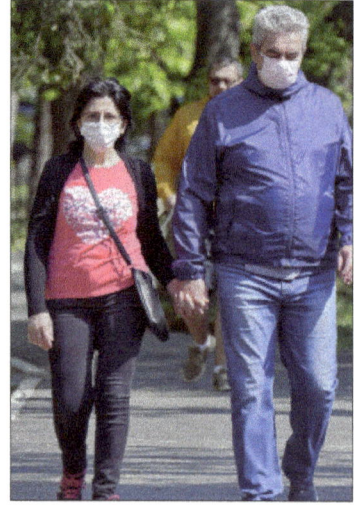

far away homes. Even when they could get to their home country, they had limited connectivity to the online resources they had grown accustomed to accessing, not to mention having to manage challenges like 'Zoom bombing' and teachers with limited technology skills who were reluctant to start anew.

Faculty who had never taught online or used virtual classrooms were caught off-guard. Student expectations exceeded faculty's ability to deliver. Communication and feedback were awkward as most faculty were unable to recreate the school-based classroom in the online environment. Everyone from the students to faculty and administrators needed to adapt to the enormous shakeup that erupted life along the medical school pathway. Everyone from kindergarten to residency education needed to be seamlessly migrated online, which was a very tall order.

Those on their undergraduate or graduate pathway toward a medical degree were forced to rethink their education and discover new ways to learn the material in a self-advocating, efficient manner despite the other obstacles they faced. Laboratory experiments could not be completed, lectures were interrupted, and collaborative projects needed a fresh lens to view project development and delivery.

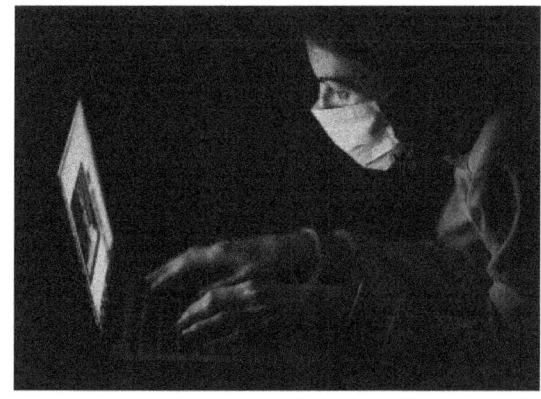

Students toward the end of applying to BS/MD programs and medical school were unable to  interview in some cases or visit their prospective schools in others. The final candidacy decisions had to be made with significantly less information.

As students struggled to make decisions, parents became more protective and cautious. Many parents started to make concrete choices about where, how, and when their children would be educated. The parents of many college bound students, preferred to keep their children closer to home due to costs, uncertainty, and support.

A change in demographics impacted the geographic diversity of many colleges across the county. While this shift occurred from 2020 to 2022, the consequences of this decision-making process lasted much longer. Decisions, decisions. Today, those in admissions continue to search for ways to empower students, even as international students face the very real possibility that their visa will not be renewed, costs at some colleges surpass $100,000 per year, and a nationwide university shakeup is altering reality. Education in 2035 and 2040 will be unrecognizable from that of 2015 or 2020.

Prospective undergraduate and graduate students may be even more dedicated to their pursuit given society's focus on medicine and health. The pandemic also instilled a curiosity about the human body, a drive to provide care for diverse, rural, and underserved communities, and a commitment to preventing the possibility of death from overshadowing life. The hunger to learn inspires many students to seek a greater understanding of how diseases and immunology impact anatomy and physiology. To be sure, the pandemic's cloud over the population clarified the real need to understand the pathophysiology of diseases and prevent their spread.

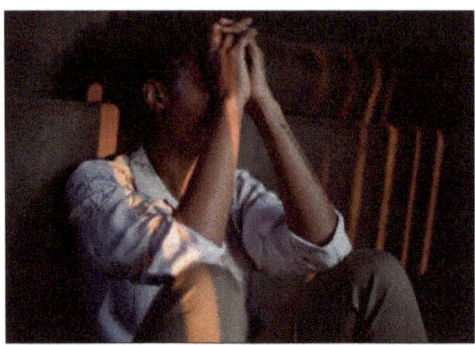

Students in the medical school pipeline faced challenges presenting themselves in the best light. Academically, they may not have been able to complete required classes, learn critical information, take summer advancement opportunities, or participate in valuable training. Other impediments blocked thoroughfares to medical school.

Research projects were discarded, disbanded, or postponed. Presentations at conferences, acceptance of papers, and delivery of proposals were put on hold or canceled altogether. Volunteer medical experiences, service projects and leadership opportunities and were hindered. Prestigious research grants were held up, not to mention the stoppage of academic travel or programs vital to service, learning, and funding. Some students had no in-person labs for either organic chemistry or physics.

Without being able to present a strong academic background, community service, dedicated hospital experiences, or teamwork through collaborative activities, students may have decided their prospects to enter BS/MD, BS/DDS programs or medical/dental schools were limited. Some counted on their SAT, ACT, MCAT, or DAT they had been studying for throughout the year to send a strong signal that they were prepared. Yet, these tests were canceled. As their pathway became disrupted, many had to rethink how to move forward with their goal.

Others may have changed course entirely, dissuaded from pursuing medicine due to the deaths of healthcare workers, lack of safety and protection, and extended hours. Those whose heart was not committed to selfless medical service may have changed their minds. Some witnessed medical practices virtually shut down for months when non-necessary procedures stopped, slowing the flow of patient appointments. Telemedicine, while offering some promise, did not make up for the number of patient appointments medical/dental professionals once had.

Quick thinking innovators, though, emerged from the smoke and rumblings of COVID-19's eruption. Their previous rigorous, but planned, course was set. They were nimble in their life choices and determined to be flexible and adaptable. 'Necessity is the mother of invention' as the saying goes, and creative acts of kindness, support, service, and healthcare during the pandemic showed tenacity and persistence. 'Walk the walk' resonates better when demonstrated rather than elegantly crafted on a personal statement.

Medical education, from pre-training in high school and skill development in college through medical school, will be different in the future. All involved in education will be more prepared. Proactive thinking will be more common on all levels. Some students will stay the course and pursue their passion with every breath in their body. Some will not. Technology will be better integrated into the curriculum. Resilience will be a sought-after attribute.

Experiential learning through shadowing, assisting, and medical practice will continue since there is no substitute for live, in-person patient care. Medical services instituted precautionary steps, changing previously held mindsets about how to care for patients while also being personally safe and healthy. Hand-sanitizing will stay, though frequent handshaking may be an anachronism of a bygone era.

After the coronavirus' tentacles were severed, widespread mental and physical recuperation was necessary. Though we survived to tell the tale, many still question whether they are better off for the transformation. Humanity stared into the face of death, reminding themselves of their mortality. Medical education from high school to residency will continue, along with the necessary adjustments needed to acclimate to new systemic changes. Rigorous education and methodological training are both necessary and powerful tools to shape talent and work ethic into skills. Some may say that learning is the most valuable tool we have to plant seeds into our new generation of physicians, fertilize them with the pandemic's dose of humility, and unite physicians, scientists, and inventors to uncover the mysteries of the human mind and body yet to be revealed.

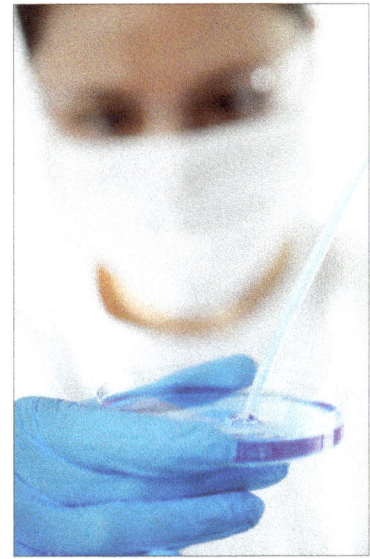

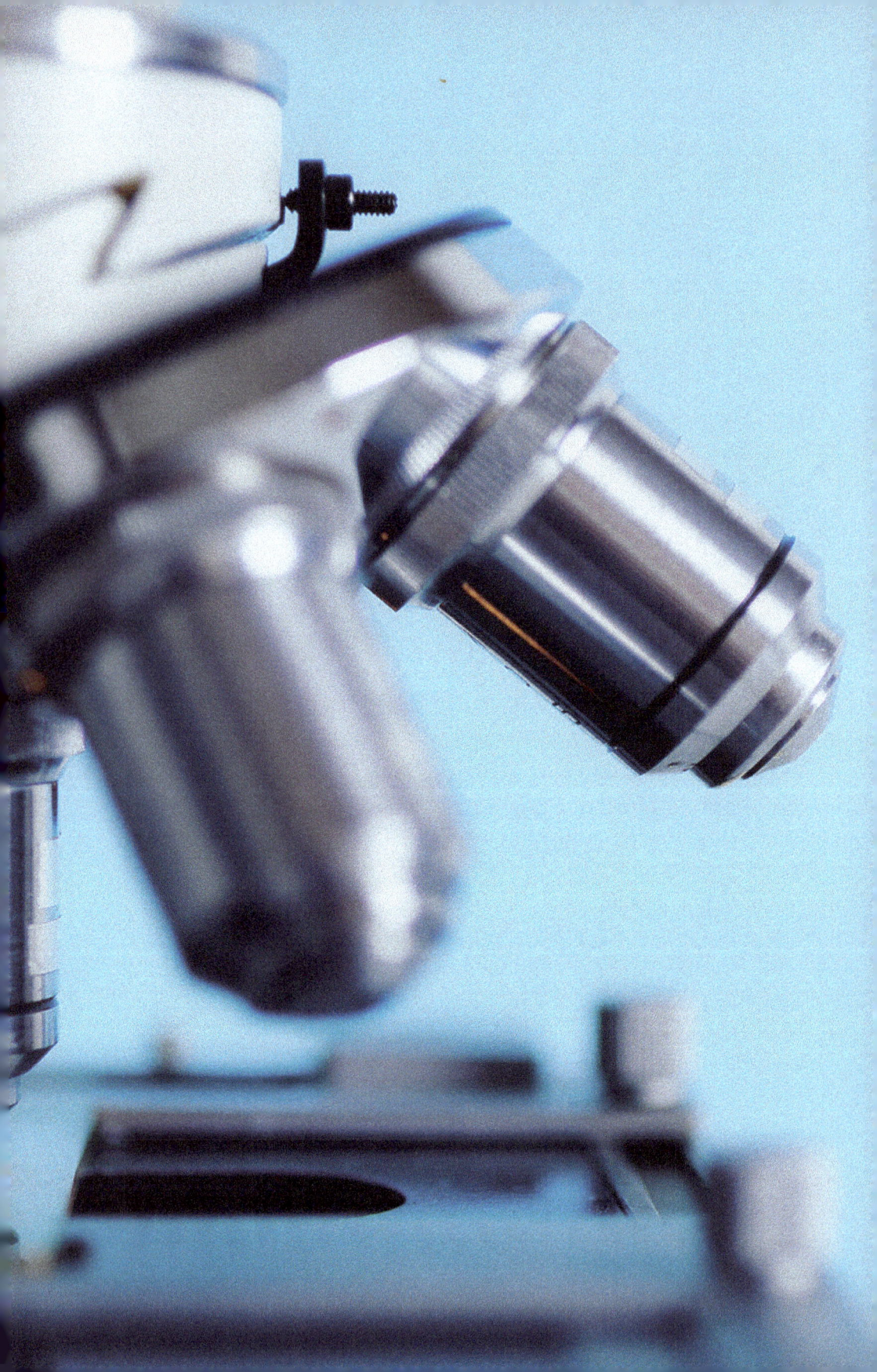

# PART TWO

# PREPARATION FOR BS/MD & BS/DDS PROGRAMS

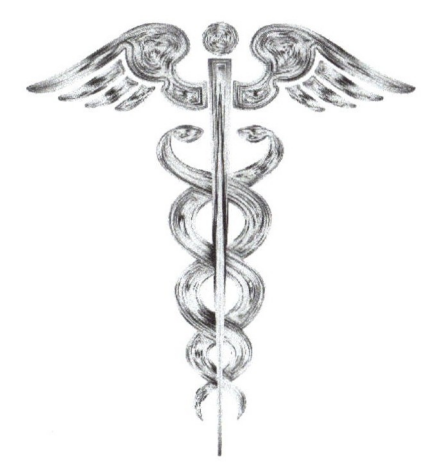

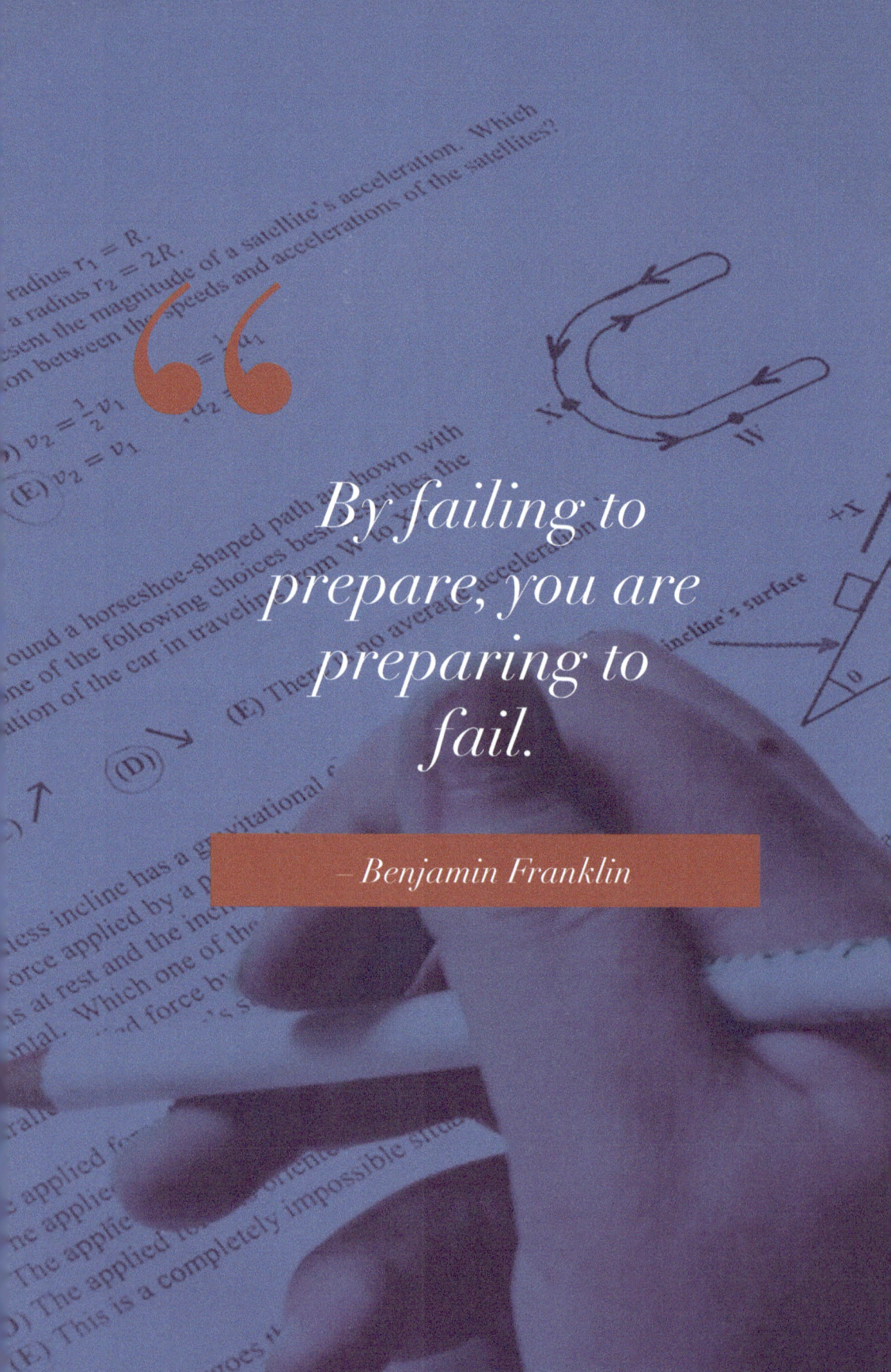

*By failing to prepare, you are preparing to fail.*

— Benjamin Franklin

# CHAPTER SEVEN

# COURSEWORK AND GPA

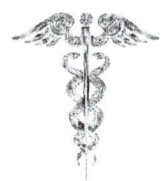

A dose of pragmatism is required in formulating a high school academic plan. You will need at least four years of high school science. Many students double science or take summer science classes at a college. More is better. That may mean taking two in your junior and senior years or taking college science classes. Two chemistry and two physics classes are preferred. Why? These two classes are the hardest and serve as your foundation. AP Environmental Science is not impressive as a science class unless you have exhausted all other AP science classes.

Most students complete AP Calculus BC, though many have a year of statistics as well. Some applicants have also taken college Multivariable Calculus, Linear Algebra, and/or Differential Equations. How do you take these if you are not far ahead in math? You can take summer bridge classes.

Science and math classes are essential components of your schedule. Why? Frequently, students begin their freshman year of college taking Chemistry, Biology, and Calculus. When graded on a curve, these classes tend to 'weed' out students who have not taken AP Chemistry, AP Biology, or AP Calculus. Imagine taking College Chemistry sitting next to a student who took two years of high school chemistry. Now imagine being told that only half of the students in your class will earn an A or a B. This is not uncommon.

I always say, "A college does not reject you because they don't like you. They reject you because they do not know enough about you to accept you."

Alternatively, "They reject you because they do not want you to fail, particularly if you are less prepared than other candidates, and you might feel overwhelmed."

Note: Since BS/MD and BS/DO programs are extremely competitive, applicants often have stronger credentials than those who pursue the traditional premedical route. On the other hand, they may also be more prepared for the rigors of college.

## COMMUNITY COLLEGE CLASSES

High school students often take community college classes to get ahead or complete lower-division requirements before attending college. Either reason is fine, though some colleges state in their admissions profile that students cannot have more than a specific number of college credits before attending a BS/MD program. UMKC comes to mind. The UMKC's six-year BA/MD program restricts applicants to no more than 24 hours of post–high school graduation college credit at the time of application. Check out any restrictions ahead of time.

If you earn AP credit or take college classes in biology, chemistry, or physics in high school, you should strongly consider retaking those classes at your college to solidify your knowledge, acclimate to the university climate, and be more fully prepared upper division classes.

Chalk off the courses you retake to experience. These classes are fundamental to your future and critical components of the MCAT. You want to master the material, particularly STEM classes, even better than the first time. Besides, earning an A by retaking the class will not hurt you. It is also very possible that your future university science classes will cover material you did not learn before. However, jumping ahead in college will only put you at a disadvantage with your classmates as you move on to higher level classes. There are no awards for bravery and precociousness. You need As. Acceptance is contingent on your GPA. So, protect it with your life. Steady your boat, dive into the material, and head for mastery. Tutor other students in your class if you feel you have learned all of the concepts.

During college, some students consider taking physics at a community college to 'dodge' a more competitive university class, finish course requirements in the summer, or choose a less expensive alternative to university classes. While the difference in difficulty may not be significant, many times community college classes, taken in required science classes, are viewed by medical schools as a red flag.

Classes taken at a community college in non-science classes could be used as GPA boosters since a student's undergraduate GPA is vitally important. Remember, a low GPA, particularly in the most challenging science classes, could thwart your plans for medical or dental school. Be prepared by taking more challenging courses in high school.

# THE IMPORTANCE OF YOUR GRADE POINT AVERAGE

### Demonstrates Academic Rigor and Consistency

BS/MD, BS/DO, and BS/DDS programs are intensely competitive and academically rigorous. A high GPA shows that a student can handle challenging coursework, especially in sciences and math, perform consistently over time, and manage a demanding academic load. Medical/dental school is rigorous. These programs want assurance that a student can thrive through 8 or more years of demanding education.

### Serves as an Initial Filter

Since thousands of students apply for relatively few spots admissions officers use GPA thresholds of 3.8+ unweighted for high school students as a screening tool to help them quickly identify applicants with a proven record of academic success. Even with strong extracurriculars or test scores, a low GPA can disqualify a candidate early in the review.

### Correlates with Future Medical School Success

GPA, especially in STEM courses, is a strong predictor of performance in college, medical/dental school, and on the MCAT/DAT. Ability to grasp complex scientific material essential for clinical decision-making. Programs seek students who will stay on track and matriculate without needing remediation.

### Reflects Key Traits of a Strong Pre-Med Student

A high GPA also signals other essential qualities for a medical career, e.g. work ethic, discipline, time management, adaptability, and resilience. These traits are critical not only for surviving medical/dental school but for thriving in a demanding healthcare environment.

### Protects the Integrity of Guaranteed Admission

BS/MD, BS/DO, and BS/DDS programs often offer conditional acceptance to medical school. To protect the reputation of the program institutions only admit students who have already proven their ability to succeed. Schools want to ensure that admitted students will not later struggle and jeopardize their matriculation into the med school portion. Maintaining a strong GPA ensures students will meet progression requirements in the undergraduate years.

GPA is evidence of a student's readiness, resilience, and capability to handle the enormous intellectual and emotional challenges of a medical/dental education and career. With so many social, academic, curricular, and financial hurdles students must overcome, GPA is an important factor in BS/MD, BS/DO, and BS/DDS admissions.

> # " "
>
> *Behind every brilliant performance, there were countless hours of practice and preparation.*

– Eric Butterworth

CHAPTER EIGHT

# TESTING

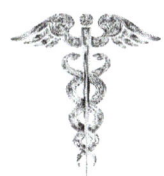

The pandemic eliminated testing requirements since test centers closed. However, many highly competitive universities and almost all BS/MD, BS/DO, and BS/DDS programs reinstated the SAT/ACT requirement. Still, check, since many colleges have flexible testing policies. This practice is slowly changing as more of the top schools either require or recommend the SAT or ACT. Direct medical/dental programs use the tests to demonstrate mastery and provide a bar for students to reach. Additional study may be required for students who have not learned the tested objectives. Khan Academy and practice tests are oft en beneficial, though there are many private tutors and organizations that assist with test preparation. Prepare, prepare, prepare!

### HERE IS A USEFUL PLAN:

### 1. Purchase Practice Test Books

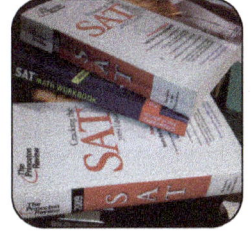

Official tests are best, straight from the testing agency. However, most of the major practice test publisher's materials are also worth getting. You do not need a book on how to do algebra since, in theory, you know algebra and the exam is intended to test what you learned. On the other hand, you do want the explanations at the end of the practice test that fully explain why the answer is right or wrong in case you missed the question. An answer of "c" is not good enough.

### 2. Establish a study schedule that you are willing to keep.

Everyone's life is different. Homework requirements vary. Clubs, sports, leadership, service, etc. take time. You know what will work for you. Decide a time that works for your schedule so you can practice.

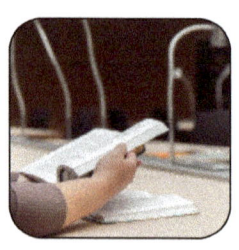

### 3. Plan to take 6 – 10 full practice tests.

Your personal game plan should include taking 6 – 10 full practice tests. Go over each question carefully to see where you made a mistake. Space out your personalized test prep schedule so that you complete as many of the ten practice tests as you can. This means that if the test is ten weeks away, plan for one a week. If the test is 20 weeks away, plan for one every two weeks. Starting early makes this process easier. If you are good at math or English, do not skip the practice test in that area since you want to get a very high score in your strong suit and not miss any of those questions.

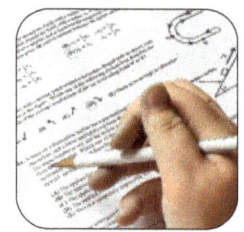

### 4. Time yourself.

You only need to take two of your practice tests as full timed tests. The others you can clock one section at a time. Sometimes you only have one hour. If so, take that one hour and do a section and check your answers. Just make sure that by the end of that week or two-week period, you have finished the entire practice test.

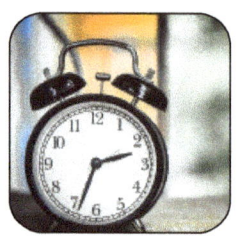

### 5. Highlight and tape flag questions you miss.

After you finish taking each full test or subsection, highlight and put a tape flag where you missed a question. Like stop lights, color-code questions with red for the questions you did not know how to solve or you skipped. Yellow (caution) for the ones in which you missed the questions but you have an idea of why it is wrong and just need to review the concept. Finally, put a green where you made a 'careless' error, and want to remember the rule that you forgot when you took the test. Whatever method you choose, make sure you identify the topics you need to review. Sometimes a pad of paper with the rules you need to remember is okay or a computer file or a sticky-note.

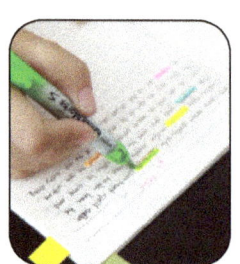

### 6. Test prep classes can be helpful.

If you do not practice, though, test prep is time consuming and inefficient. You have very little time if you are actively involved in school. Figure out what makes sense so you do not sacrifice your classwork and GPA. The cost for test prep is not as much of a problem as driving back and forth on a schedule that does not always fit your busy set of activities.

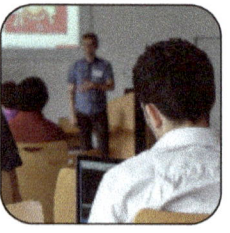

Some test prep classes are helpful and offer valuable training. However, often with test prep classes, you watch and listen to lectures on material you already know. In other cases, the test prep company times you while you take a test. You can really do that at home with a stopwatch or timer. However, if you choose to study on your own, you may find that after every test you take, you may want to hire a private tutor for an hour or two to go over the questions you missed.

Delaying the test-taking until the fall of your senior year is unwise unless absolutely necessary. Yet, you should not take a test in which you are unprepared or not in the test-taking mindset. Thus, the best time to take the SAT or ACT is when you are ready. However, do not delay. Typically, juniors take the SAT in March and ACT in April. May and June of your junior year is likely to be challenging with multiple AP tests and finals. Pace yourself. You need to take the tests, but this is not a good time to cram for the exam. Spread apart your preparation and test-taking. Prepare in the summer before your junior year or Christmas break when you have some time to take practice tests.

## SAT AND ACT

Almost all schools profiled in this book require either SAT or ACT. Some BS/MD programs, like Brown, George Washington, and Case Western expect to see AP test scores as well, especially in the biology, chemistry, physics, and mathematics.

Higher than average test scores are required since these programs are designed for the best and brightest students. Some programs have lower requirements for

entry, particularly those whose focus is on attracting students who are committed to working in rural areas or with disadvantaged communities. However, for the most competitive programs, students who matriculate have ACT scores of above 34 and SAT scores higher than 1450, though 1500 or higher is standard for those who are accepted in the admissions process.

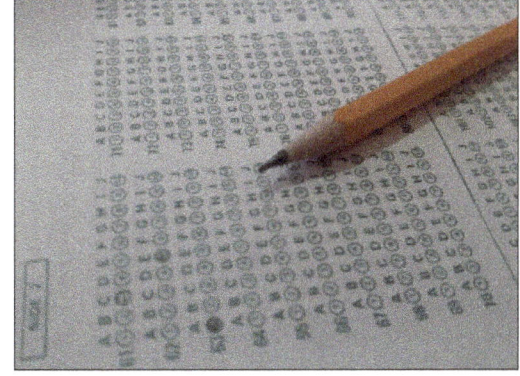

Minimum scores are often given so students do not spend considerable time working on an application in which they have virtually no chance of being accepted. Keep in mind, if this is your dream and you have the courses, grades, test scores, and determination to earn your medical degree while you are in high school the BS/MD, BS/DO, or BS/DDS route is a phenomenal opportunity.

As you might expect, admissions committees must have some cutoffs for applicant requirements to evaluate the best candidates. For Brown University's Program in Liberal Medical Education entering class of 2024 there were:

* Applicants: 4,251
* Offers of Admission: 94
* Matriculants: 63
* SAT Evidence-Based Reading and Writing (Average): 748
* SAT Mathematics (Average): 779
* ACT Composite (Average): 35

While super-scored tests are common in admissions processes that consider standardized testing, it is less common for BS/MD, BS/DO, and BS/DDS programs. Since super-scoring is not done in medical school admissions for the MCAT or DAT, in general, medical schools would prefer to see a test score in one sitting.

## AP TESTS

Self-reported AP test scores are used to determine mastery and official scores are only sent to colleges after the admissions process is concluded for verification. Planned AP tests are also self-reported. Most students applying to BS/MD, BS/DO, and BS/DDS programs have taken six AP or IB tests by the end of their junior year and have four to five planned for their senior year. Typically, AP scores include Chemistry and Biology and Calculus AB or BC. Senior AP tests frequently include Physics C.

## NATIONAL AP AWARDS (REVISED IN 2024)

**AP Scholar:** Scores of 3 or higher on three or more AP Exams.

**AP Scholar with Honor:** An average score of at least 3.25 on all AP Exams taken, and scores of 3 or higher on four or more of these exams.

**AP Scholar with Distinction:** An average score of at least 3.5 on all AP Exams taken, and scores of 3 or higher on five or more of these exams.

**Seminar and Research Certificate:** 3 or higher in both AP Research & AP Seminar

**Capstone Diploma:** Earn a 3 or higher in AP Research, AP Seminar, & 4 additional AP exams

**Discontinued awards include:** State AP Scholar, DoDEA AP Scholar, National AP Scholar, and International AP Scholar

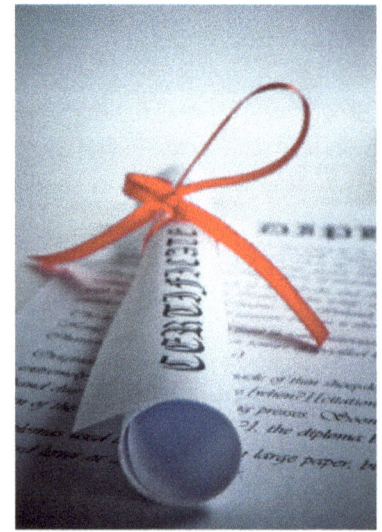

At this point, though some colleges remain test-optional, many schools are returning to standardized test requirements. Check first. While test optional means you are not required to take the SAT or ACT, if you have a good score, submit! Your test results may make all the difference in gaining admission. College admissions officers are studying this topic and reconsidering their policies.

Meanwhile, some colleges proclaim that test-optional truly means the test is not considered. Yet, evidence proves otherwise. Thus, many students still take the test and work around test preparation and test site hurdles amid the confusion. Data show that students who submitted scores within the college's range were accepted at a higher rate than those without a score. Meanwhile, some schools are test blind, meaning they do not consider test scores. Even so, a few of these same colleges still provide a place to input scores. Thus, they are not truly blind.

Nevertheless, the decision regarding whether you should take the test and/or submit your scores is yours. If the school does not require an admissions test, you can choose to take and submit the test as you like. If your academics are solid and you are willing to prepare for the test, you should take the test.

Competition continues to drive students to present evidence demonstrating they are worthy candidates. In the end, colleges need to make a final decision between very good students. If one student has a high standardized test score, that student may have a higher likelihood of acceptance depending upon the admissions committee's formal or subliminal decision-making process.

If you are taking AP classes, you are undoubtedly working diligently and mastering volumes of material tailored to valuable college skillsets. AP test scores give colleges a numerical score designed to tell whether you learned the material required in the curriculum. Though factors like sleep, practice, and mastery play a part in your outcome, many colleges believe your score is an important test of your subject matter knowledge.

Self-study is an option, but this requires discipline. Staying on track is tough through April and May with spring break, sports, service, clubs, school, and responsibilities. Cram sessions are helpful since most students take more than one AP test back-to-back in May. Practice tests and strategy workshops are helpful too. Many AP teachers work hard to ensure their students are prepared. Others do not, so take responsibility rather than blame others. Where there's a will, there's a way.

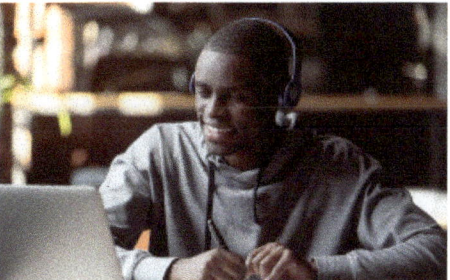

**Success is not the key to happiness. Happiness is the key to success. If you love what you are doing, you will be successful.**

–Albert Schweitzer

## CHAPTER NINE
# VOLUNTEER & SERVICE ACTIVITIES

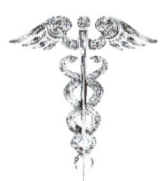

C olleges look at more than just grades and test scores. A holistic review is particularly true for BS/MD, BS/DO, and BS/DDS programs since a small group of students work together independently and collaboratively, fostering relationships throughout the program. Yet, another major factor is that students in these programs are considered the best and brightest. They are often in the honors program and are looked to as leaders. Their habits are likely to be emulated by other pre-med hopefuls. Thus, school involvement and leadership are considered highly in the application process.

If you cannot join a club or a club is defunct, take responsibility for its resurgence or start a new one. Many students will quit clubs because "nobody is doing anything." That is a red flag. When people are no longer participating, and there are no activities planned, it takes leadership to get the club up and running again. If you were working on a team project and your elected group leader got sick, would you quit? If the leader of your group project did not respond to e-mails, would you decide not to finish the assignment and fail to deliver your class presentation? If your club is inactive, breathe life into the group. Find a list of members, invite new members, and revive the heart of the group's activities.

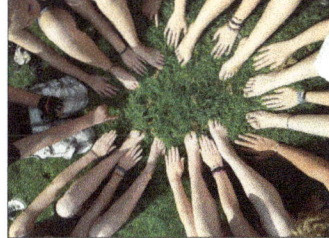

Getting involved in student body leadership on a school-wide scale is valuable, since holding an elected office and serving as a representative identifies those who may also pursue student body leadership in college as well. Furthermore, the role of a doctor in a clinic or hospital is, in many ways, a leadership position. Thus, whether you are the leader of a club, sport, student group, or team, you are demonstrating the skills needed to progress as a leader in the healthcare industry.

Community service is essential to understanding the world around you. There are dozens of places to serve with public and private organizations. Tutoring kids at a local elementary or junior high school, volunteering at the YMCA, coaching a kids camp, helping build homes in Mexico, or spending a week at Vacation Bible School are just a few of the volunteer opportunities with children. You can work with the elderly at a nursing/retirement home or at a soup kitchen or homeless shelter. Some in admissions consider the absence of community service a deal-breaker.

Here are a few options:

| | | | |
|---|---|---|---|
| 5K Walks | Drug Awareness | Medical Missions | Salvation Army |
| Africa Cries Out | Elder/Hospice Care | Medical Research | Schools |
| Animal Shelters | Feed America | Musical Events | Soup Kitchens |
| Beach Cleanup | Fire Prevention | Nursing Homes | Special Olympic |
| Boating Safety | Food Banks | Operation Smile | Sports Camps |
| Carnivals | Forest Renewal | Park Cleanups | Suicide Prevention |
| Charity Events | Habitat for Humanity | Political Campaigns | Theater Docent |
| Church Events | Homeless Shelters | Red Cross | Veterans Events |
| Club Dust | Human Trafficking | Refugee Centers | Wetlands Conservation |
| Doctors w/o Borders | International Service | Rescue Missions | Working Wardrobes |
| Domestic Violence Ctrs | Marine Life Asst | Ronald Mcdonald | Youth Action Teams |

... along with organizations supporting conditions like Alzheimer's, cancer, cleft palate, cystic fibrosis, dementia, diabetes, Ebola, heart disease, HIV/AIDS, leukemia, multiple sclerosis, muscular dystrophy, Parkinson's, polio, and TB. By starting now and accumulating hours, you can earn one of the following Presidential awards.

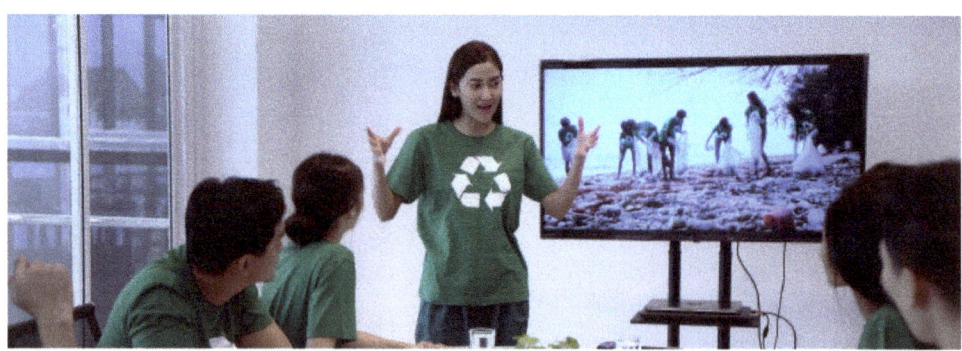

# PRESIDENT'S VOLUNTEER SERVICE AWARD

**Hours Required to Earn Awards in Each Age Group**

| Age Group | Bronze | Silver | Gold | Lifetime Achievement Award |
|---|---|---|---|---|
| Kids (5–10 years old) | 26–49 hours | 50–74 hours | 75+ hours | 4,000+ hours |
| Teens (11–15) | 50–74 hours | 75–99 hours | 100+ hours | 4,000+ hours |
| Young Adults (16–25) | 100–174 hours | 175–249 hours | 250+ hours | 4,000+ hours |
| Adults (26+) | 100–249 hours | 250–499 hours | 500+ hours | 4,000+ hours |

# LEARNING OBJECTIVES

Community service teaches numerous lessons that can be applied to the practice of medicine and dentistry.

**Communication** – In service activities, students learn to listen carefully, follow directions, and communicate instructions to others. Clarity is essential, but compassion is equally important. Similarly, physicians must communicate appropriately, respectfully, and empathetically. However, effectively explaining complex scientific topics is not as easy as it sounds, especially since many patients have no technical or scientific background. Attentive listening is equally important. By working alongside others on community service projects, students improve their communication.

**Teamwork** - Serving with others at a 5K, orphanage, or a kids sports camp provides opportunities to communicate, cooperate, and integrate, while developing the necessary skills for collaboration, leadership, and inclusivity. As such, students discover other's strengths and weaknesses while establishing goals, dividing tasks, and creating a plan of action.

**Creativity** – In serving others, students harness creativity, problem-solving, and critical thinking. In a research internship, students might compile statistical data in charts, articles, and Powerpoint presentations. Similarly, physicians test, analyze, and evaluate, making decisions based on a multitude of factors.

**Problem Solving** – When serving at a nursing home, homeless shelter, or food bank, there are always more people to help and ways to serve. Identify opportunities along with challenges that need to be resolved. With a solutions-oriented approach, money can be raised or friends can be invited to help at the next event. Physicians constantly solve problems since many cases are unique and emergencies arise.

**Ethics** – When finding a person's wallet during a beach clean up, locate the nearest responsible party. When two kids are fighting over a ball, cultivate a sense of trust and fairness. When you are asked to post the hours you work, do not overinflate them. Likewise, physicians have an ethical responsibility to society and a professional responsibility to patients, colleagues, and clinic leaders.

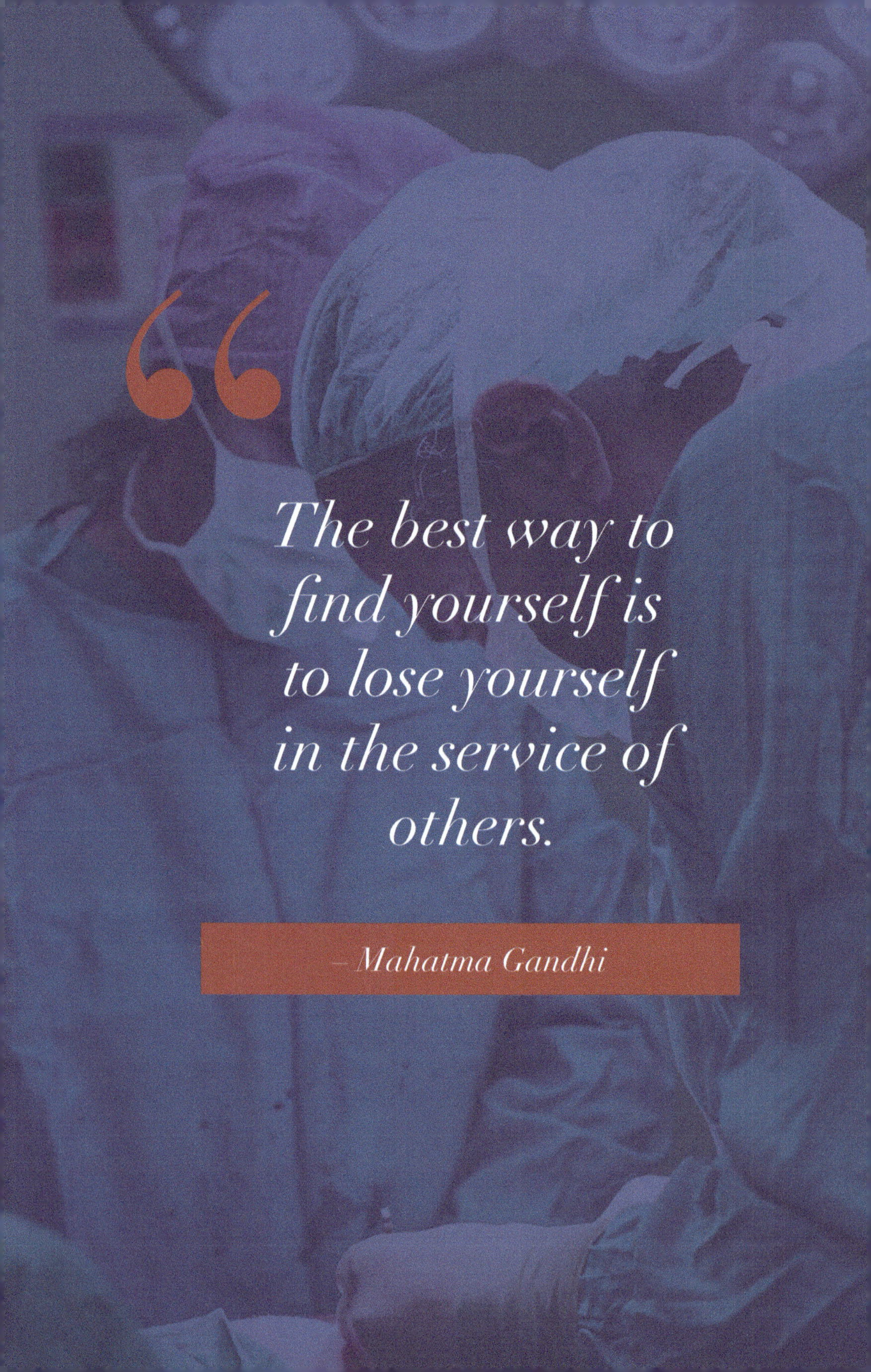

"

The best way to
find yourself is
to lose yourself
in the service of
others.

– Mahatma Gandhi

CHAPTER TEN

# RESEARCH & HEALTHCARE EXPERIENCES

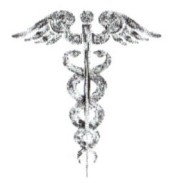

## RESEARCH

Experience with scientific research allows you to better understand not only the scientific method but the process scientists undergo to understand the complexity of the human mind, body, and behaviors. Whether you are involved in stem-cell research, neuroscience development, virus testing, or the demographic study of disease spread, you have embarked on uncovering problems yet to be resolved. Knowing how this process works in university or private laboratories provides you with a deeper understanding of medicine's advancement through the research process.

Some universities place a high priority on students who conducted literature reviews, worked in research laboratories, or developed their own research projects. The Regeneron Science Talent Search, often referred to as the "Junior Nobel Prize," is the oldest and most prestigious research-based science competition for high school seniors, giving out $3.1 million each year with a first-place prize of $250,000.

There are numerous competitions and many are included in this book. However, conducting research at a university, pharmaceutical company, or government facility is valuable. Obtain these opportunities by contacting researchers, asking neighbors if they know anyone who can get you an interview, or talking to your school counselor. There are also internships, summer programs, and laboratory assistantships. Some have training or apprenticeship programs.

## SUMMER RESEARCH PROGRAMS (SHORT LIST)

**Applications of Nanoscience Summer Institute** – 2-week residential research program held at UCLA.

**Caltech - Summer Research Connection** - Hands-on STEM - Pasadena Jrs & Srs

**CeBA - Cell Biology Academy @ Duke U.** - Summer research for HS Jrs & Srs

**Clark Scholars Program** – Texas Tech's 7-week research program w/stipend. Cold **Spring Harbor Lab Partners for the Future** - Competitive HS research prog.

**COSMOS** - The University of California's Summer STEM Program.

**GL4HS - NASA GeneLab** for HS Jrs & Srs - Space biosciences, 12 weeks virtual

**HRSA** - UT Austin HS Research Academy - 5-weeks biochem, neurosci, & genetics

**HSHSP** – Michigan State University's High School Honors STEM Program – 7-week intensive summer research program (MI residency not required).

**Jackson Laboratory Summer Student Program** -10-wks (18+) research internship.

**MITES** – Minority Introduction to Engineering and Science - Free 6-week intensive program; 80 students chosen.

**MMSS** – Michigan Math and Science Scholars (MMSS) – 2- research program

**NSA** - Cybersecurity, Data Science, National Security - HS Juniors & Seniors

**NIH Summer Internship Program (SIP)** - HS-College-Grad in biomed research.

**RABS** – Cornell University's Research Apprenticeship in Biological Sciences – 6-week medical/ research program.

**RIBS** - University of Chicago's Research in the Biological Sciences

**RISE** – BU Research in Science & Eng – 6-week practicum or internship track.

**Rochester Young Scholars in Immunology** - Biomedical sciences research at UR

**RSI** – Research Science Institute - Free, 6-weeks applied science; 70 students.

**SAMS** – Carnegie Mellon's Summer Academy for Math & Science – 6-week residential program.

**SIMR** – Stanford Institutes of Medicine Summer Research Program – 8-week intensive for rising junior or senior.

**SPARK** - Cedars Sinai's California Institute of Regenerative Medicine – Stem Cell Internship – 7-week mentorship program for HS juniors - 8 students chosen.

**SSP** – Summer Science Program is a 6-week prestigious summer research experience for high school students, hosted at 14 university campuses in 2025.

**WTP** – Women's Technology Program – 4-week hands-on engineering labs/ projects; 60 students chosen.

Research universities look for talented students who will bring curiosity and skills to their projects. Many are difficult to obtain, so some creativity may be needed to land you a clinical or academic research opportunity. If you do pursue a research project, be able to explain why you got involved, the lab procedures you undertook, what the study aimed to discover, and what you learned from the experience.

# SECURING A VOLUNTEER RESEARCH INTERNSHIP

For students interested in careers in medicine, biotechnology, neuroscience, or immunology, obtaining early research experience can be a powerful step. Internships, especially volunteer opportunities, open doors to mentorship, technical skills, and a deeper understanding of scientific inquiry. Yet, for many students, the biggest question is: *how do I get started if I don't know anyone?*

## Step 1: Define Your Interests

Before you reach out to anyone, clarify your focus. Are you more interested in wet lab biology, computational immunology, clinical trials, or public health applications of biotech? Defining your interests allows you to target your outreach efforts effectively.

## Step 2: Research Professors, Labs, and Institutions

To find

* University professors who conduct research in your interest area use university department websites or platforms like Google Scholar.

* Pharmaceutical companies, consider internship or volunteer programs with AbbVie, Allergan, Eli Lilly, Genentech, Johnson & Johnson, Merck, Pfizer, etc.)

* Biotech Companies, review opportunities with Amgen, Biogen, Gilead Sciences, Regeneron, Vertex, etc.

* Research hospitals and medical centers with summer student research programs

* Nonprofits or think tanks in health policy or biotechnology

Use keywords like "immunology lab," "biotech internship for high school students," or "volunteer research in medicine" along with the names of local universities or institutions.

## Step 3: Prepare a Targeted Email

If your family does not have a contact name, cold emailing is your best option. Your message should be concise and professional. Include:

1. A short introduction (name, grade/year, school)
2. A statement of interest (why their work caught your eye)
3. A brief academic background (relevant classes, skills, GPA if strong)
4. A polite request to volunteer or assist in ongoing research
5. Your resume (attached as a PDF)

Example:

"Dear Dr. Lee, I am a high school junior who is interested in pursuing immunology. I was fascinated by your recent work on T-cell therapies published in *Nature Immunology*. I am writing to you today to ask whether I might be able to volunteer in your lab this summer to gain experience and contribute in any capacity."

## Step 4: Explore Formal Programs

Many universities and labs offer structured summer research programs for high school and undergraduate students. Apply early since many have deadlines between January and March.

## Step 5: Follow Up and Stay Professional

If you have not heard back after 10–14 days, it is okay to send a polite follow-up email. If the lab or researcher declines, thank them and ask if they can refer you to anyone else who might be looking for assistance.

Start local. Many labs are open to curious, driven students, especially those who show initiative. Persistence, professionalism, and passion sets you apart even without connections. Do not be discouraged by a few rejections. One yes starts your journey into research.

## CLINICAL

Volunteer healthcare service demonstrates five qualities: (1) Empathy, (2) Care, (3) Awareness, (4) Commitment, (5) Passion. It takes more than intellect and knowledge to be an excellent physician. It takes a large dose of humanity. Selflessness is an essential ingredient as well. During the coronavirus pandemic, physicians compassionately treated patients, even though their lives were in jeopardy. Many doctors died just to save their patients. Service is a mindset. Altruism is highly valued.

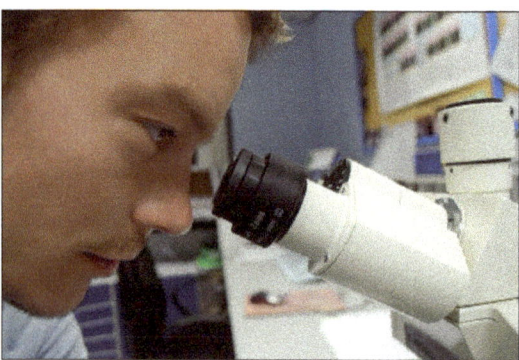

Thus, clinical experiences are essential to understanding the practice of medicine. BS/MD, BS/DO, and BS/DDS admissions officers want to know if you are serious about medicine. Remember, accepting you is their promise to support you through this process on some level. This is both a commitment and an investment. They could choose someone else. Admissions decision-makers also want to know that you are dedicated to helping people and passionate about serving your community.

Experiences in medicine provide a chance to know whether you enjoy helping the weak, challenged, ill, or dying. Patients and their families tend to be anxious, concerned their condition may be serious and wanting immediate answers. They may be upset, in pain, or frustrated with the environment, the food, or just waiting.

Common clinical opportunities include hospital volunteer programs, physician shadowing, hospice volunteering, medical assistant internships, and participation in pre-health summer programs hosted by universities or hospitals. Shadowing a physician, even for a few days, provides exposure to the daily routines, challenges, and ethical decisions faced by medical professionals.

More extensive, sustained experiences show a consistent commitment. The primary underlying reason is for you to learn more about healthcare and whether or not you are a good fit for this field, its demands, and the importance of empathy and compassion for those whose health and possibly life is in question. Many students who apply have 50 – 100 hours of clinical experience.

To find opportunities, students can start by contacting local hospitals, community clinics, or private practices and inquiring about youth volunteer programs. Many hospitals have structured high school volunteer tracks that allow students to assist with non-clinical tasks, interact with patients, and observe healthcare settings. Students should also ask family doctors or specialists if they allow high school observers. Additionally, organizations such as HOSA-Future Health Professionals or local Red Cross chapters offer health-related volunteer roles.

Volunteering in a hospital, clinic, or dental office helps you learn more about the field and determine your commitment. You will develop a reasonable expectation of what you might experience in the medical/dental field. BS/MD, BS/DO, and BS/DDS admissions officers seek students who fully demonstrate their determination to pursue medicine through service and describe this commitment in an interview.

Strong communication, professionalism, and persistence are essential when requesting opportunities. Write a concise email expressing their interest in medicine/dentistry, availability, and willingness to comply with privacy regulations and health screenings. These early experiences help applicants understand patient care and clarify their commitment to a future in medicine or dentistry.

> ## If your actions inspire others to dream more, learn more, do more, and become more, you are a leader.

— *John Quincy Adams*

# CHAPTER ELEVEN
# ACADEMIC PREPARATION & COMPETITIONS

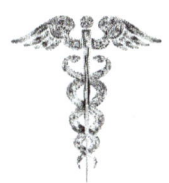

S tudent-centered competitions inspire a sense of purpose. With each round, students grow, learn, and improve. As the level of competition rises, races, games, or problems get harder and participants become more formidable opponents. Resilience and persistence are essential. The lessons learned in competition remain throughout life, helping individuals continue when they want to quit, work harder at improving themselves, and staying true to themselves even when challenges are not always fair.

Whether participating in art, chess, debate, speed cubing, Scrabble, poetry, or Science Olympiad, the lessons are valuable. Academic competitions test knowledge, but they also serve as powerful platforms for growth, discovery, and inspiration. Students ignite their innate curiosity and push self-imposed boundaries. With practice, organization, and regrouping, they read their textbooks and apply what they have learned in exciting, real-world contexts. These events stretch thinking and resolve problems, allowing students to explore their passions in ways that are deeply rewarding and personally transformative.

Beyond academics and social assimilation, competitions build confidence and character. They teach perseverance in the face of setbacks, while cultivating discipline, fostering collaboration, and developing communication skills. When students prepare for and compete with their peers, they learn how to handle pressure, speak with conviction, and adapt quickly. Win or lose, every participant walks away with something valuable: a sharper mind, a stronger spirit, and a deeper understanding of what it means to challenge themselves.

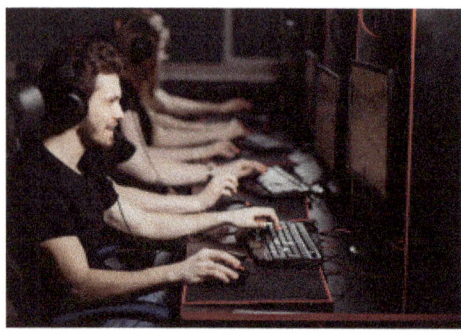
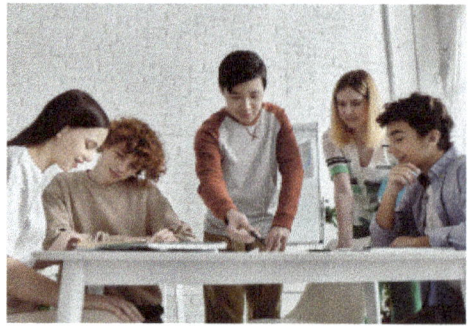

Most importantly, students connect to a broader community of thinkers, dreamers, and doers who share their excitement for and interests in international affairs, law, science, robotics, or rocketry. In these vibrant, competitive environments, students discover their willingness to spend sleepless nights on the floor of a massive hackathon or in conference center halls reciting information for a debate. These experiences spark lifelong interests. For any student looking to grow intellectually and personally, stepping into the world of student-centered competitions is one of the most empowering and enriching choices of their high school experience.

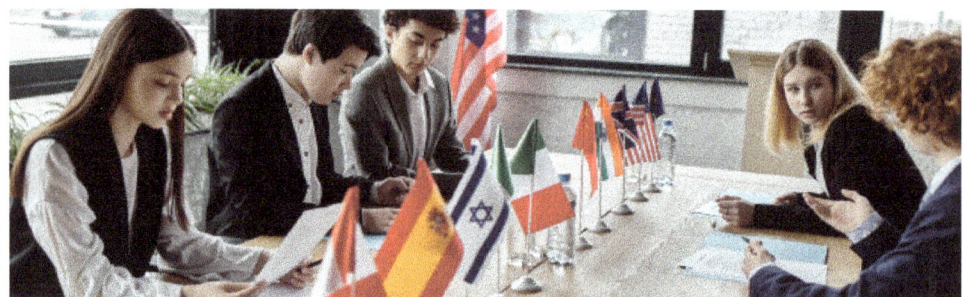

## COMPETITIONS AND PRIZES

***3M Young Scientist Challenge*** – Sponsored by 3M and administered by Discovery Education, this middle school competition inspires students to improve people's lives. Ten finalists are chosen based on communication, originality, potential, and a short video explaining their project. Finalists are paired with 3M scientists who mentor them in the development process. One national winner is selected.

***American Rocketry Challenge*** – The Design/Build/Fly rocketry contest is the world's largest student rocket contest. First sponsored in 2002 by the Aerospace Industries Association and the National Association of Rocketry, events seek to increase interest in STEM subjects in middle and high school students. The top 100 teams are invited to the National Finals where prizes are awarded. The American Institute of Aeronautics & Astronautics holds Design/Build/Fly  contests on the collegiate level.

***American Society of Human Genetics Essay Contest*** – This high school competition considers topics related to human genetics.  The 2025 DNA Essay Contest asked, in 750 words, "What risks or harms do you think using AI could pose in healthcare?"

***Bioethics Essay Contest*** – This STEM writing competition allows high school students to explore ethical issues in science and technology.

***BioGENEius Challenge*** – This internationally recognized competition  focused on STEM solutions to biotechnology problems in Healthcare, Agriculture-Biotech, and Industrial-Environmental Biotechnology. Winners are chosen in each category.

***Breakthrough Junior Challenge*** – This science video competition encourages students 13 to 18 to create short videos that explain complex scientific ideas in engaging ways. Participants compete for prizes, including a $250,000 college scholarship, a $50,000 award for their teacher, and a $100,000 school science lab.

***Broadcom MASTERS (Math, Applied Science, Technology, and Engineering for Rising Stars)*** – Since 2011, this prestigious middle school science and engineering competition awards students for innovative STEM projects and teamwork. Thirty finalists are selected to participate in a team-based, hands-on STEM competition which showcases the most practical and extraordinary science fair projects.

***Conrad Challenge*** – This competition continues the legacy of astronaut Charles "Pete" Conrad Jr. (third to walk on the Moon). This multi-phase competition focuses on innovation and entrepreneurship. Teams of 2-5 students pitch ideas to solve global challenges. Winners present their ideas to judges at the Innovation Summit. Winners develop a viable, scalable solution with real-world impact.

***eCYBERMISSION*** – The U.S. Army Educational Outreach Program sponsors this STEM competition for middle school students. Teams propose a solution to a real-world challenge with regional winners in 6,7,8, and 9 grades and one national winner.

***Engineer Girl Writing Contest*** – This writing contest, sponsored by the National Academy of Engineering focuses on how engineering impacts the world.

***ExploraVision Science Competition (Toshiba & the National Science Teaching Assn)*** Students use futuristic thinking to develop technology that may exist in 20 years in one of the world's largest K-12 science competitions. National, regional, and honorable mention winners are selected each year in four grade-level categories.

***FIRST Robotics Competition (FRC)*** – FIRST (For Inspiration and Recognition of Science & Technology) sponsors the international high school FRC. Teams design, build, and program robots for competitions, promoting teamwork and innovation.

***Genius Olympiad*** – This high school competition, coordinated by the Terra Science Education Foundation, focuses on environmental issues. Based in New York, students compete worldwide in the areas of science, visual and performing arts, writing, business, and robotics. Awards are given in each category.

***Google Science Fair*** – This online science/engineering competition is for students 13 to 18 who pose a question, develop a hypothesis, and conduct research. Regional finalists compete to be global finalists who are invited to Google's headquarters for the final round. Prizes are given in different age-specific and thematic categories.

***International Biology Olympiad (IBO)*** – Since 1990, more than a million students have competed in preliminary  competitions. On the international level, this prestigious event includes up to four of the top competitors selected from their National Biology Olympiad's local, regional, and national competitions.  Students from more than 75 countries come together each year to compete for the world prize.

***International Chemistry Olympiad (IChO)*** - This annual high school competition started in 1968 with three European teams and now represents 90+ countries. Each participating country selects its national team and two team leaders through its internal competition process. Team selection process varies by country. The IChO includes a 5-hour laboratory practical exam and a 5-hour written theoretical and experimental exam. Individual and team awards are presented.

***International Olympiad on Astronomy & Astrophysics (IOAA)*** – The annual IOAA high school competition, which started in 2007, recently, included 52 countries. National teams of up to five members (two team leaders) are selected by the participating country, typically from its national competition. The IOAA includes theoretical, observational, and practical exams. Individual and team awards are presented.

***International Physics Olympiad (IPhO)*** – This high school competition, started in 1967, recently hosted students from 90 countries. Each participating country selects its national team and two team leaders through its internal competitions. The team selection process varies by country. The IPhO tests knowledge and problem-solving in theoretical and experimental exams. Individual and team awards are presented.

***Junior Science and Humanities Symposia (JSHS)*** – Established in 1958 by the U.S. Army, Navy, & Air Force, this program challenges high school students to conduct STEM research in regional events. Winners advance to the national competition. Students present original research. The winners receive scholarships.

***Lexus Eco Challenge*** – The goal of the Land & Water Challenge and Air & Climate Challenge is to develop/implement programs that provide real-world environmental solutions to communities. Sixteen winning teams (eight middle school and eight high school) are awarded prizes and given the opportunity to participate in the Final Final Challenge, where the grand prize winners are selected.

***Living Rainforest International Schools Essay Competition*** – This essay contest challenges students to write about sustainable living and human's relationship with nature. In 2025, the topic considers "Eco-Anxiety to Eco Action & Empowerment".

***MATE ROV (Remotely Operated Vehicle)*** - This event brings students, educators, and professionals globally to compete in underwater robotics (categories for different skill/age groups). Participants design and build ROVs to complete mission tasks that simulated real-world scenarios, emphasizing problem-solving in marine technology.

***Microsoft Imagine Cup Junior*** – Introduced in 2020, this high school technology and innovation competition was created as part of Microsoft's broader Imagine Cup for university students. The junior level seeks to encourage students to pursue technology and computer science by developing global solutions for social impact. Winners are selected by their participation and development of technology like machine learning, virtual reality, artificial intelligence, and augmented reality.

**Moody's Mega Math (M3) Challenge** – M3, started in 2005, is a mathematics competition for high school students. Over a 14-hours, teams use models to solve real-world challenges. The top four to six teams are awarded scholarships.

**NASA Competitions** - Cube Quest, Break the Ice, Deep Space Food, and Watts on the Moon – These offer prizes totaling $5,000,000 to teams.

**NASA Scientist for a Day Essay Contest** – Students are challenged to write an essay about a topic related to space and planetary science. The 2025 Power to Explore topic was, "If you could plan an RPS-powered mission to any moon in our solar system, which moon would you choose to unravel its mysteries?"

**National Bioethics Bowl** – In this U.S. intercollegiate competition, students debate ethical issues in medicine, biotechnology, and healthcare. In each round, teams are given a case and present arguments to the other team and judges.

**Ocean Awareness Contest (Bow Seat Ocean Awareness Program)** – This high school student competition invites students to present art, research, and essays to win awards.

**Regeneron ISEF - International Science & Engineering Fair** – Over 175,000 students compete for $1.8 million in 400+ regional, state, and national science fairs worldwide with finalists representing 70 countries, regions, and territories. ISEF the largest intl HS STEM competition. Students present research/discoveries to win prizes in multiple categories. Grand Awards: 17 categories; each with first, second, third, and fourth place. There are also special awards given by public and private organizations.

**Regeneron Science Talent Search** – Started in 1942 by Westinghouse and Intel, this is the oldest U.S. science talent competition. From 300 scholar semifinalists, 40 finalists are chosen to present their research in D.C. and compete for awards.

**RoboCup** –This is the world's largest international robotics/AI competition. The long-term goal is to create a fully autonomous humanoid robot capable of winning in soccer against the reigning human World Cup champions.

**Samsung Solve for Tomorrow** – In this middle and high school student contest, participants use STEM solutions to address real-world issues. State winners are selected. National finalists are chosen to receive prizes, technology, and resources.

**Science Olympiad** - This STEM competition engages students from middle and high schools across the country. Teams participate in various events that involve building devices, experimenting, solving problems, and answering written tests.

**Shell Science Lab Challenge** – In 2010, the Shell Oil Company began sponsoring this contest, administered by the National Science Teaching Association for middle and high school science teachers who approach science in an innovative way. Approximately 18 winners receive a lab makeover with equipment and resources.

**Society for Technical Communication High School Writing Contest** – This contest challenges students to write essays on topics regarding science and technology.

**Wiki Science Competition:** – This photo contest encourages the creation of science imagery. Categories include People in Science, Microscopy, Non-Photographic Media, Image Sets, and Wildlife & Nature, Astronomy. Winning national-level images go on to the international level; unaffiliated countries are considered "other".

*Young Naturalist Awards (American Museum of Natural History)* – This essay competition is for middle and high school students with scientific research/writing.

# 21 PROGRAMMING CONTESTS

Good Luck!!! "May the force be with you!"

**ACM International Collegiate Programming Contest (ICPC)** - The ICPC is a prestigious, global programming competition; 3-member teams that solve algorithmic problems, showcasing programming skills. The ICPC holds regional contests in six continents.
*Notes*: Teams have three students and one coach. Over 50,000 students, 3,000 universities, 110 countries; about 140 teams compete in the World Finals. The fee is about $100/team. The prizes may include trophies, medals, or cash prizes.

**AtCoder Grand Contest (AGC)** - AGC is a programming contest organized by AtCoder, a Japanese platform. AGC tests data structure, algorithm, and problem-solving skills
*Notes:* All age groups, from beginner to expert, can participate w/no entry fee. Most of the 3,000 participants are advanced high school or college students. Register on the AtCoder website. Winners receive cash prizes/certificates. The finals are held online.

**Baidu Star** - Baidu Star is a Chinese programming contest organized by Baidu and open to students and professionals.
*Notes:* College students or professionals enter at no cost. The contest, which draws thousands of participants, is open to anyone with knowledge of algorithms and data structures. The winners receive cash prizes, job offers, or internships.

**CodeChef Long Challenge** - CodeChef's Long Challenge is a 10-day online programming contest. Participants have ample time to solve a series of problems.
*Notes:* All ages are invited, though most of the 20,000 – 25,000 participants are advanced high school and college students. Some are hobbyists seek to sharpen their skills. Register on CodeChef. Winners receive cash prizes, merchandise, or certificates.

**Codeforces Contest** - Codeforce participants solve timed programming problems and is known for both its dynamic ranking system and large global community.
*Notes:* Teams of 2-6 students, take part in rounds. National winners receive awards, scholarships, and trophies. Cost: about $200/team; over 6,000 teams participate.

*Codeforces Global Rounds:* These free events have more challenging problems. Fierce competition attracts 10,000-15,000 top coders from around the world.

**CyberPatriot (National Youth Cyber Defense Competition)** - CyberPatriot is a U.S. cybersecurity competition for middle/high school students. Teams compete to secure computer systems and networks in simulated environments.
*Notes:* Teams of 2-6 students and a coach, take part in rounds. National winners receive scholarships, trophies, or recognition. Cost: about $200/team; over 6,000 teams participate.

**Educational Computing Organization of Ontario (ECOO) Contest**- ECOO hosts a HS programming contest in Ontario, Canada focused on algorithmic problem-solving.
*Notes:* Hundreds of teams enter (~$100) with a coach. Winners receive medals, trophies, or recognition.

**Facebook Hacker Cup** - This annual competition challenges participants to solve algorithmic problems in multiple rounds; the top coders advance to the finals.
*Notes:* All ages are invited. Free. Individual registration (about 20,000 participate). Cash prizes, t-shirts, or plaques for winners.

**Google Code Jam** - This annual coding competition invites programmers globally to solve algorithmic problems in several rounds, culminating in a world final.
*Notes:* All ages are invited. Free. Individual registration (about 50,000 participants). Cash prizes up to $15,000, t-shirts, or plaques.

**Google Hash Code** - In this team-based programming competition coders work together to solve a real-world engineering problem within a fixed time frame.
*Notes:* All ages are invited. Free. Register in 2-4 person teams. With over 100,000 participants, Google offers winning teams cash, t-shirts, or plaques.

**Hackerrank Contests** - Regular timed programming contests, including algorithms, data structures, and AI, help to improve coding skills.
*Notes:* All ages are invited. Free. Individual registration on Hackerrank. Prizes include cash, swag, or job opportunities.

**ICPC for Women (ICPCW)** - ICPCW is a programming contest encourages women to compete in programming.
*Notes:* Female college students compete in teams of three students and one coach. Prizes can include trophies, medals, and cash.

**International Olympiad in Informatics (IOI)** - IOI is a prestigious computer science competition for high school students, testing skills in algorithmic problem-solving, programming, and informatics.
*Notes:* About 400 high school students worldwide compete in individual contests for medals, certificates or scholarships.

**Kaggle Competitions** - This data science/machine learning competition offers real-world predictive modeling w/prizes & recognition in the data science community.
*Notes:* Individual or team - varies based on the contest. Thousands compete for cash prices up to $100,000, along with job opportunities and recognition.

**Kick Start(Google Coding Competition)** - This online coding competition helps participants improve their coding skills and prepare for technical interviews.
*Notes:* All ages are invited. Free. Individual competition with 10,000-15,000 participants. Prizes include recognition and t-shirts.

**Microsoft Imagine Cup** - Student developers/entrepreneurs create innovative solutions to real-world problems using Microsoft technology.
*Notes:* Students 16+ compete in teams of 1-3 members for cash, mentorship, and project funding up to $100,000. Thousands compete annually.

**NASA Space Apps Challenge** - In this global hackathon, participants develop solutions to challenges related to space exploration, Earth science, and technology. *Notes:* Teams of all ages compete in coding, design, and engineering. Over 40,000 participants compete for recognition, NASA items, and free invites to NASA events.

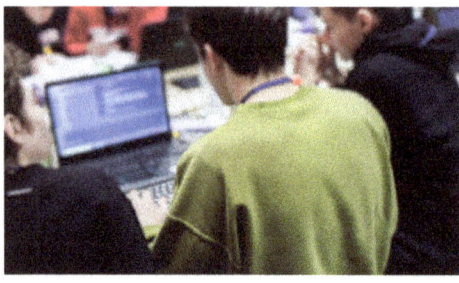 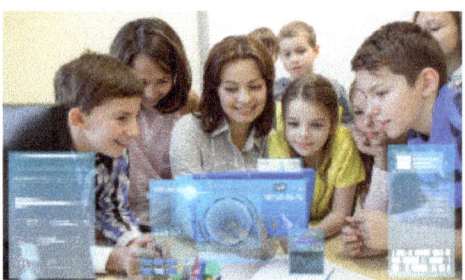

**picoCTF** - Middle/high school students, participate in free, fun, online game-like cybersecurity challenges developed by CMU with 700,000 participants worldwide. *Notes:* Free event with 1-4 student teams. Over 20,000 students compete for scholarships, cash, and recognition.

**TopCoder Open (TCO)** - In TCO's intl programming competition, participants compete in coding challenges, including algorithms, data science, and marathon matches. *Notes:* All ages can join this free individual event. Register on TopCoder. Prizes up to $15,000, merchandise, and recognition.

**USA Computing Olympiad (USACO)** - U.S. high school students participate in USACO's progressively challenging algorithmic problem-solving competition. *Notes:* Free for enrolled HS students in this individual event with 5,000-7,000 participants. Prizes include medals, certificates, and qualification for the IOI.

**Yandex Algorithm Contest** - This annual competition challenges participants with difficult algorithmic problems. *Notes:* Popular among Russian-speaking programmers, in this free individual event, all ages are welcome. Prizes include cash, merchandise, and certificates.

## 11 POPULAR CAPTURE THE FLAG COMPETITIONS

**ASIS CTF -** One of the largest and most popular online CTF competitions, this worldwide event is known for its difficult and creative challenges.

**Boston Key Party CTF** - BKP is a large, well-known, and highly regarded online CTF competition with innovative challenges and participation from top teams globally.

**DEF CON CTF -** The most famous CTF competitions worldwide, held annually at the DEF CON hacker conference. Elite teams come from around the globe and feature highly complex challenges. Winning this competition is considered a major accomplishment. **Location:** Las Vegas, NV

**Facebook CTF -** In this online cybersecurity competition, participants solve security challenges, including cryptography, reverse engineering, and web security. All ages are invited. Free. Register in teams (hundreds compete). Cash prizes and recognition in the cybersecurity community.

**Google CTF -** This global online competition offers both beginner and advanced challenges, drawing thousands worldwide. Cybersecurity topics include reverse engineering, cryptography, and web exploitation.

**Hack-A-Sat CTF –** This space-focused competition is hosted by the U.S. Air Force and Space Force. This major event involves hacking satellite systems and defending against cyberattacks. **Location:** Online and DEF CON Las Vegas, NV

**Hack-In-The-Box CTF –** The HITB CTF cybersecurity competition draws global participants, featuring advanced challenges and attracting top teams. **Location:** HTB conferences in Amsterdam, Dubai, Singapore, etc.

**PlaidCTF -** Plaid Parliament of Pwning CTF, centered at Carnegie Mellon University, is one of the most competitive and well-regarded online CTF events globally, attracting teams worldwide with challenging cybersecurity problems covering areas such as web hacking, reverse engineering, exploitation, forensics, and cryptography.

**RuCTF -** This major CTF competition is known for its unique challenges and high level of difficulty. Universities/companies compete. **Location:** Yekaterinburg, Russia

**UCSB iCTF (International CTF) -** The UCSB iCTF is one of the longest-running academic CTF competitions, with offensive/defensive challenges that attract students/professionals from around the world. **Location:** UCSB and online

**VolgaCTF -** This international competition attracts high-level teams from various countries in high-impact challenges. **Location:** Russia

## 25 TOP HACKATHONS

**AngelHack –** This online hackathon series fosters entrepreneurship, encouraging participants 18 and older to turn their ideas into startups.

**Cal Hacks -** UC Berkeley hosts Cal Hacks, one of the largest college hackathons in the world for about 2,000 students, fostering innovation in various fields.

**Dragon Hacks -** Drexel's hackathon, with about 300 college students, focuses on innovation and technology development.

**DubHacks –** In Seattle, U-Dub hosts the largest Pacific Northwest event for college students, with about 800 students.

**ETHDenver –** This free event is a leading blockchain hackathon and conference focusing on decentralized applications and Web3 technologies for about 2,000 participants ages 18 and up.

**Hack the North –** In Canada's largest hackathon, hosted at the University of Waterloo, college students focus on building innovative tech solutions. The event is free and hosts about 1,500 participants.

**Hack the Planet –** Planet Labs, a company specializing in satellite imagery and Earth data, hosts this free event for about 1,000 entrants on climate change and environmental sustainability challenges using satellite data and geospatial analysis.

**HackDuke** - Known as "Code for Good", HackDuke focuses on social innovation and using technology to solve societal problems with about 600 college students.

**HackGT** - Georgia Tech's fall hackathon attracts about 1,500 college students to work on tech-driven projects.

**HackIllinois** - Hosted at the University of Illinois with tracks for software development, hardware, design, and data science, about 1,000 students create innovative solutions to real-world problems – prizes and networking.

**HackKU** – This University of Kansas-sponsored event brings about 200 students together to create innovative projects in 36 hours.

**HackMIT** – Hosted by MIT, this is one of the largest free undergraduate hackathons, attracting around 1,000 students globally to solve real-world challenges.

**HackNY** – This free NYC-based college student hackathon with about 300 participants promotes creativity and innovation in technology.

**HackNYU** - NYU's global hackathon is held simultaneously in New York, Abu Dhabi, and Shanghai, focusing on innovative tech solutions. The spring event is free for the 500 college students who attend.

**HackRU** - Rutgers offers about 600 college students a chance to work on exciting tech projects over 24 hours.

**HackUMass** – Held at UMass, this free event for college students brings 1,000 students together to create tech solutions in a collaborative environment.

**HackZurich** – At Europe's largest free hackathon, more than 500 participants 18 and up focus on creating innovative and impactful digital solutions.

**Junction** - Europe's leading hackathon with about 1,300 participants, hosted in Finland, focuses on building digital and hardware projects.

**LA Hacks** – In the largest hackathon in Southern California, UCLA hosts this free event for about 1,500 college students focusing on creating impactful tech solutions.

**Major League Hacking (MLH) Hackathons** – MLH organizes a series of free hackathons primarily for 200-500 college students worldwide. This competition is known for promoting student innovation and learning.

**MHacks** – The University of Michigan hosts one of the largest and most influential student hackathons in the U.S. for college students.

**PennApps** – This was one of the first hackathons. PennApps' competitive environment brings about 1,500 college students to this free event.

**TechCrunch Disrupt Hackathon** – This free popular hackathon for about 1,000 participants 18 and up focuses on innovative tech solutions.

**TreeHacks** – Stanford hosts its premier hackathon in the winter for about 1,000 participants. College students solve pressing societal challenges.

**Yale Hack** – Yale's hackathon encourages around 300 college students to create innovative solutions in various fields.

# ARTISTIC, WRITING, AND PHILOSOPHY COMPETITIONS

### *Adroit Journal* - Gregory Djanikian Scholarships (Poetry and Short Story)

- Eligibility: Emerging writers who have not published full-length collections or novels, regardless of age, geographic location, or educational status
- Prizes: $100-$200 and publication of their portfolios of poems or short stories in a future issue of the *Adroit Journal.*

### American Foreign Service Association (AFSA) High School  Essay Contest

- Topic: Changes annually, with the 2024 topic focusing on how U.S. diplomats can adapt and mitigate global challenges
- Eligibility: High school students
- Prizes: $2,500, an all-expense-paid trip to Washington, D.C., a voyage on Semester at Sea, and the winner's school receives 10 copies of an AFSA publication on diplomacy

### American Legion Oratorical Contest

- Topic: U.S. Constitution (varies annually)
- Format: 8-10 minute speech delivered without technology
- Eligibility: High school students
- Prizes: Travel and lodging expenses covered for department winners and their chaperones

### American Philosophical Association

- Topics: Various (bioethics, climate, democracy, film, health, law, policy, race, etc.)
- Eligibility: High school, college, and graduate students
- Prizes: Vary by submission type

### Ayn Rand Essay Contests

- Books: *Anthem, The Fountainhead, and Atlas Shrugged*
- Eligibility: Students in grades 8-12 and, for *Atlas Shrugged*, also college students
- Prizes: Up to $25,000

### Bennington Young Writers Awards

- Categories: Poetry, Fiction, Nonfiction
- Eligibility: High school students in grades 9-12
- Prizes: $250, $500, $1,000

### Bill of Rights Institute – We the Students  Essay Contest

- Topic: Natural rights
- Eligibility: High school students
- Prizes: $500-$7,500

### Bow Seat Ocean Awareness Art, Poetry, and Writing Contest

- Categories: Art, Poetry, Writing
- Eligibility: Students aged 11-18 worldwide

- Prizes: $100-$1,500

## Columbia Scholastic Press Association (CSPA) Contests

- Categories: Six categories, four award categories (Gold Circles)
- Eligibility: High school and college students

## Concord Review

- Focus: Academic research papers on history
- Eligibility: High school students
- Prizes: Emerson Prize

## Daughters of the American Revolution (DAR) Essay Contests

- Middle School: American History  Essay Contest
- High School: Patriots of the American Revolution Contest
- Prizes: Certificates, medals, monetary awards

## David McCullough Essay Prize

- Topics: American history
- Eligibility: High school students
- Prizes: $10,000, $5,000, $1,000

## Elie Wiesel Prize in Ethics Essay Contest

- Topic (2025): "What challenges awaken your consciousness?"
- Eligibility: College students
- Prizes: $10,000, $5,000, $3,000, and $1,000

## EngineerGirl Writing Contest

- Topics: Engineering and global impact
- Eligibility: Students in grades 3-12
- Prizes: $100-$500

## Girls State, Girls Nation,  Boys State, Boys Nation – American Legion & Auxiliary

- Focus: Leadership, government learning
- Eligibility: Top high school students in each state
- Prizes: Varies by event

## Great History Challenge

- Focus: History passion and interest
- Eligibility: Middle school students
- Prizes: National championship qualification

## Holocaust Art & Writing Contest

- Categories: Art, film, poetry, prose
- Eligibility: High school students
- Prizes: 1st, 2nd, and 3rd place awards

## International History Olympiad

- Qualification:  National History Bee & Bowl Tournaments, U.S. History Bee, Qualifying Exam
- Divisions: Varsity, JV, Middle School, Intermediate, Elementary

- Prizes: Varies by event

## Jane Austen Society of North America  Essay Contest

- Categories: High school, college/university, graduate school
- Prizes: $1,000, $500, $250

## John F. Kennedy Center for the Performing Arts VSA  Playwright Discovery Program

- Eligibility: Students ages 14-19 with disabilities
- Prizes: Playwrights program participation at the Kennedy Center

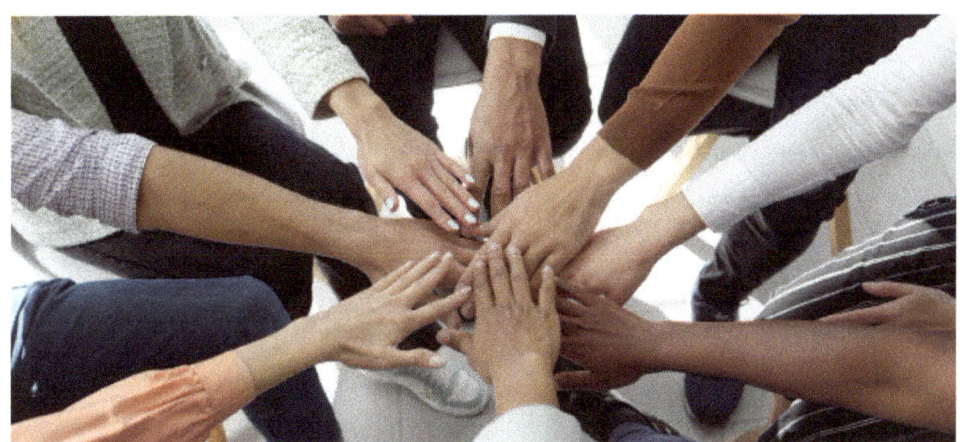

## John Locke Global Essay Competition

- Categories: Philosophy, Politics, Economics, History, Psychology, Theology, Law
- Eligibility: Students
- Prizes: Varies by category

## Nancy Thorp Poetry Contest

- Eligibility: Female high school and college students
- Prizes: $350, publication, scholarships

## National Council of Teachers of English (NCTE) Contests

- Achievement Awards in Writing: Sophomores and juniors
- The Humanities and a Freer Tomorrow: Juniors and seniors
- Prizes: Certificates, $500-$1,000

## National History, Geography, Science,  Political Science Bee

- Eligibility: Individual students
- Prizes: National and international competition qualification

## National History Day Contest

- Focus: Historical events or figures
- Eligibility: Students
- Prizes: National Contest participation at the  University of Maryland

### National History Bowl – International Academic Competitions (IAC)

- Focus: Global history quiz competition
- Eligibility: Teams of up to four students
- Prizes: National championship qualification

### National Society of High School Scholars  Creative Writing Scholarship

- Categories: Poetry, Fiction
- Eligibility: High school students
- Prizes: $2,000

### New York Public Library Young Lions Fiction Award

- Eligibility: Writers younger than 35.
- Prizes: $10,000.

### Princeton's Lewis Center of the Arts – Leonard Milberg HS Poetry Prize

- Eligibility: 11th-grade students
- Prizes: $1,500, $750, $500

### Princeton University's Lewis Center of the Arts –  10-minute Play Contest

- Eligibility: 11th-grade students
- Prizes: $100-$500

### Profiles in Courage  Essay Contest

- Eligibility: U.S. students in grades 9-12
- Prizes: $100-$10,000

### Rachel Carson Landmark Alliance – Sense of Wonder/ Sense of the Wild Contest

- Eligibility: Teams of two or more people of different generations
- Prizes: Varies by submission

### Saint Mary's College of California  River of Words Contest

- Focus: Natural world topics
- Eligibility: Students aged 5-19
- Prizes: More than 100 prizes

### Scholastic Art and Writing Competition – Alliance for Young Artists & Writers

- Categories: Various art and writing categories
- Eligibility: Teens in grades 7-12
- Prizes:  Scholarships up to $12,500

### Society of Prof. Journalists/Journalism Education Assn. HS Essay Contest

- Focus: Journalism and societal issues
- Eligibility: Students in grades 9-12
- Prizes: $1,000, $500, $300

### Sons of the American Revolution (SAR) Contests

- Categories: Writing, Oration, Poster, Eagle Scout
- Prizes: Cash prizes

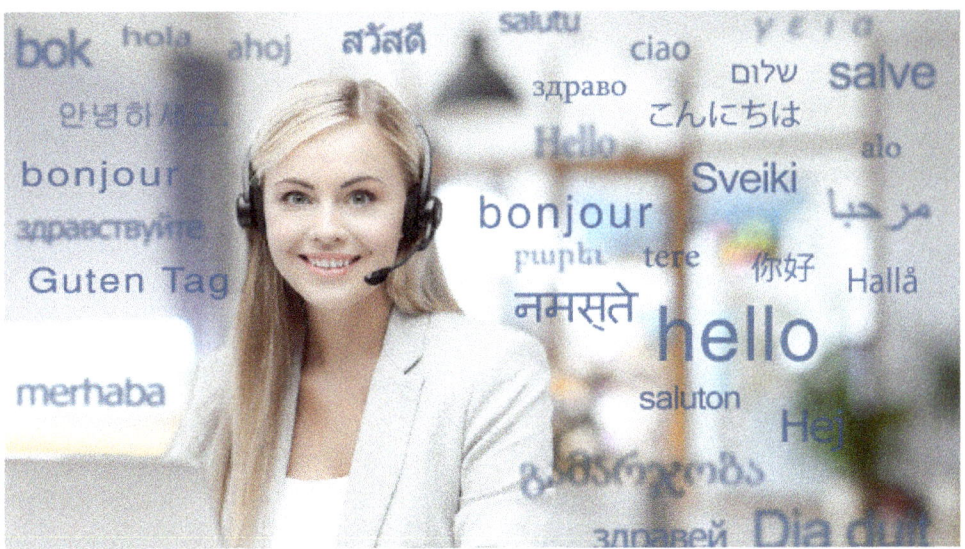

## Veterans of Foreign Wars – Voice of Democracy Youth Scholarship Essay

- Eligibility: Middle and high school students
- Prizes: $1,000-$35,000

## World Historian Student Essay Competition

- Eligibility: K-12 students
- Prizes: $500

## Writopia Lab Worldwide Play Festival

- Eligibility: Playwrights aged 6-18
- Prizes: Prizes for performed plays

## YoungArts National Writing Competition – The National Foundation for the Advancement of Artists

- Categories: Visual, literary, performing arts
- Eligibility: High school students
- Prizes: Varies by category

## Young Playwright's Festival - The Blank Theatre

- Eligibility: Students aged 9-19
- Prizes: Professional production of plays

## Young Writers' Annual Showcase

- Eligibility: Students aged 4-18
- Prizes: $100, trophy, publication

# BUSINESS COMPETITIONS

**Blue Ocean High School Entrepreneurship Competition** – Business pitch competition based on the Blue Ocean Strategy.

**DECA (Distributive Education Clubs of America)** – Events Competitive events in business, marketing, finance, and entrepreneurship.

**Diamond Challenge for High School Entrepreneurs** – Global entrepreneurship competition.

**Enactus World Cup (High School Division)** – Social entrepreneurship.

**FBLA (Future Business Leaders of America)** – Business and leadership.

**High School Fed Challenge** – A competition by the Federal Reserve focused on monetary policy and economics.

**Junior Achievement National Student Leadership Summit** – Business and entrepreneurship pitch competition.

**MIT Launch X** – Business and entrepreneurship competition.

**National Economics Challenge** – Tests economic knowledge in micro, macro, and international economics.

**Wharton Global High School Investment Competition** – Stock market simulation and investment challenge.

# HISTORY COMPETITIONS

**American Foreign Service National High School Essay Contest** – A diplomatic history and foreign policy essay competition hosted by the U.S. Foreign Service.

**Concord Review** – A prestigious competition where students submit high-quality research papers for publication on historical topics.

**Davidson Fellows Scholarship (History Category)** – A prestigious award for students who complete an advanced historical research project.

**International History Olympiad** – A global history competition featuring quiz-style events, exams, and simulation-based challenges.

**John Locke Institute History Essay Competition** – A high-level history essay competition where students write essays on major historical themes.

**Gilder Lehrman Lincoln Essay Competition** – Students write essays about Abraham Lincoln's legacy and impact on American history.

**National History Day (NHD)** – A nationwide research-based competition where students create papers, exhibits, documentaries, performances, and websites.

**National History Bowl** – A team-based history competition with buzzer-style quiz rounds on a wide range of historical topics.

**SPJ/JEA High School Essay Contest (Journalism History Focus)** – A competition where students analyze the historical role of journalism in society.

**World Scholar's Cup (History Section)** – An academic competition that includes a history category in its Team Debate and Scholar's Challenge events.

## PSYCHOLOGY COMPETITIONS

**American Psychological Association (APA) TOPSS Essay Competition** – High school students write essays on psychology topics.

**Behavioral Economics Challenge** – Psychology/economics decisions.

**Brain Bee at the Regional and National Levels** – Tests knowledge in neuroscience and psychology.

**CogSci High School Research Competition** – Cognitive science research.

**International Brain Bee** – Neuroscience competition for HS students.

**Psi Chi National Honor Society in Psychology High School Research Competition** – Psychology research awards.

**Psychology Science Fair (Regeneron ISEF, Google Science Fair, etc.)** – Conduct research in psychology and behavioral sciences.

**Society for Neuroscience (SfN) Next Generation Award** – Recognizes high school students for outreach in neuroscience.

**The Brain Awareness Video Contest** – Students create videos about neuroscience topics.

**The Neuroscience Research Prize** – Sponsored by the American Academy of Neurology for outstanding research in neuroscience.

## POLITICAL SCIENCE COMPETITIONS

**American Legion Oratorical Contest** – Constitutional speech contest.

**Constitutional Rights Foundation's Mock Trial Competition** – Simulated court trials for aspiring lawyers and policymakers.

**Harvard Model Congress** – A government simulation for students interested in politics.

**International Public Policy Forum (IPPF)** – Global debate competition focused on public policy issues.

**Junior Statesmen of America (JSA) Debate Competitions** – Public policy and government debate contests.

**Model United Nations (MUN)** – International relations, diplomacy, and debate competitions.

**National Speech & Debate Association (NSDA)** – Includes policy debate, public forum, and congressional debate.

**Princeton Moot Court** – Legal and policy debate competition.

**We the People: The Citizen and the Constitution** – A civics and constitutional law competition.

**Yale Model Congress** – Government simulation where students take on roles in a mock legislature.

## FILM & VIDEO COMPETITIONS

**All American High School Film Festival -** The largest scholarship-granting high school film festival globally, featuring screenings in NYC.

**Austin Film Festival (Young Filmmakers Competition) -** A free contest for high school students, showcasing films during the festival.

**C-SPAN's StudentCam -** A national documentary competition inviting students to explore issues of national importance.

**Meridian Stories -** Offers digital storytelling competitions across various subjects, encouraging creativity and collaboration.

**One Earth Young Filmmakers Contest -** An international contest focusing on environmental themes (students up to age 25).

**OUR PRIDE Education & Film Competition -** Young filmmakers create stories documenting LGBTQ+ people, places, & events.

**Student Television Network Contests -** Hosts competitions in broadcast journalism, video production, & filmmaking.

**Very Short Film Festival -** Encourages students to create short films, offering awards, mentoring, & prizes.

**YoungArts (Film Discipline) -** A national competition for excellence in narrative, documentary, experimental, & animation.

## JOURNALISM & WRITING CONTESTS

**JEA Journalist of the Year Scholarships -** Recognizes outstanding high school journalists with scholarships & national recognition.

**NSPA Individual Awards** – Honors excellent journalism (writing, design, & photography).

**Quill & Scroll Contests -** Offers competitions for student journalists, including writing, photography, & design.

**Pulitzer Center Student Contests -** Invites students to engage with global issues through writing and multimedia projects.

**New York Post Scholars Contest** - A writing competition for New York high school students (winners published in the *New York Post*).

## IMPORTANCE & VALUE OF COMPETITIONS

Competitions inspire new ideas while developing adaptability, creativity, and teamwork. Start by understanding the rules and stepping back to determine the tools, skills, and unique approaches they might take to separate themselves from the pack. Winners display motivation, inspiration, and perseverance.

In the process of diving into a project, students typically learn how to devise a plan, organize a set of procedures, and implement the requirements to succeed. In knowledge-based competitions, students also acquire vast amounts of information.

Similarly, physicians must incorporate diverse information sets and contemplate mitigating circumstances that may confound or alter a treatment plan. New tools and solutions are envisioned, helping to develop scientifically sound, repeatedly tested, and effectively administrated methods. Whether you compete individually or in a group, you will obtain valuable skills. In groups, you will implement innovative projects, programming strategies, and evaluation processes. The point is not to copy previous teams but to re-imagine possibilities and build upon the seeds of success.

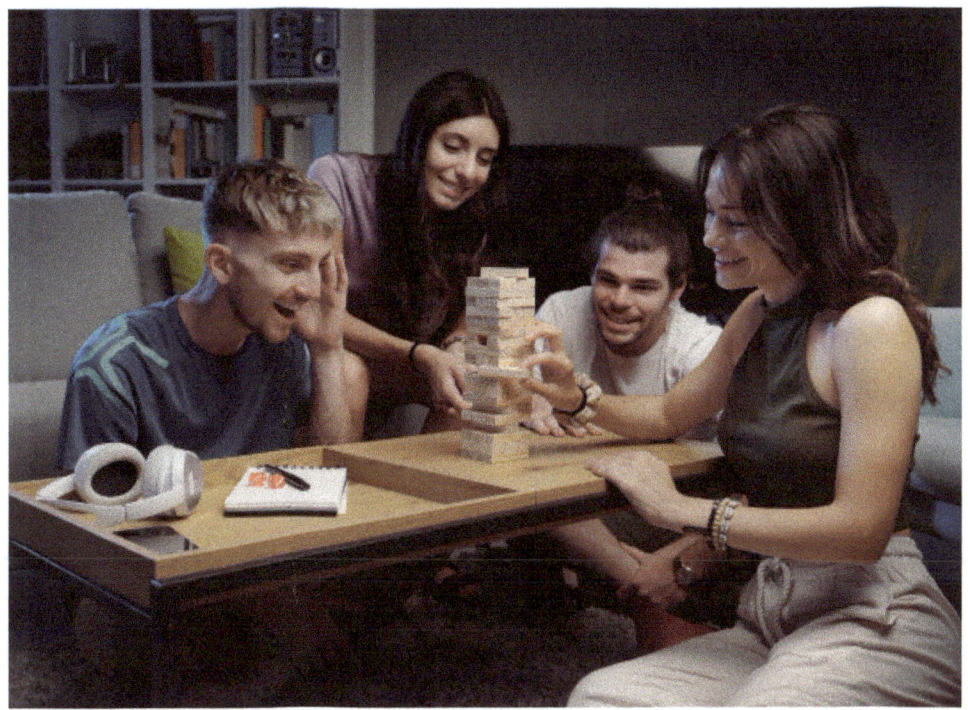

*Courage doesn't always roar. Sometimes courage is the quiet voice at the end of the day saying, 'I will try again tomorrow.*

— Mary Anne Radmacher

CHAPTER TWELVE

# ATHLETICS, CLUBS, INVOLVEMENT

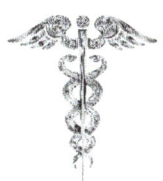

When students and parents consider college admission, especially for medical school, academic excellence dominates the conversation. However, medical schools seek students who are involved. Activities like athletics, arts, clubs, service, or research are vital to becoming a well-rounded, compassionate, and culturally-aware future physician.

Involvement tells a story, demonstrating your interests when you are not in a classroom. These commitments reveal your passion, persistence, and ability to connect with others. Medical schools want more than just students who can ace chemistry, though scientific knowledge is essential. They want students who know how to work in a team, lead with humility, manage time under pressure, and commit to serving others. High school is a training ground where your journey toward a career in medicine quietly begins.

## WHY EXTRACURRICULARS MATTER

Engaging in clubs, sports, and service teaches lessons not found in a textbook. In soccer, you may learn how to think fast, push through discomfort, and rely on teammates, just like doctors must do in an emergency room. In a school club, you may learn how to plan events, collaborate across differences, and stay organized under stress. These are the same skills you will need in medical school rotations, research labs, and patient care.

Moreover, extracurricular activities offer a chance to demonstrate skills, leadership, and initiative. Start a future physicians club, organize a fundraiser for a medical cause, or tutor peers. Take ownership of your interests. Initiative says, "I can learn, but I also lead, act, and build."

Participation teaches empathy and teamwork, qualities central to medicine. Volunteering with special needs kids or mentoring younger students shows that you value connection and service, which admissions committees hold in high regard.

## HOW TO GET INVOLVED

You do not need to be a jack of all trades. You just need to do a few things well and be consistent, responsible, and reliable. Choose what excites you. Maybe you prefer sports, public speaking, or robotics. You might run for a leadership position or be a person people want to follow. However, true leadership does not require a title, but is instead grounded in humility, character, and the ability to inspire others through quiet strength. Lao Tzu once said, "A leader is best when people barely know he exists. When his work is done and his aim fulfilled, they will say, 'We did it ourselves.'" Influence is earned, not enforced.

Remain involved. Colleges prefer sustained commitment. Take on a meaningful project or help grow an organization. Most students suddenly figure out in their junior year they really should get involved. However, with a difficult academic workload, sustained effort is hard. Then, SAT/ACT preparation takes over just before AP exams. Many take action after their junior year. Unfortunately, in the fall, with applications, scholarships, interviews, and academics, many students put activities aside. So, start earlier. If nothing on campus seems interesting, create your own club. Partner with a local hospital. Write a blog. Start a podcast about mental health. Authenticity and creativity are powerful, demonstrating your true interests.

## THE VALUE OF ATHLETIC PARTICIPATION

Participation in sports requires significant time, but also demonstrates profound benefits aligning closely with the demands of a medical career. By participating in practices, training, and competitions, athletes develop discipline, resilience, and the ability to work under pressure. A team's camaraderie fosters communication, mutual trust, and collective responsibility. Whether bouncing back from a loss or pushing through a tough game, student-athletes develop emotional stamina and a solution-oriented mindset that translates seamlessly to clinical environments.

Sports instill an awareness of physical health, nutrition, and body mechanics, key components of medicine. Athletes gain firsthand experience with performance optimization, injury prevention, and recovery, making them more attuned to the physiology they will study. Understanding the relationship between mental focus, diet, and physical condition enhances their appreciation of holistic health.

A winning mindset forged on the field and rooted in persistence, preparation, and accountability. This way of thinking helps students excel academically and professionally. For aspiring doctors, the lessons learned in athletics provide an early education in the discipline, empathy, and teamwork required to care for others.

## POSSIBLE EXTRACURRICULAR ACTIVITIES

4-H Youth Development Program
Audio/Visual Team
Best Buddies
Boy Scouts & Girl Scouts
Boys State & Girls State
Civil Air Patrol Cadet Program
Congressional Award Program
Cultural or Language Clubs
CyberPatriot
Health or Mental Wellness Clubs
HOBY Leadership & Service
Hospital or Clinic Volunteer
Junior State of America
Key Club
Mock Trial
Model United Nations
Morning Announcements
National Honor Society

Orchestra or Band
Peer Tutoring
Red Cross Club
Religious/Community Leadership
Robotics & Rocketry
Science Olympiad
Science Fair/Research
Shadow Physicians
Special Olympics
Speech and Debate
Sports (JV, Varsity, Club)
STEM Summer Programs
Student Government
Theater or Drama
Yearbook or School Newspaper
Yoga/Meditation Group
Youth Advisory Boards
Youth & Government (YAG)

## BALANCE ACADEMICS AND ACTIVITIES

Some students and their parents worry that activities take away from studying. Possibly, but involvement sharpens student's ability to manage time and focus. Pursuing genuine interests provides inspiration, energy, motivation, and purpose, connecting academic work to real life. Participation in school and community activities shows colleges and future medical schools you are more than a grade point average, you are a driven individual capable of leadership and meaningful impact.

Thus, involvement is not a distraction, but the difference between memorizing medical terminology and living core values. Extracurricular activities help students grow, while testing resilience and discovering the kind of doctor they want to be.

Start now. Join. Serve. Lead. Not only will your involvement strengthen your school and community, but your applications will highlight what you enjoy and what inspires you. Interacting with students and being part of a team also shapes the way you see others and the role you hope to play in your community.

"

*Your talents and abilities will improve over time, but for that, you have to start.*

— Martin Luther King Jr.

## CHAPTER THIRTEEN

# SUMMER PROGRAMS

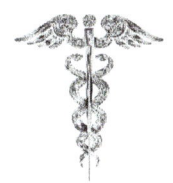

Start early to gain medical, research, engineering, software, and design, experiences. Internships and summer programs are as important in your educational pathway as coursework. The lessons you learn from working collaboratively with mentors is equally important. Historian and scholar, W.E.B. DuBois (1868-1963), the first Black American to earn a Harvard Ph.D. said, "Education must not simply teach work - it must teach life." Your college and life education will go hand-in-hand, driven by purpose and foresight since life truly is a journey, not a destination.

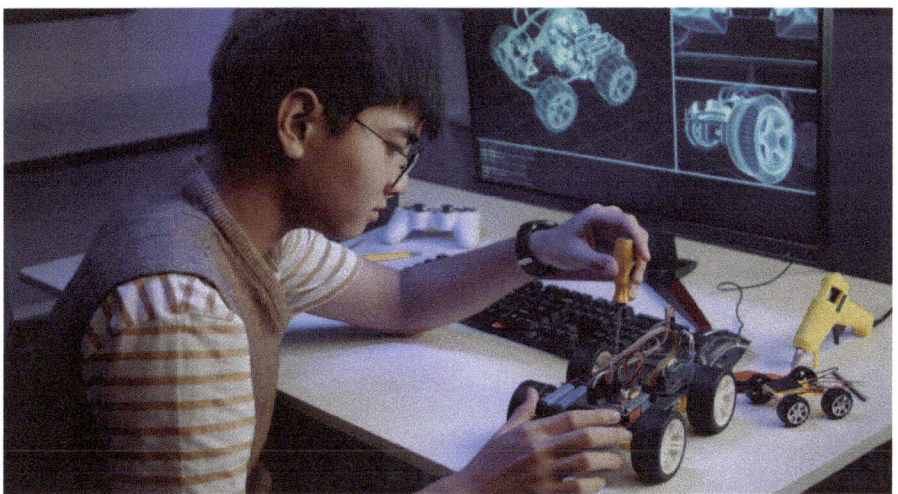

## WHY PARTICIPATE IN SUMMER PROGRAMS/INTERNSHIPS?

Although some students participate to look good and show dedication, the real reason should be to develop skills and obtain feedback. Discussions, seminars, and portfolio development are immensely valuable for any future pursuit. However, merely living on a campus and getting a feel for college life cannot be understated. Some immersions like Girls Who Code, Code Connects, Veritas AI Scholars, NextGen Boot Camp are completely online. Other programs like the iD Tech camps offer robotics, AI, and tech programs at 65 locations. You might consider interning with the National Parks Service, NASA, or Departments of Defense, Energy, Labor, or Treasury.

Consider attending  MIT's Splash November weekend event, where high school students choose from 250+ hands-on classes. The cost was $50 in 2025.

Note: The following list is not exhaustive nor an endorsement of any program. Dates, camps, internships, descriptions, and length may change yearly.

## SUMMER CAMPS & PROGRAMS FOR ART, ARCHITECTURE, COMPUTER SCIENCE, ENGINEERING, & SUSTAINABILITY

### Alabama

**Auburn University – Engineering Camps - STEM - Architecture Camp –  Creative Writing – Industrial Design - Multiple Sessions/Scholarships Available**

Work w/professors. Counselors support/supervise students. Engineering Summer Expo (9th-11th); Senior Engineering Expo (12th); Computing/ Robotics for All (7th-8th) Minority Intro to Engineering (11th- 12th); Paper & Bioresource Engineering Camp (12th); Computer Science, AI, Cybersecurity (9th-12th)

**Cyberpatriot - Air Force Assn National Youth Cyber Education Program - 1 Week**

HS Students - Multiple camp locations, incl Calhoun CC & the Univ. of Alabama

**Defense Intelligence Agency Summer College Internship-Engineering/Technology**

10-14 Week Summer Internship Program Intelligence/Tech Apply in Feb Huntsville, AL - College Jr/Sr or Grad Student

**GenCyber – 5-day Nat Security Agency-Sponsored Cybersecurity Camp for HS Students - Univ. of Alabama, Huntsville - Taught by Cyber Industry Professionals**

Engaging & Dynamic - Role-playing, visual aids, activities, discussions: Computer networking, systems security, cyber operations, defense, AI, virtual reality

### Alaska

**GenCyber – 5-day Nat Security Agency-Sponsored Cybersecurity Camp for HS Students - Univ. of Alaska, Anchorage – Taught by Cyber Industry Professionals**

Engaging & Dynamic - Role-playing, visual aids, activities, discussions: Computer networking, systems security, cyber operations, defense, AI, virtual reality

# Arizona

### Arcosanti – Re-Imagined Urbanism – 6-week discussion-based classes - AZ

Architecture & ecology (arcology). Learn in the World's First Prototype Arcology. Core values: (1) Frugality & Resourcefulness, (2) Ecological Accountability, (3) Experiential Learning, (4) Leaving a Limited Footprint, Arcosanti is juxtaposed to mass consumerism, urban sprawl, unchecked consumption, & social isolation.

### Bank of America Student Leaders Program - 3+ AZ Cities - HS Students - 8 Wks

Paid internships with nonprofits. Work experience & leadership development. Week long all-expense-paid Student Leaders Summit in Washington, DC in July. Submit application essays, recommendations, and resume in January.

### Cyberpatriot - Air Force Assn National Youth Cyber Education Program - 1 Week

HS Students - Multiple camp locations, incl Cochise CC & the Univ. of Arizona

### Earthwatch Teen Expeditions - 15-18 year olds - Portal, AZ - 8 days

*Following Forest Owls in the Western U.S.* - Learn how climate change threatens the routine of species as tree cavities and food sources disappear. study habitats

### Engineering Education Outreach - at ASU - 1-wk day camp for 11th/12th Graders

Train, collaborate, & compete in the National Underwater Robotics Competition Fun, hands-on training ground in buoyancy, electricity, & autonomy. No Exp Nec.

### GenCyber – 5-day Nat Security Agency-Sponsored Cybersecurity Camp for HS Students - Grand Canyon University – Taught by Cyber Industry Professionals

Engaging & Dynamic - Role-playing, visual aids, activities, discussions: Computer networking, systems security, cyber operations, defense, AI, virtual reality

### National Institute of Health – 8-week Paid Internship Program – Phoenix, AZ

Biomedical research internship for students 17 years or older by June. HS-SIP for high school juniors & seniors June to August hands-on research.

### Science and Engineering Apprenticeship Program (SEAP) – US Navy - Flagstaff

8-weeks, 300 openings, 30 research labs nationwide, $4,000-$4,500 salary. HS students must be 16+ years old. Apply starting in August for following summer.

### University of Arizona Summer Engineering Academy - HS Students - Hands-on

3-day and week-long residential camps; ChallENGe Accepted, Engineer Society Apply Feb-March; projects, mentorship, networking, engineering exploration

# Arkansas

### Bank of America Student Leaders Program - Pulaski - HS Students - 8 Wks

Paid internships with nonprofits. Work experience & leadership development. Week long all-expense-paid Student Leaders Summit in Washington, DC in July. Submit application essays, recommendations, and resume in January.

### University of Arkansas – FREE In Person & Virtual Design Camp – Fayetteville, AR

Grades 9-12 - Projects, studio groups, & meetings w/local designers; students are paired w/faculty members. Advanced Design Camp for students in Grades 11-12.

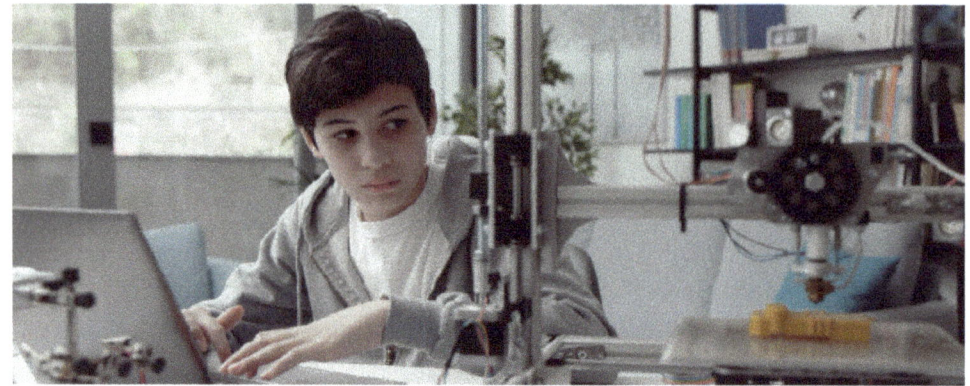

# California

**Academy of Art University – 4-6 Week Pre-College Art/Design/Fashion/Film - SF**

Advertising, Animation/VFX, Architecture, Fashion, Game Devt, Graphic Design. Illustration, Ind Design, Motion Pictures, Music Prod, Photo, Writing for Film/TV

**Bank of America Student Leaders Program - 25+ CA Cities - HS Students - 8 Wks**

Paid internships with nonprofits. Work experience & leadership development. Week long all-expense-paid Student Leaders Summit in Washington, DC in July. Submit application essays, recommendations, and resume in in January.

**Boeing Summer Internship – High School & College – Seal Beach & Palmdale, CA**

Hands-on Industry Experience - Aviation and Engineering Internships

**California State Summer School of the Arts (CSSSA) Sacramento - Grades 9–12**

Rigorous 4-week, visual/ perf arts - 2D & 3D, painting, printmaking, sculpture, ceramics, digital media, & photography; scholarship opp for CA residents.

**Cal Poly Pomona Engineering Summer Program - On-Campus, Hands-On**

Workshops, labs, team projects, lectures & speakers - mechanical, civil, electrical

**Canon Insights Summer Internship – Canon USA – Irvine, CA**

Computer Science Major – 2nd or 3rd year; Position: Computer Vision Tech Assist with Quality Assurance Engineers; Digital Imaging Solution Division

**COPE Scholars Program – Healthcare Internship – 280 Training/Experience Hrs**

Anaheim/Orange, Bakersfield, Covina/Glendora, Hanford, Irvine, LA, Mendocino, Mission Viejo, Newport, Oxnard, Riverside, Simi Valley, Tulare, Woodland Hills Health Scholars must be 18+. Students assist w/basic healthcare for medical or nursing school, etc. Certificate of Completion - Keck Graduate Institute.

**COSMOS – UC - California State Summer School for Math & Science – 4 weeks**

Hands-on research program for California high school students (9-12) pursuing STEM fields; students live on campus and work with UC researchers. Application opens in January and closes in Feb. Topics from biomedical to space science.

**Cyberpatriot - Air Force Assn National Youth Cyber Education Program - 1 Week**
HS Students - Multiple camp locations, including Consumnes River Col & LBCC

**Edwards Air Force Base - Lancaster, CA - Air Force Research Labs - 8-12 Weeks**
Students participate in mentored ongoing research. Paid internship: comp sci, physics, materials science, & aerospace. Workshops, seminars, presentations.

**Edwards Lifesciences Summer Internship Program – BS, MS, Ph.D., MBA - Irvine, CA**
Currently enrolled in college - Interested in healthcare related programs
Proficient in engineering drafting software, writing, or business/leadership

**GenCyber – 5-day Nat Security Agency-Sponsored Cybersecurity Camp for HS Students at CSU Bakersfield & CSU San Bernardino – Taught by Cyber Industry**
Engaging/Dynamic: Role-playing, visual aids, activities, & discussions: Computer networking, systems security, cyber operations, defense, AI, & virtual reality

**Getty Museum – Paid Student Gallery Guide - Summer internship– LA, CA**
Learn about museums and public speaking while leading visitors around the grounds. Also, Open Call for teen photographers to share images, 8-week paid STEAM internship, Summer Latin Academy at the Getty Villa to learn Latin.

**Great Books Summer Program - Stanford University - Grades 6-8 and 9-12**
Great Books & Big Ideas, Writer's Workshops, and Literary Travel Programs Read, Write, & Discuss Big Ideas in Literature and Philosophy with scholars

**Golden Gate National Parks Conservancy - Linking Individuals to their Natural Community (LINC) 6-Week Summer Program for HS Students - San Francisco, CA**
Trail work, habitat restoration, community clean up, wildlife monitoring, outdoor fun

**Harvey Mudd Annual Future Achievers in Science & Technology (FAST) Program**
All-expenses paid fly-in program for high-achieving college-bound HS seniors
September or October weekend. Apply in August - speakers, presentations

**Keck Graduate Institute (KGI) - 3-Week High School Summer STEM Program & Summer Undergrad Research Experience (SURE) - Claremont, CA - 16+ yrs old**
Hands-on research experience w/KGI faculty mentor; seminars & workshops

**Laguna College of Art & Design Pre-College Program – Laguna Beach, CA**
Animation, Sculpture, Drawing Fundamentals, Figure Drawing, Graphic Design

**Los Angeles Air Force Base - L.A., CA - Air Force Research Labs - 8-12 Weeks**
Students participate in mentored ongoing research. Paid internship: comp sci, physics, materials science, & aerospace. Workshops, seminars, presentations.

**Los Angeles County Office of Education's Career Technical Education Internships**
This 6-8 week summer internship is for HS students to gain real-world experience and technical training in 15 industry sectors.

**NASA Jet Propulsion Laboratory – Pasadena, CA (Apply by March 31)**
Paid Internship - Must be in an undergraduate in a STEM subject

**NatureBridge Summer Programs - Yosemite National Park - 1-2 weeks**
Environmental science education, & hands-on fieldwork while backpacking for students in 7th - 12th grades. Connect to nature with trail building, habitat restoration, and wilderness exploration.

**Otis College of Art and Design Summer of Art Intensive - 4 Weeks - Los Angeles**
Portfolio/studio training for students 15+ - art, architecture, design, digital and printmaking; lectures and critiques. Merit/ need-based scholarships available.

**Parker Hannifin Corporation – Paid Summer Internship – Irvine, CA**
Mechanical or Industrial Engineering Major – Flight Control, Aircraft Systems

**Pathway Summer Program Dept of Energy RENEW Initiative-HS/College Students**
Mentorship, hands-on engineering/technology - Lawrence Berkeley National Lab

**Rady Children's Hospital - Summer Medical Academy - San Diego, CA**
Students 15-19 years old can apply to attend this 2-week medical training camp.

**Rosetta Institute for Biomedical Research - 2-Week Middle/High School - Alameda**
Molecular Biology of Aging, Cancer, Immunology, Neuroscience, Medicinal Chemistry, Bioinformatics of Cancer, Intro to Cellular & Molecular Medicine

**Salk Institute - Heithoff-Brody HS Summer Scholars Program - San Diego Schools**
8-Week hands-on biological research/paid internship in La Jolla - Mentorship Seminars, workshops, biotech site visits, research, presentations. Apply Dec-March

**Sandia National Labs - Livermore, CA - Engineering/Tech Internship - HS/College**
* Ages 16+ - FT HS Student - Work on STEM Projects with mentors
* 10-12 Week College Summer Internship, Year-Round Internship, & Co-Ops

**Santa Clara University Summer Engineering Seminar (SES) – 10th and 11th Grade**
4-day program introduces students to engineering practice, research, and education

**School of Creative & Performing Arts ( SOCAPA)–Occidental College (13-18-yr-olds)**
2-week, 3-week - learn Filmmaking, Screenwriting, Dance, Music, Photography

**SCI-Arc ( Southern California Institute of Architecture) Immersive 4-week Summer Program (Design Immersion Days) – Los Angeles**
Introduction to the academic and professional world of architecture – Grades 9-12

**Science and Engineering Apprenticeship Program ( SEAP) – US Navy Camp Pendleton, Port Hueneme, Pt. Mugu, San Diego, Monterey, Corona**
8-weeks, 300 openings, 30 research labs nationwide, $4,000-$4,500 salary. HS students must be 16+ years old. Apply starting in August for following summer.

**Sierra Club's Summer Outings - Channel Islands**
Kayaking and hiking - families can go together to explore scenic areas

## SpaceX – Summer Engineering/Co-op – Hawthorne, Irvine, & Vandenberg AFB
Paid Internship - Must be in an undergraduate in a STEM subject.

## Stanford University Summer Programs for HS Students - Apply by March
**Art & Architecture Exploration Program** - 3 Weeks - Architecture, Art,  Drawing, Dance,  Creative Writing, Music, and Photography

**Earth & Environmental Sciences** - HS research, labs, field trips, discussions, speakers, & research methodology at the Doerr School of Sustainability.

**Humanities Institute** - 3-Weeks On-Campus, 11th & 12th Grade - Explore politics, literature, and philosophy with Stanford professors and graduate students.

**ID Tech (on-campus, not sponsored by S.U.)** - Courses in coding, Minecraft game design, and other aspects of computer, VR, AR, & AI technology.

**Math Circle** - 10-Week Accelerated Math Program - Online w/groups for advanced students in grade levels from 1st to 12th grade - year round.

**Middle School Scholars Program (SMSSP)** - Free - Low-income, grades  6 & 7 - Selective & rigorous for exceptional students - 3 Weeks

**Psychology & Neuroscience Pre-College Summer Institute - 2-3 Weeks** Intensive hands-on study in psychology/neuroscience; lectures, & discussions.

**Stanford Anesthesia Summer Institute (SASI)** - 2 Week medical internship for HS students & pre-med undergrads seeking careers in clinical medicine.

**Stanford Institutes of Medicine Summer Research Program (SIMR)** 8-Week internship for HS juniors/seniors interested in biomedical research (Bioeng, Cancer, Cardiovascular, Genetics, Immunology, Neurobiology) Apply Dec - Feb.

**Stanford Medical Youth Science Program (SMYSP)** 5-Week Medical Research Program for Juniors & Seniors (US Citizens or Permanent Res) - Highly competitive

**Stanford Summer Engineering Academy (SSEA)** - 4 weeks  - Fully Funded Exceptional students engage in hands-on engineering - highly competitive

**SUMaC – Stanford University Mathematics Camp** - Highly selective & intensive program in advanced mathematics & problem solving.

## TeenNat - Grades 10-12, 6-Week, Hands-On Research - Pepperwood Preserve
Scientific inquiry, data collection, & statistical analysis. The program develops a sense of stewardship and appreciation for the natural environment.

## Tesla Internships – – More than $35/hour – Dozens of FT Positions Throughout CA
Automotive Design, Engineering Technologies, Vehicle Service Research/Training

## University of California, Berkeley Summer Programs for HS Students
**Academic Talent Development Program (ATDP) & Explorations** - Students can take 2 Berkeley courses w/small classes & hands-on activities.

**AI4ALL @ UC Berkeley** - 9th & 10th Grade Underrepresented Students - Learn about computer programming & artificial intelligence - Free, On Campus

**Computer Science Academy** - 2 Weeks - Rigorous immersion into coding, & problem-solving. Intense exploration of "big ideas". Apply by March.

**Environmental Design (CED) Program** - Students pursue environmental studies hands-on, immersive experiences in urban planning & sustainable design.

**ID Tech (on-campus, not sponsored by UCB** - Courses in coding, Minecraft game design, and other aspects of computer, VR, AR, & AI technology

**Psychology Pre-College Summer Institute** - 3-6 Weeks Students take college-level psychology courses and engage in discussions and activites related to cognitive science, neuroscience, and social psychology.

## University of California, Davis - Young Scholars Program (YSP) - Apply in March

6-week STEM Summer Research Program - Rising juniors and seniors

## University of California, Irvine Engineering Summer Academy & 1-WkAI Camp

On-campus engineering academy: guest speakers, interactive workshops in robotics, computer science, mechanical engineering; NSF funded "Privacy IoT and AI" - Create Alexa-like assistants using Raspberry Pi, Python, & OpenAI.

## UCLA Computer Science Intro Track - 6 Week Boot Camp - Apply by June 1

College-level coding classes & labs in computer science, design (strings, lists, structures, & functional decomposition). No experience necessary.

## UCLA SummerJumpstart Summer Art Inst, Digital Media Arts Inst, Digital Filmmaking Institute, Game Lab Institute. Computer Science Summer Institute

2-week program - Portfolio development– college credit available
Drawing, Painting, Photography, Sculpture, Video Art, Animation, and Game Design

## University of California, San Diego - Academic Connections - HS Students

Lab and academic programs/projects in STEM subjects - 3-week program

## University of California, Santa Barbara - Research Mentorship Program

6-week STEM Summer Research Program - Rising juniors and seniors

## University of California, Santa Cruz HS Student Science Internship Program

10-week research internship for high school students in STEM fields. Conduct research with a faculty/doctoral student mentor. Apply in March.

## USC Psychological Science & Society - 4 Weeks - June/July Los Angeles

This summer program for HS students explores classic and contemporary psychological theories with real-world hands-on activities.

## University of Southern California Viterbi Discover Engineering - HS Students

Hands-on; design, 3D print, build, & test; Field trips to JPL & Hyperion. Aerospace, biomedical, chemical, computer science, electrical, environmental, industrial, & mechanical engineering. Also, SHINE Biomedical/Robotics Prog.

## USC Summer Film, Writing, Drama, and Architecture Programs – 2-4 Weeks

Creative Writing Workshop, Comedy Performance, Exploring Architecture

# Colorado

### Bank of America Student Leaders Program - 10+ CO Cities - HS Students - 8 Wks

Paid internships with nonprofits. Work experience & leadership development. Week long all-expense-paid Student Leaders Summit in Washington, DC in July. Submit application essays, recommendations, and resume in January.

### Catalyst Campus - Colorado Springs, CO - Air Force Research Labs - 8-12 Weeks

Students participate in mentored ongoing research. Paid internship: comp sci, physics, materials science, & aerospace. Workshops, seminars, presentations.

### Colorado School of Mines Summer Programs for HS Students - Golden, CO

**Engineering Design Camp** - 10th - 12th  - Real world problem solving and engineering design while living on the Mines campus.

**SUMMET (Summer Multicultural Engineering Training)** - 11th & 12th  - Program for ethnic/racial minorities, women, and first-gen college students.

### Cyberpatriot - Air Force Assn National Youth Cyber Education Program - 1 Week

HS Students - Training at the National Cybersecurity Center, Colorado Springs.

### Defense Intelligence Agency Summer College Internship- Engineering/Technology

10-14 Week Summer Internship Program Intelligence/Tech Apply in Feb Colorado Springs, CO - College Jr/Sr or Grad Student

### GenCyber – 5-day Nat Security Agency-Sponsored Cybersecurity Camp for HS Students - Univ. of CO Denver & Colorado Springs – Taught by Cyber Industry

Engaging & Dynamic - Role-playing, visual aids, activities, & discussions. Computer networking, systems security, cyber operations, defense, AI, & virtual reality

### Mentorship for Environmental Scholars (MES) Program - 10 Wk Paid - HS/College

Grand Junction Dept of Energy Site - Research in Environmental Science & STEM

### National Security Agency (NSA) – Paid Computer Internship – Aurora

Students must be at least a junior in high school with interest in business, engineering, or computer science. Apply between September 1 and October 31.

### University of Colorado, Boulder - Summer STEM Program - K-12 Options

All age levels - AI, comp sci, DNA, biomedical eng, biotech, geology, technology design, LEGOs, math, medicine, programming, rockets. microbes, & video games.

### University of Colorado Summer Science Program Intensive - HS Students 5-6 Wks

Biochemistry and molecular biology research - experimental design/synthesis; advanced lab techniques, lectures, collaborative workshops - highly competitive

## Connecticut

### Bank of America Student Leaders Program - 3+ CT Cities - HS Students - 8 Wks

Paid internships with nonprofits. Work experience & leadership development. Week long all-expense-paid Student Leaders Summit in Washington, DC in July. Submit application essays, recommendations, and resume in January.

**GenCyber – 5-day Nat Security Agency-Sponsored Cybersecurity Camp for HS Students - Univ. of New Haven – Taught by Cyber Industry Professionals**

Engaging & Dynamic - Role-playing, visual aids, activities, discussions. Computer networking, systems security, cyber operations, defense, AI, virtual reality

**Jackson Laboratory's Summer Student Program - 12th Grade & College Students**

Farmington, CT - Develop & execute research, analyze data, present findings; $6,500 stipend along with room, board, and travel to and from the lab

**Science and Engineering Apprenticeship Program (SEAP) – US Navy – Groton**

8-weeks, 300 openings, 30 research labs nationwide, $4,000-$4,500 salary. HS students must be 16+ years old. Apply starting in August for following summer.

**Summer Studio: Discovering Graphic Design – Free 4-Weeks in Bridgeport, CT**

11th, 12th; Week 1 – Music Festival Poster, Week 2 – Digital Media Poster Week 3 – Animating Your Ideas, Week 4 – Portfolio Art for College Applications

**Yale Summer Program in Astrophysics (YSPA) - Rising HS Seniors**

Research/enrichment at the Leitner Family Observatory & Planetarium; 2-week online preliminary & 4-week on-campus program w/a final research project

**Yale Young Global Scholars - 2-Week On-Campus HS Program; June, July, & August**

Apps due in Jan - Solving Global Challenges, Environmental Issues, Innovations in Science & Tech, Literature, Philosophy, & Culture, Politics Law & Economics. The Biological & Biomedical Science prog reviews topics in psychology, neuroscience, and biomedical sciences in lectures and seminars with renowned faculty.

## Delaware

**Bank of America Student Leaders Program - 3+ DE Cities - HS Students - 8 Wks**

Paid internships with nonprofits. Work experience & leadership development. Week long all-expense-paid Student Leaders Summit in Washington, DC in July. Submit application essays, recommendations, and resume in January.

## District of Columbia

**American Chemical Society - Project SEED Summer Program - 8-Week, Hands-on**

Research/mentor, 11,000 low income students; virtual opp. in 40 U.S. states

**Bank of America Student Leaders Program - DC - HS Students - 8 Wks**

Paid internships with nonprofits; work experience & leadership development. With week long all-expense-paid Student Leaders Summit in Washington, DC in July. Submit application, essays, recommendations, and resume in January.

**Catholic University School of Architecture and Planning**

Summer High School Program - 2-week Residential (Two Session Options)

**Defense Intelligence Agency Summer College Internship-Engineering/Technology**

10-14 Week Summer Internship Program Intelligence/Tech Apply in Feb Washington, D.C. - College Jr/Sr or Grad Student

### Federal Summer Internship Program - Paid - High School & College Students

**National Institutes of Health (NIH)** - Biomedical, behavioral, & social science research for 11th grade to grad school. Interns work w/a Principal Investigator.

**Pathways Internship Program** - HS to grad school - Hands-on w/govt agencies.

**U.S. Fish & Wildlife Service Internships** - Work in wildlife conservation and visitor services. Practical experience may lead to permanent federal positions.

### GenCyber – 5-day Nat Security Agency-Sponsored Cybersecurity Camp for HS Students - Gallaudet University – Taught by Cyber Industry Professionals

Engaging & Dynamic - Role-playing, visual aids, activities, discussions: Computer networking, systems security, cyber operations, defense, AI, virtual reality

### George Washington University Digital Storytelling Pre-College Program – July

Produce stories w/smartphones, learn storyboarding, & social media broadcast craft ideas, capture images, & create compelling content, w/character devt.

### Georgetown University – 1-week – Creative Writing – Publishing

Fiction, Short Story, Poetry, and Professional Writing; visit literary hubs

### National Air and Space Museum in Washington, D.C. – HS and College Students

The Explainers Program offers ~$15/hr year-round paid position for students to help visitors better understand the Museum and its artifacts and exhibitions.

### U.S. Department of Education - Internships for HS & College - Fall, Winter, Spring, & Summer; Must be 16+; 8-Week Program

Human Resources/Project Mgmt, Educational Policies, Data Analytics, Training/Development; Grants Management; Communications; Information Technology

## Florida

### Bank of America Student Leaders Program - 20+ FL Cities - HS Students - 8 Wks

Paid internships with nonprofits. Work experience & leadership development. Week long all-expense-paid Student Leaders Summit in Washington, DC in July. Submit application essays, recommendations, and resume in January.

### Cyberpatriot - Air Force Assn National Youth Cyber Education Program - 1 Week

HS Students - Multiple camp locations, incl FL SW Col, DoD StarBase, & USF

### Defense Intelligence Agency Summer College Internship-Engineering/Technology

10-14 Wk Program Intelligence/Tech Apply in Feb Miami/Tampa - College Jr/Sr

### Disney Dreamers Academy - 4-Day HS Program - Walt Disney World - Apply in Oct

Mentorship program w/workshops & seminars; connect students with Disney executives, celebrities, and educators. Apply w/essays and video introduction.

### Earthwatch Teen Expeditions - 8 days - 15-18 year olds - Sarasota, FL

*Tracking Sharks & Rays* - Conduct research alongside scientists; Students consider overexploitation & environmental threats. Mote Marine Laboratory & Aquarium.

### Eglin Air Force Base - Valparaiso, FL - Air Force Research Labs - 8-12 Weeks

Students participate in mentored in ongoing research. Paid internships: comp sci, physics, materials science, & aerospace. Workshops, seminars, presentations.

### Florida Atlantic University School of Architecture– Boca Raton & Ft. Lauderdale

July 3-weeks; HS & first 2 years of college - Portfolio development, fabrication, architectural education, portfolio display, & critiques; Certificate of Completion

### Florida International University - Journalism Jumpstart - FREE - Miami, FL

Diverse national showcase working w/media professionals; Partnership & grant from the Dow Jones News Fund. Student work on Jumpstart Journal Webpage.

### GenCyber – 5-day Nat Security Agency-Sponsored Cybersecurity Camp for HS Students - Florida Tech, FIU, Innovation Tech Academy, U of West FL

Engaging & Dynamic - Role-playing, visual aids, activities, discussions: Computer networking, systems security, cyber operations, defense, AI, virtual reality

### Ringling College of Art and Design –Sarasota, FL - Intensive 4-week Program

Animation, VR, creative writing, digital sculpting, entertainment design, film, game art, game design, illustration, painting, photography, and storyboarding

### Science and Engineering Apprenticeship Program (SEAP) – US Navy Patrick SFB, Jacksonville, Orlando, Panama City

8-weeks, 300 openings, 30 research labs nationwide, $4,000-$4,500 salary. HS students must be 16+ years old. Apply starting in August for following summer.

### SpaceX – Summer Engineering/Co-op Program – Cape Canaveral, FL

Paid Internship - Must be an undergraduate in a STEM subject.

### University of Florida Design Exploration Program (DEP) - 3 Weeks - On Campus

Architecture theory & design, studio projects, teamwork, seminars, field trips

### University of Florida - Student Science Training Program (SSTP) 6-Weeks

Rising seniors; 16+ years old; UF-SSTP is a rigorous, fast paced program for academically talented, and self-motivated students.

### University of Miami Summer Scholars, Explorations in Architecture & Design

3-week Residential program; 6 college credits; Design, Graphics, and Theory. Architecture, Landscape Architecture, Historic Preservation; Urban Planning. Studio experience with drawing, model making, drafting, CAD, visual analysis.

## Georgia

### Bank of America Student Leaders Program - 10+ GA Cities - HS Students - 8 Wks

Paid internships with nonprofits. Work experience & leadership development. Week long all-expense-paid Student Leaders Summit in Washington, DC in July. Submit application essays, recommendations, and resume in January.

**Centers for Disease Control - Atlanta, GA - CDC Disease Detective Day Camp**

11th & 12th Grade - Lectures on global health, interventions, infectious diseases, chronic disease, & injury prevention. Students participate in mock press conferences, re-created outbreaks, lab sessions, & disease surveillance.

**Cyberpatriot - Air Force Assn National Youth Cyber Education Program - 1 Week**

HS Students - Multiple camp locations, including GA Cyber Innovation/Training Center, Middle GA State U., Ft Valley State U., & Wesley Community College

**Emory University – Atlanta, GA – 2-, 4-, 6-Week Writing Programs**

Journalism, Dramatic Writing, Media & Politics, Psychology & Fiction

**GenCyber – 5-day Nat Security Agency-Sponsored Cybersecurity Camp for HS Students - Columbus State Univ., Savannah State Univ. , Univ. of North Georgia, Westminster Schools of Augusta - Taught by Cyber Industry Professionals**

Engaging & Dynamic - Role-playing, visual aids, activities, discussions: Computer networking, systems security, cyber operations, defense, AI, virtual reality

**Georgia Institute of Technology Pre-College Design Program – Atlanta, GA**

2-week Residential program – College of Design – Grades 11 & 12 (Two Sessions); Architecture, Building Construction, Industrial Design, and Music Technology

**Georgia Tech Summer Engineering Institute - Atlanta, GA - 3-Week**

Residential engineering/tech prog. Grades 11-12, underrepresented students

**Mentorship for Environmental Scholars (MES) Program - 10 Wk Paid - HS/College**

Savannah State Univ. - Dept of Energy - Research in Environmental Science/STEM

**National Security Agency (NSA) – Paid Computer Internship – Augusta**

Students must be at least a junior in high school with interest in business, engineering, or computer science. Apply between September 1 & October 31.

**Savannah College of Art & Design – 2-5-Wk Rising Star On-Campus SCAD Courses**

Grades 11 & 12 - Advertising, animation, fashion, film, graphic design, illustration, nidustrial design, painting, photography, storyboarding, & virtual reality,

**University of Georgia - Women Experience Creativity, Excitement, & Learning (ExCEL)**

1-Week - Engineering Discovery Laboratory & Fabrication Studio

# Hawaii

**COPE Scholars Program – Healthcare Internship – 280 Hrs Training in Kailua**

Health Scholars must be 18+. Students assist w/basic healthcare for medical or nursing school, etc. Certificate of Completion -  Keck Graduate Institute.

**Defense Intelligence Agency Summer College Engineering Internship 10-14 Weeks**

Intelligence/Tech Apply in February Honolulu - College Jr/Sr or Grad Student

GenCyber – 5-day Cybersecurity Camp for HS Students - UH, Hilo, UH Kahului, UH Kaunakakai, UH Lihue-UH Wahiawa: Taught by Cyber Industry Professional

Engaging & Dynamic - Role-playing, visual aids, activities, discussions: Computer networking, systems security, cyber operations, defense, AI, virtual reality

Maui Optical & Super Computing Site - Maui, HI - Air Force Research Labs: 8-12 Wks

Students participate in mentored ongoing research teams. Paid internship: comp sci, physics, materials science, & aerospace. Workshops, seminars, presentations.

National Security Agency (NSA) – Paid Computer Internship – Oahu

Students must be at least a junior in high school with interest in business, engineering, or computer science. Apply between September 1 and October 31.

Science and Engineering Apprenticeship Program (SEAP) – US Navy – Honolulu

8-weeks, 300 openings, 30 research labs nationwide, $4,000-$4,500 salary. HS students must be 16+ years old. Apply starting in August for following summer.

Science Camps of America - Land & Sea Camp - 9-day HS Residential Camp

Practical exploration of volcanos, turtles, fish, & geological/marine conservation

STEMworks Innovation Internship Program - HS Students - $2,000 stipend

Focus areas include: 3D design, architecture, biomedical tech & engineering

University of Hawaii, Manoa College of Engineering Summer HS Student Program

Hands-on engineering & STEM program in robotics and interactive learning.

## Idaho

Bank of America Student Leaders Program - 3+ ID Cities - HS Students - 8 Wks

Paid internships with nonprofits; work experience & leadership development. With week long all-expense-paid Student Leaders Summit in Washington, DC in July. Submit application, essays, recommendations, and resume in January.

GenCyber – 5-day Nat Security Agency-Sponsored Cybersecurity Camp for HS Students - Boise State University – Taught by Cyber Industry Professionals

Engaging & Dynamic - Role-playing, visual aids, activities, discussions: Computer networking, systems security, cyber operations, defense, AI, virtual reality

Idaho National Laboratory Internships - Idaho Falls, ID - 6-Week Paid Program

Nuclear Energy, Renewable Energy, and/or National Security. Interns apply STEM to solve real-world problems with experts in the nuclear field.

## Illinois

After School Matters - 6-8 Wk Summer Internship/Apprenticeship Prog - Chicago

Internships include science, sports, technology, and communications.

Argonne National Laboratory - 8-Week - College Bound Research Program

STEM Lab/lecture w/interactive  programs. Students take part in real-world problem-solving. This program is FREE, plus $500 per week stipend.

### Bank of America Student Leaders Program - 5+ IL Cities - HS Students - 8 Wks

Paid internships with nonprofits. Work experience & leadership development.
Week long all-expense-paid Student Leaders Summit in Washington, DC in July.
Submit application essays, recommendations, and resume in January.

### Cass County CEO Program - HS Summer & Academic Year - Cass County

HS students work w/business owners to develop/implement business ideas.

### Cyberpatriot - Air Force Assn National Youth Cyber Education Program - 1 Week

HS Students - Camp locations include Elmhurst University

### Defense Intelligence Agency Summer College Engineering Internship - 10-14 Weeks

Intelligence/Tech Apply in Feb; Scott Air Force Base - College Jr/Sr, Grad Student

### GenCyber – 5-day Nat Security Agency-Sponsored Cybersecurity Camp for HS Students - College of Dupage – Taught by Cyber Industry Professionals

Engaging & Dynamic - Role-playing, visual aids, activities, discussions: Computer
networking, systems security, cyber operations, defense, AI, virtual reality

### Great Books Summer Program - Northwestern University - Grades 6-8 and 9-12

Great Books & Big Ideas, Writer's Workshops, and Literary Travel Programs
Read, Write, & Discuss Big Ideas in Literature and Philosophy with scholars

### Illinois Institute of Technology - HS Summer Introduction to Architecture

2-week - Comprehensive overview; 1-week Exploration in Architecture for middle
school students – studio-based, firm visits, field trips, projects.

### Northwestern University Center for Talent Development Rigorous/Accel - Grades 9-12

Medical Pharmacology, Neuroplasticity, Cybersecurity, Data Science,
Astrophysics, Quantum Mechanics, IoT, Build Your Own Computer, & Machine Learning

### Northwestern University – National High School Institute

5-week Film & Video, Music, Speech & Debate, Theatre, and Dramaturgy

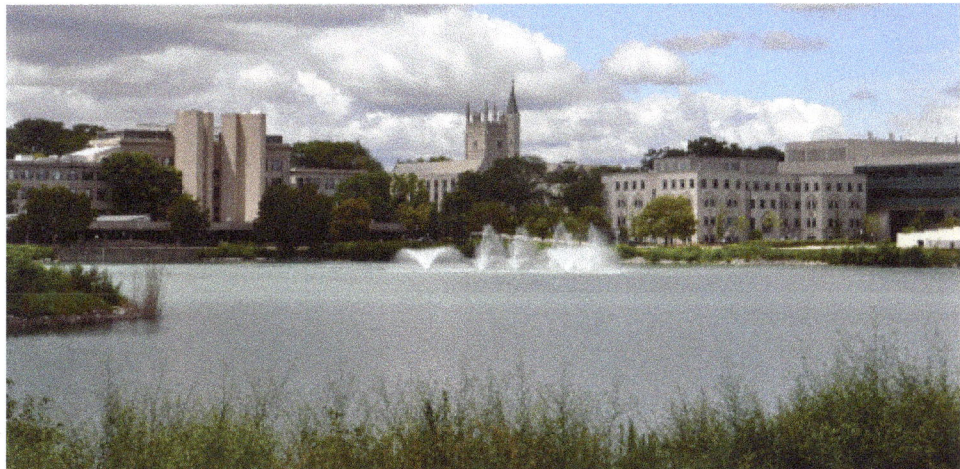

**Pathway Summer Program Dept of Energy RENEW Initiative-HS/College**
Mentorship, hands-on engineering/technology - Argonne National Lab

**School of the Art Institute of Chicago – HS Students - 1-, 2-, 4-Wk on-campus**
Painting, drawing, animation, comics/graphic novels, & fashion design. Portfolio devt; earn  college credit. Full-tuition  scholarships are available.

**Southern Illinois University Carbondale – Kid Architecture**
1-week Elementary Grades, Middle School & High School Architecture Camp

**University of Chicago Creative Writing Immersion - HS Writing Program**
"Collegiate Writing: Awakening Into Consciousness"

**University of Chicago - 3-4 Weeks - Psychology Summer - Understanding the Mind**
Explore cognitive psychology & neuroscience to understand the mind.

**University of Chicago Research in the Biological Sciences (RIBS) 4 week Intensive**
Highly competitive project-based training in molecular, microbiological, & cell biology; weekly writing assignments & lunch seminars; intependent project

**University of Illinois at Chicago Architecture - HiArch Summer HS Program**
1 & 2-week (July) - Culture of architecture, design, thinking, and artmaking.

**University of Illinois at Urbana-Champaign - Women in Engineering - 6th-12th**
The Grainger College of Engineering introduces engineering to teenage girls.

**Univ of Illinois, Urbana-Champaign - HS Students Discover Engineering Camp**
STEM-focused camps - 7th-12th grade - Specialized Aerospace, Chemical  Electrical, Computer, Mechanical, Nuclear, Radiological, Materials Science, AI, Programming, Molecule Making camps. 20+ camps from June to August

**Young Scholars Summer STEMM Research Programs at Univ of Illinois (UIUC)**
6-weeks, Rising 10th-12th graders collaborate on cutting-edge research in cancer, immunology, neuroscience, artificial intelligence, physics, quantum mechanics, bioengineering, electrical engineering - Final Symposium held in early August.

## Indiana

**Bank of America Student Leaders Program - 5+ IN Cities - HS Students - 8 Wks**
Paid internships with nonprofits. Work experience & leadership development. Week long all-expense-paid Student Leaders Summit in Washington, DC in July. Submit application essays, recommendations, and resume in January.

**Cyberpatriot - Air Force Assn National Youth Cyber Education Program - 1 Week**
HS Students - Camp locations include Ivy Tech Community College

**GenCyber – 5-day Nat Security Agency-Sponsored Cybersecurity Camp for HS Students - Purdue Univ. Northwest – Taught by Cyber Industry Professionals**
Engaging & Dynamic - Role-playing, visual aids, activities, discussions: Computer networking, systems security, cyber operations, defense, AI, virtual reality

### Indiana University Bloomington Summer Science Program - HS Students 5-6 Wks

Biochemistry and molecular biology research - highly competitive, hands-on, collaborative; mentors; student teams; analysis, scientific writing, presentations

### Purdue University Summer Programs for HS Students

**Seminar for Top Engineering Prospects (STEP) - 1 Week**
Program for rising seniors to explore engineering opportunities.
**Minority Engineering Program - 7th - 9th Grade Students**
This summer camp introduces to engineering careers and the design process.
**Summer Science Program - HS Students 5-6 Wks**
Biochemistry and molecular biology research - highly competitive, hands-on, collaborative; mentors; student teams; analysis, scientific writing, presentations

### Rose-Hulman Institute of Technology - Operation Catapult - 2 Weeks

Engineering projects, robotics, research, and STEM design projects - Rising HS juniors or seniors participate in hands-on engineering activities.

### Science and Engineering Apprenticeship Program (SEAP) – US Navy – Crane

8-weeks, 300 openings, 30 research labs nationwide, $4,000-$4,500 salary. HS students must be 16+ years old. Apply starting in August for following summer.

### University of Notre Dame Summer Scholars Program - 2-weeks HS Students

Film, Photography, Performing Arts - studios, seminars, and field trips STEM: Climate Change, Artificial Intelligence, Engineering, Chemistry, Medicine

## Iowa

### Bank of America Student Leaders Program - Polk County - HS Students - 8 Wks

Paid internships with nonprofits. Work experience & leadership development. Week long all-expense-paid Student Leaders Summit in Washington, DC in July. Submit application essays, recommendations, and resume in January.

### Iowa State University – College of Design - Design Camps - HS Students

1-week – Architecture, Studio/Fine Arts, Graphic, Interior, & Industrial Design

## Kansas

### Bank of America Student Leaders Program - 2 KS Cities - HS Students - 8 Wks

Paid internships with nonprofits. Work experience & leadership development. Week long all-expense-paid Student Leaders Summit in Washington, DC in July. Submit application essays, recommendations, and resume in January.

## Kentucky

### Bank of America Student Leaders Program - 10+ KY Cities - HS Students - 8 Wks

Paid internships with nonprofits. Work experience & leadership development. Week long all-expense-paid Student Leaders Summit in Washington, DC in July. Submit application essays, recommendations, and resume in January.

GenCyber – 5-day Nat Security Agency-Sponsored Cybersecurity Camp for HS Students - Big Sandy Community & Technical College – Taught by Cyber Industry

Engaging & Dynamic - Role-playing, visual aids, activities, discussions: Computer networking, systems security, cyber operations, defense, AI, virtual reality

## Louisiana

Bank of America Student Leaders Program - 20+ LA Cities - HS Students - 8 Wks

Paid internships with nonprofits. Work experience & leadership development. Week long all-expense-paid Student Leaders Summit in Washington, DC in July. Submit application essays, recommendations, and resume in January.

Barksdale Air Force Base - Bossier Parish, LA - Air Force Research Labs - 8-12 Weeks

Students participate in mentored ongoing research. Paid internship: comp sci, physics, materials science, & aerospace. Workshops, seminars, presentations.

GenCyber – 5-day Nat Security Agency-Sponsored Cybersecurity Camp for HS Students - Louisiana Tech University – Taught by Cyber Industry Professionals

Engaging & Dynamic - Role-playing, visual aids, activities, discussions: Computer networking, systems security, cyber operations, defense, AI, virtual reality

Science and Engineering Apprenticeship Program (SEAP) – US Navy – New Orleans

8-weeks, 300 openings, 30 research labs nationwide, $4,000-$4,500 salary. HS students must be 16+ years old. Apply starting in August for following summer.

## Maine

Bank of America Student Leaders Program - Cumberland - HS Students - 8 Wks

Paid internships with nonprofits. Work experience & leadership development. Week long all-expense-paid Student Leaders Summit in Washington, DC in July. Submit application essays, recommendations, and resume in January.

Earthwatch Teen Expeditions - Acadia National Park, Maine - 1 week students must be 16+ years old. Apply starting in August for following summer.

*Climate Change:* Sea to the Trees science exploration program; understand patterns and make observations regarding how humans are changing the ecosystem; wildlife diversity, bird migration, ocean acidification, sea warming

GenCyber – 5-day Nat Security Agency-Sponsored Cybersecurity Camp for HS Students - Northeastern Univ Portland, Maine – Taught by Cyber Industry Prof

Engaging & Dynamic - Role-playing, visual aids, activities, discussions: Computer networking, systems security, cyber operations, defense, AI, virtual reality

Jackson Laboratory's Summer Student Program - 12th Grade & College Students

Bar Harbor, ME - Develop & execute research, analyze data, present findings; $6,500 stipend along with room, board, and travel to and from the lab

# Maryland

### Bank of America Student Leaders Program - 10+ MD Cities - HS Students - 8 Wks

Paid internships with nonprofits. Work experience & leadership development. Week long all-expense-paid Student Leaders Summit in Washington, DC in July. Submit application essays, recommendations, and resume in January.

### Defense Intelligence Agency Summer College Internship - Engineering/Technology

10-14 Week Summer Internship Program Intelligence & Technology. Apply in February Ft. Meade, MD - College Jr/Sr or Grad Student

### GenCyber – 5-day Nat Security Agency-Sponsored Cybersecurity Camp for HS Students - Anne Arundel CC, Harford CC, PGCC – Taught by Cyber Industry

Engaging & Dynamic - Role-playing, visual aids, activities, discussions: Computer networking, systems security, cyber operations, defense, AI, virtual reality

### Goddard Space Flight Center (NASA) - High School & College

Summer Aerospace and Climate Change Internship at GISS - Greenbelt, MD Research, Mentorship, Experiential Learning Opportunities

### Johns Hopkins Engineering Summer Programs in Innovation Sustainable Energy, and Biomedical Engineering - Online and In-Person

Biomedical, chemical, civil, electrical, environmental, and mechanical

### Maryland Institute College of Art (MICA) – 2-, 3-, 5-week - HS Students

Live studio workshops, artist talks, collaboration, feedback, critique, evaluation

### National Institute of Health – 8-week Paid Internship– Bethesda, Baltimore, and Frederick. MD Research Group Locations - Apply by mid February

Biomedical research internship for students 17 years or older by June 15th. HS-SIP for high school juniors & seniors - June to August - hands-on research.

### National Security Agency (NSA) – Paid Computer Internship – Ft. Meade

Students must be at least a junior in high school with interest in business, engineering, or computer science. Apply between September 1 and October 31.

### Naval Academy Summer STEM Program - Annapolis, MD - HS Students

Three week-long sessions for students interested in coding, game design computer projects, robotics, & engineering. Collaborate in world-class labs.

### Science and Engineering Apprenticeship Program (SEAP) – US Navy – Bethesda, Patuxent River, Silver Spring, Indian Head, and Annapolis

8-weeks, 300 openings, 30 research labs nationwide, $4,000-$4,500 salary. HS students must be 16+ years old. Apply starting in August for following summer.

### Terp Young Scholars - University of Maryland - 3-Week High School Program

Immersion into computer science with projects, exams, and collaboration.

### University of Maryland – 4-week ESTEEM/SER-Quest Summer Program

Rising seniors undertake engineering-focused projects while conducting research

**University of Maryland - Discovering Engineering - 1 week (additional programs also)**

Exploration of engineering with faculty to learn about the various disciplines.

**United States Naval Academy - Summer STEM Program for Students in 9th - 11th**

Design and build STEM projects with USNA Faculty and Midshipmen
1 week residential program, $700, includes lodging, meals, transport from airport

## Massachusetts

**Bank of America Student Leaders Program - 5+ MA Cities - HS Students - 8 Wks**

Paid internships with nonprofits. Work experience & leadership development.
Week long all-expense-paid Student Leaders Summit in Washington, DC in July.
Submit application essays, recommendations, and resume in January.

**Bentley University - Wolfram Math/Computer -2 Week - HS Summer Program**

Intensive training in programming, computation, & technology. Students
produce a project from ideation to completion (Wolfram Emerging Scholars).

**Boston College - Cognitive & Affective Neuroscience Lab (CANLab)**

One HS Student is chosen each year to intern in the lab learning aging, memory,
brain health, sleep, and both cognitive and affective neuroscience.

**Boston College - Boston, MA – Creative Writing Seminar Program**

3-week (July) Residential Program – HS Students – nonfiction, fiction, poetry
Create & edit the class literary journal and present writings at a public reading.

**Boston University Math, Engineering, Technology, Media, and Journalism**

**AMP - Academy of Media Production** – Cinematic/journalistic in visual
storytelling (Grades 10 – 12)
**Code Breakers** – 10th & 11th Grade Females - Cybersecurity, Cryptography,
Computer Programming, and Ethical Hacking (Free)
**Girls Get Math@BU** – 5-day Non-residential summer program for enthusiastic
10th – 11th graders
**Neuroscience** - 6-Weeks - 11th & 12th Grade - Lectures and discussions cover
psychology, neuropharmacology, neurology, and neuropsychology.
**Journalism Academy** – 2-week Writing, Photography, Reporting ages 14-18
**PROMYS – Program in Mathematics for Young Scientists** – 6 weeks 80 high
school students 14+ years old (scholarships available); seminars in number
theory, cryptography, linear algebra, matrices, graphs, and data visualization.
**RISE – Research in Science & Engineering** - 6-week Research in Science &
Engineering program in astronomy, chemistry, neuroscience, and medicine.
Engineering Research Options: Biomedical, Computer, Electrical, Mechanical
**U-Design** – 2-week Engineering Design Prog – hands-on workshop - 6th - 10th

**Forsyth Student Scholars Summer Internship Program - 8-Weeks - 11th & 12th grades**

Science research mentor program for underserved Massachusetts HS students.

**GenCyber – 5-day Nat Security Agency-Sponsored Cybersecurity Camp for HS
Students - Assumption University & Cape Cod CC – Taught by Cyber Industry**

Engaging & Dynamic - Role-playing, visual aids, activities, discussions: Computer
networking, systems security, cyber operations, defense, AI, virtual reality

### Great Books Summer Program - Amherst College - Grades 6-8 and 9-12

Great Books & Big Ideas, Writer's Workshops, and Literary Travel Programs
Read, Write, & Discuss Big Ideas in Literature and Philosophy with scholars

### Harvard Medical School - MEDscience Simulation Lab - Grades 9-12

Students learn biotech/medicine in an immersive, hands-on clinical research lab. This 1-week program offers medical simulations and research with DNA extraction, PCR, Gel Electrophoresis, ELISA, and disease diagnosis and treatment

### Harvard University GSD Design Discovery– Cambridge, MA (Ages 18+)

3-week Residential Program – Architecture, Landscape, Urban Planning & Design
Students participate in physical modeling, fabrication, and assembly.

### Harvard Summer Program for High School Students Credit/Non Credit Classes

7-week college credit (campus dorms) include: Creating Comics & Graphic Novels; Advertising, Visual Imagery, Creative Writing, Physics, Chemistry, Biology, Medicinal Topics, Calculus, Economics, and Computer Science

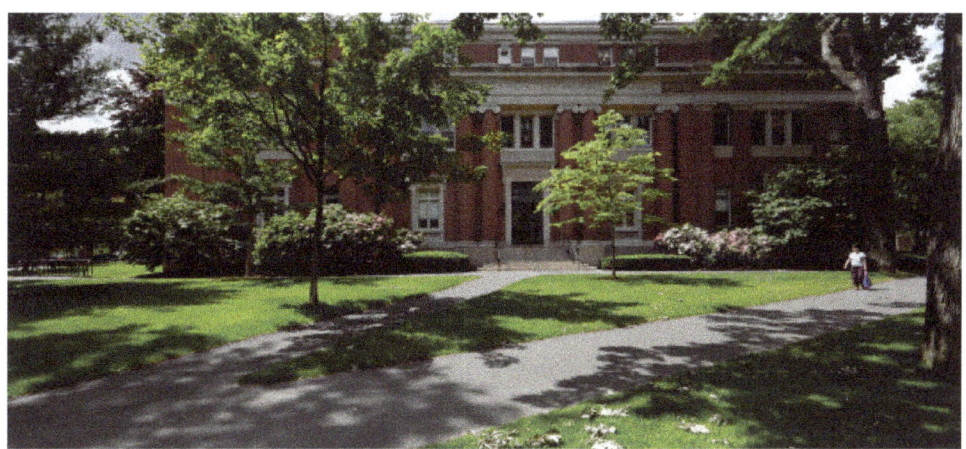

### Massachusetts College of Art & Design – 4-Week Art Immersion Program

Students take 3 foundation courses and participate in a closing exhibition.

### Massachusetts Institute of Technology – HS Students – Cambridge

**Beaver Works Summer Institute** – 4-week intensive program for first-generation high school juniors. Programs include Autonomous Underwater Vehicles to Quantum Software and to Serious Game Design with AI.

**Lincoln Laboratory Radar Introduction for Student Engineers (LLRISE)** - FREE 2-week  project-based workshop to teach students how to build small Doppler and range radar systems. HS Juniors. Applications open in January.

**MITES – Minority Introduction to Engineering and Science** – Intensive 6-week residential program for 80 high school juniors who intend to enter STEM programs, especially from underrepresented groups. The program is free.

**MOTSTEC** - Hands-on, in-depth STEM mentorship for HS seniors; courses/projects; present research at 5-day event (FREE) Work w/MIT faculty/researchers. Six-month hybrid learning program with 2-week STEM Immersion June-August.

**RSI – Research Science Institute** – Free. Competitive/Intensive 6-week program for 70 HS juniors who research/study advanced theory in math, science, & engineering. Distinguished Lectures/Alumni Network. Apply by early December.

**THINK Scholars Program** - 4 months HS students apply between Nov 1-Jan 1, accepted in Feb, join program in June. Pair with MIT researcher. Summer 4-days at MIT, All Expenses Paid + $1,000. Submit detailed proposals for novel ideas.

**WTP – Women's Technology Program** – 4-wk engineering focus - EE, ME, EECS

**Urbanframe Summer Design** - Build Project - CAD, drafting, sketching, mapping and context study, historical research, carpentry & construction.

**Additional MIT Hosted Programs:** LaunchX, OSC, iD Tech Camps, National Geographic Student Expeditions

## National Institute of Health – Paid Internship - Apply in Feb– Framingham, MA

8-week - Biomedical research internship for students 17 years or older by June. HS-SIP for high school juniors & seniors June to August hands-on research.

## Northeastern University - Drug Discovery to Clinical Care - 2 Weeks - HS Students

Hands-on ,interactive - medication life cycle from drug discovery to human use. Students visit facilities, compound, and learn therapeutics & toxicology.

## Northeastern Univ Young Scholars Program w/field trips - Rising HS Seniors

Intro to Engineering - Chemical, Civil, EE, Computer, Mechanical & Industrial Radar, batteries, energy, robotics, lasers, microwave, biotech, medicine, bldgs

## Tufts University – 6-Week Writing Intensive - HS Students - Develop Papers

Writing exercises, evaluation from professors, revise, and build on a theme.

## Tufts University Summer Accelerator - 2-Weeks for HS Students in 10th-12th

Take 2 college seminars: AI, neuroscience, coding, physiology, intl affairs, criminal justice, chaos theory, engineering, astrochemistry, & mythology.

## University of Massachusetts Amherst Pre-College – Amherst, MA

1-, 2-, 3-week Residential Intensives Grades 10-12; 3-D Design, 3-D Animation, Building & Construction Technology; Combatting the Climate Crisis Summer Engineering Institute, Design Academy, Programming for Aspiring Scientists

## Wellesley College – 2-week Residential Program - Wellesley, MA

EXPLO Pre-College + Career for Grades 10-12 Three session options; Topics include – AI, Entrepreneurship, Engineering, Medicine, Law, CSI

## Wentworth Institute of Technology - 2-4 Week Impact Lab - HS 11th & 12th

On-Campus Comp Sci, Engineering, Info Technology, Architecture, & Construction

## WPI Frontiers Program - Worcester Polytechnic Institute - Two 2-Week Sessions

This residential program allows HS students to explore comp sci & data science.

## Youth Design Boston (AIGA) – Boston, MA

Summer Graphic Design Internship & Mentoring Program

# Michigan

## Andrews University School of Architecture & Interior Design - Renaissance Kids
Virtual Studio Projects; lecture; community build projects

## Bank of America Student Leaders Program - 5+ MI Cities - HS Students - 8 Wks
Paid internships with nonprofits. Work experience & leadership development.
Week long all-expense-paid Student Leaders Summit in Washington, DC in July.
Submit application essays, recommendations, and resume in January.

## GenCyber – 5-day Nat Security Agency-Sponsored Cybersecurity Camp for HS Students - Northern MI U. & Oakland U. – Taught by Cyber Industry Professionals
Engaging & Dynamic - Role-playing, visual aids, activities, discussions: Computer networking, systems security, cyber operations, defense, AI, virtual reality

## Interlochen Center for the Arts – Summer Arts Camp – 1-6 Weeks
Creative Writing, Dance, Art, Motion Picture, Music, Theatre, Visual Arts

## Michigan State University - HS Honors Science, Math, Engineering Program
7-week intensive, hands-on summer research program & engineering projects.

## National Institute of Health – 8-week Paid Internship - Apply in Feb– Detroit
Research biomedical internship for students 17 years or older by June.
HS-SIP for high school juniors & seniors June to August hands-on research.

## University of Michigan – Stamps School of Art & Design – 3-Week BFA Preview
HS Students – Creative retreat w/state-of-the-art facilities & museum excursions

## University of Michigan – Summer Engineering Exploration (SEE) - 1 Week
On-campus - engineering design challenges - Apply Jan-Feb – Grades 10-12

# Minnesota

## Bank of America Student Leaders Program - 10+ MN Cities - HS Students - 8 Wks
Paid internships with nonprofits. Work experience & leadership development.
Week long all-expense-paid Student Leaders Summit in Washington, DC in July.
Submit application essays, recommendations, and resume in January.

## GenCyber – 5-day Nat Security Agency-Sponsored Cybersecurity Camp for HS Students - Alexandria Tech & CC & Lake Superior College – Cyber Industry Prof
Engaging & Dynamic - Role-playing, visual aids, activities, discussions: Computer networking, systems security, cyber operations, defense, AI, virtual reality

## Summer Liberal Arts Institute (SLAI) Computer Science Program - HS Jr & Sr
Hands-on, project-based residential program in computational solutions to problems, research, and a final symposium to present findings.

# Mississippi

### GenCyber – 5-day Nat Security Agency-Sponsored Cybersecurity Camp for HS Students - Univ. of Southern MS – Taught by Cyber Industry Professionals

Engaging & Dynamic - Role-playing, visual aids, activities, discussions: Computer networking, systems security, cyber operations, defense, AI, virtual reality

### Science and Engineering Apprenticeship Program (SEAP) – US Navy – Stennis

8-weeks, 300 openings, 30 research labs nationwide, $4,000-$4,500 salary. HS students must be 16+ years old. Apply starting in August for following summer.

# Missouri

### Bank of America Student Leaders Program - 10+ MO Cities - HS Students - 8 Wks

Paid internships with nonprofits. Work experience & leadership development. Week long all-expense-paid Student Leaders Summit in Washington, DC in July. Submit application essays, recommendations, and resume in January.

### GenCyber – 5-day Nat Security Agency-Sponsored Cybersecurity Camp for HS Students - Univ. of MO, Kansas City – Taught by Cyber Industry Professionals

Engaging & Dynamic - Role-playing, visual aids, activities, discussions: Computer networking, systems security, cyber operations, defense, AI, virtual reality

### Univ of Missouri Kansas City – Dept of Architecture, Urban Planning & Design

Design Discovery Program – Architecture, Interior Design, Landscape Architecture 3-day (July) Non-Residential Program – HS Students/Current College Students

### Washington University in St. Louis - HS Programs

**Biology of the Brain** - 4-5 week summer - Grades 11, 12 - Students learn brain anatomy, composition, changes, development, memories, and injury
**Creative Writing Program** – 2-weeks - fiction, nonfiction, and poetry. Morning writer's workshops. Students edit, share ideas, and discuss work
**Arts & Journalism Program** - 5-8 week – Dance, Journalism, Photography, Music, Drama, Photojournalism
**Young Scientist Program** - Rising Seniors - Summer Focus is an 8-week paid summer research internship.
**Shaw Institute for Field Training** (SIFT) and Tyson Environmental Research **Apprenticeship** (TERA) programs.
**BOLD@Olin** - 1-week Business Leadership/Entrepreneurship Program

### Whiteman Air Force Base - Knob Noster, MO - Air Force Research Labs - 8-12 Weeks

Students participate in mentored ongoing research teams. Paid internship: comp sci, physics, materials science, & aerospace. Workshops, seminars, presentations.

# Montana

### Cyberpatriot - Air Force Assn National Youth Cyber Education Program - 1 Week

HS Students - Camp locations include Montana State University

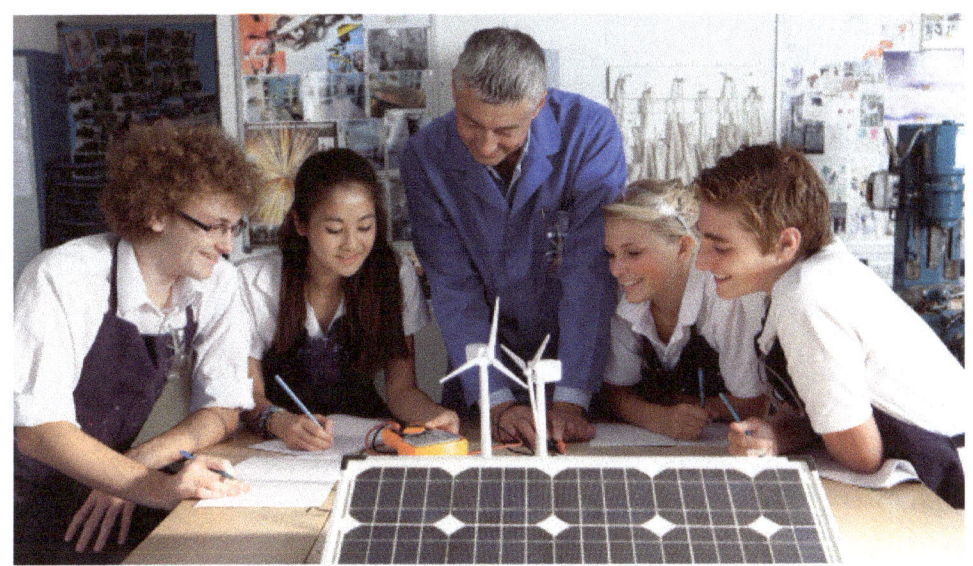

**GenCyber – 5-day Nat Security Agency-Sponsored Cybersecurity Camp for HS Students - Univ. of Montana, Missoula – Taught by Cyber Industry Professionals**

Engaging & Dynamic - Role-playing, visual aids, activities, discussions: Computer networking, systems security, cyber operations, defense, AI, virtual reality

**National Institute of Health – 8-week Paid Internship – Hamilton, MT**

Biomedical research internship for students 17 years or older by June. HS-SIP for high school juniors & seniors June to August hands-on research.

## Nebraska

**Bank of America Student Leaders Program - 3+ NE Cities - HS Students - 8 Wks**

Paid internships with nonprofits. Work experience & leadership development. Week long all-expense-paid Student Leaders Summit in Washington, DC in July. Submit application essays, recommendations, and resume in January.

**Cyberpatriot - Air Force Assn National Youth Cyber Education Program - 1 Week**

HS Students - Multiple camp locations include Bellevue University.

**GenCyber – 5-day Nat Security Agency-Sponsored Cybersecurity Camp for HS Students - Univ. of Nebraska, Omaha – Taught by Cyber Industry Professionals**

Engaging & Dynamic - Role-playing, visual aids, activities, discussions: Computer networking, systems security, cyber operations, defense, AI, virtual reality

**University of Nebraska College of Architecture – 6-day (June) - Grades 11-12**

6-day (June) Residential Program – Grades 11 & 12 – Studio training; architectural design;  scholarships

## Nevada

### AFWERX - Las Vegas, NV - Air Force Research Labs - 8-12 Weeks

Students participate in mentored ongoing research teams. Paid internship: comp sci, physics, materials science, & aerospace. Workshops, seminars, presentations

### Bank of America Student Leaders Program - 3+ NV Cities - HS Students - 8 Wks

Paid internships with nonprofits. Work experience & leadership development. Week long all-expense-paid Student Leaders Summit in Washington, DC in July. Submit application essays, recommendations, and resume in January.

### GenCyber – 5-day Nat Security Agency-Sponsored Cybersecurity Camp for HS Students - University of Nevada, LV – Taught by Cyber Industry Professionals

Engaging & Dynamic - Role-playing, visual aids, activities, discussions: Computer networking, systems security, cyber operations, defense, AI, virtual reality

### University of Nevada - Hands-On Engineering & Cybersecurity Camps - HS Students

UNR Engineering Exploration - Projects/activities - design, engineer, build, & test UNLV Cybersecurity Camp - Interactive labs/projects on cyber threats & defense.

## New Jersey

### Bank of America Student Leaders Program - 10+ NJ Cities - HS Students - 8 Wks

Paid internships with nonprofits. Work experience & leadership development. Week long all-expense-paid Student Leaders Summit in Washington, DC in July. Submit application essays, recommendations, and resume in January.

### New Jersey Institute of Technology – Hillier College of Architecture & Design

1-week (July) Residential Program – HS Students – Architecture, Interior Design, Industrial Design, Digital Design - Architecture + Design Programs (2 Start Dates)

### Pathway Summer Program Dept of Energy RENEW - HS & College Students

Mentorship, hands-on engineering/technology - Princeton Plasma Physics Lab

### Princeton Summer Journalism Program (PSJP) - FREE Residential Program for HS Jrs

Year-long college prep program for HS juniors from low-income backgrounds. Summer intensive at Princeton University (10 days); tours, seminars, writing project.

### Princeton University Laboratory Learning Program 5-6 Weeks, 16+ years old

Summer science/engineering research for HS students; lab experience; write paper

### Science and Engineering Apprenticeship Program (SEAP) – US Navy – Lakehurst

8-weeks, 300 openings, 30 research labs nationwide, $4,000-$4,500 salary. HS students must be 16+ years old. Apply starting in August for following summer.

## New Hampshire

### Bank of America Student Leaders Program - 2 NH Cities - HS Students - 8 Wks

Paid internships with nonprofits. Work experience & leadership development. Week long all-expense-paid Student Leaders Summit in Washington, DC in July. Submit application essays, recommendations, and resume in January.

**Sustainable Summer @ Dartmouth - Environmental Leadership Academy**
Students ages 15-18 attend 2-week program; bootcamp, research/development environmental problem, and then convert abstract ideas into real initiatives.

**University of New Hampshire InterOperability Lab - HighTech Bound - 4-6 Weeks**
Paid summer program for rising HS seniors pursuing careers in technology. Real-world mentored projects, visit tech companies, Apply between Jan & Feb

## New Mexico

**Bank of America Student Leaders Program - 2 NM Cities - HS Students - 8 Wks**
Paid internships with nonprofits. Work experience & leadership development. Week long all-expense-paid Student Leaders Summit in Washington, DC in July. Submit application essays, recommendations, and resume in January.

**Cyberpatriot - Air Force Assn National Youth Cyber Education Program - 1 Week**
HS Students - Multiple camp locations include San Juan College

**GenCyber – 5-day Nat Security Agency-Sponsored Cybersecurity Camp for HS Students - San Juan College – Taught by Cyber Industry Professionals**
Engaging & Dynamic - Role-playing, visual aids, activities, discussions: Computer networking, systems security, cyber operations, defense, AI, virtual reality

**Kirtland Air Force Base - Albuquerque, NM - Air Force Research Labs - 8-12 Weeks**
Students participate in mentored ongoing research. Paid internship: comp sci, physics, materials science, & aerospace. Workshops, seminars, presentations.

**Mentorship for Environmental Scholars (MES) Program - 10 Wk Paid - HS/College**
Sandia Nat Lab Dept of Energy Albuquerque - Environmental Science & STEM

**New Mexico State Summer Science Program - 5-6 Weeks - HS Students**
Astrophysics calculations, astronomy, original research program; mentors, workshops; collaborative community - highly selective - transformative

**Pathway Summer Program Dept of Energy RENEW Initiative-HS & College Students**
Mentorship, hands-on engineering/technology - Sandia National Laboratories

**Sandia National Labs - Albuquerque - Engineering/Tech Internship - HS/College**
* Ages 16+ - FT HS Student - Work on STEM Projects with mentors
* 10-12 Week College Summer Internship, Year-Round Internship, & Co-Ops

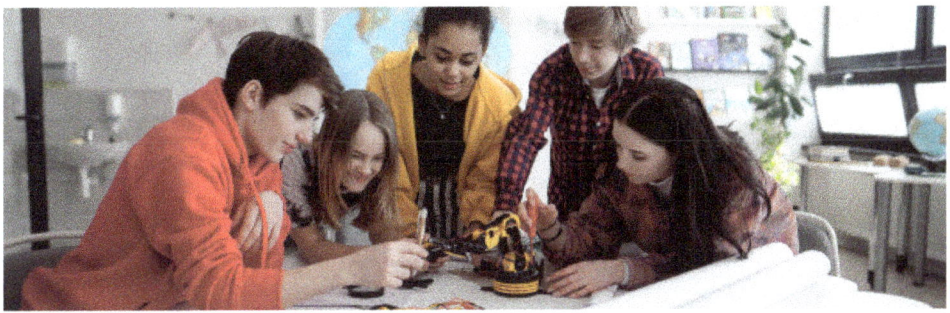

# New York

### AIA New York – Center for Architecture 1-week (July) – HS Students
Grades 3-12 include Architectural Design Studio, Drawing, Rooftop Dwelling, Dream House, Treehouses, Skyscrapers, Green Island Home, Neighborhood Design, Subway Architecture, Waterfront City, Parks & Playground Design

### Bank of America Student Leaders Program - 10+ NY Cities - HS Students - 8 Wks
Paid internships with nonprofits. Work experience & leadership development. Week long all-expense-paid Student Leaders Summit in Washington, DC in July. Submit application essays, recommendations, and resume in January.

### Brookhaven National Laboratory - Upton, NY - US Dept of Energy - Rising HS Seniors
Ensure America's energy security, environment, nuclear challenges by researching solutions. 6-week High School Research Program (HSRP) STEM research

### Brooklyn College STEM Research Academy - Urban Ecology & Design for HS Students
This 6-week environmental science research program includes lab, fieldwork, and methodology. Students dive into data collection and analysis.

### Canon Insights Summer Internship – Canon USA – PR/Marketing - Huntington, NY
Public Relations & Marketing Majors – 10 Week Paid Position

### City College of New York - STEM Institute Research/Project for HS Students
Build 3D Printers, Robot, Rockets, & Drones - Free Supercharged Program

### Cold Spring Harbor Laboratory - Partners for the Future Program - HS Students
Long Island HS seniors engage in biomedical research - min 10 hrs/wk from Sept - March of their senior year. State-of-the-art molecular biology - present findings.

### Columbia University Summer Programs for HS Students
**BRAINYAC** - Zuckerman Institute's Brain Research Apprenticeships for HS students in NYC. Weekends and 7 weeks in the summer.
**Neuroscience of Psychiatric Disorders** - Grades 9-12 - Students learn brain anatomy  and explore case studies of neuropsychiatric disorders.
**School of Engineering** - HS Maker Lab - 6-Weeks - Free - Students address a health problem - design, prototype, & test a biomedical device. Final presentation given to leading biomedical executives.
**SHAPE** (3-Wk - Summer HS Program in Technology & Engineering) - Build 3D Printers, Robots, Rockets, & Drones - Free Supercharged  Program - This engineering program is for HS students pursuing technology-focused subjects.
**Science of Psychology** - Introduction to the theory & science of psychology.
**Summer Art Immersion** - 3-week July-August Residential Program – Drawing Architecture, Creative Writing, Filmmaking, Photography, Theater, Visual Arts

### Cooper Union - New York, NY – Summer Art Intensive - 4-Week July-August
Residential Prog – Portfolio Devt, Exhibition, Anthology Publication; Drawing Animation,  Creative Writing, Photography, Graphic Design, & Stop Animation

## Cornell University – 3-Week Transmedia: Image, Sound, Motion Program

3-, 6-, 9-week June-August Residential Program; Drawing and New Media (collage, drawing, digital photography, screen printing, & video)
Architecture: Design Studio, Culture, and Society, Architectural Science & Technology

## Cornell University – CURIE Academy High School females entering 11th and 12th

Students who excel in math & science break the rules to make new discoveries.

## Cornell University - CATALYST Scholars - 1-Week STEM Academy (diverse students)

Cornell Engineering faculty/students participate in ten field sessions.

## Corning Summer Internships for College Students – Corning, NY

Advanced optics, Gorilla Glass, emerging innovations, life sciences, pharmaceuticals. Internships offered in engineering, science, & business

## Environmental Studies Summer Youth Inst-Hobart & William Smith Colleges

2-week, college experience for HS Students - Immerse in discussions, fieldwork in the Adirondacks, and projects on the environment and sustainability.

## Federal Bureau of Investigation - Future Agents in Training - Teen Academy

FBI classes on terrorism, cyber crime, public corruption, polygraph exams, evidence response, and SWAT. Meet w/special agents and intelligence analysts.

## GenCyber – 5-day Nat Security Agency-Sponsored Cybersecurity Camp for HS Students - Mohawk Valley CC, RIT, & SUNY Buffalo – Taught by Cyber Industry

Engaging & Dynamic - Role-playing, visual aids, activities, discussions: Computer networking, systems security, cyber operations, defense, AI, virtual reality

## Goddard Institute for Space Studies (GISS) New York City - Climate Change Research Initiative (CCRI) Summer Internship - High School & College

Research, Mentorship, and Experiential Learning Opportunities

## Hofstra University Summer Science Research Program (HUSSRP) - 5-Week HS Prog

Students conduct research with matched faculty mentors, culminating in a poster session; students attend weekly seminars.

## Jacobs Institute 8-week Paid Biomedical Internship (Apply Nov.-Jan.)

HS Jr/Sr or College Student – Gates Vascular Institute, Buffalo, NY Niagara Medical Campus; Lunch and Learn, weekly grand rounds, research, presentations

## John Jay College of Criminal Justice - 4 week - Introduction to Psychology

New York high school students - Learn research methods in thought, memory, learning, personality, socialization, development, disorders, and the biological basis of behavior.

## Lamont-Doherty Earth Observatory Secondary School Field Research Program

6-week - research, lab, and fieldwork - HS students - $1,400 stipend. Students follow through a research process to resolve environmental problems.

## Manhattan College Engineering Summer Camp - 1-Week - HS Students

Campers explore five engineering specialties: mechanical, electrical, civil, chemical, and environmental engineering.

**Mount Sinai - Icahn School of Medicine - Internship Program - FREE - Rising Senior**

African-American/Black or Hispanic/Latino w/demonstrated interest in medicine
6-Week summer program. Dept of Neurosurgery. Applications open in January

**New York University Engineering Innovation and Computer Science Programs**

**Applied Research in Science and Engineering (ARISE)** - ARISE is a Free 7-week
STEM program focused on Biomedical, Chemical Civil, Computer, Electrical,
Mechanical, & Aerospace Engineering
**Cyber Security Awareness Week (CSAW)** - Cybersecurity Games & Conference
NYU Center for Cyber Security - World's largest student-run event for students of
all ages, evolving to keep pace w/the changing threat landscape & innovations.
**Computer Science for Cyber Security (CS4CS)** - 3-week Immersive CS Intro for
HS students w/no cybersecurity/programming exp - Learn data usage, hacking,
digital forensics, privacy, cryptography, steganography & relevant cyber issues
**Innovation, Entrepreneurship and the Science of Smart Cities (ieSoSC)**
**- Advancing Technology & Engineering** - FREE 5-week program focused on
'smart city' design, prototypes, & research Lessons: circuits, electronics, coding,
complex tasks, team projects/presentation
**SPARC - Summer Prog in Automation, Robotics, & Coding** - Three 2-week,
programs for HS Students in robotics, mechatronics, AR, AI, IoT, computer
science, electrical engineering, mechanical engineering, machine learning

**Pace University - 2-Week STEM Summer Institute for HS Students - In-Person**

Coding w/Python, Data Analytics, Design Thinking

**Parsons School of Design – New York and Paris - 4-Week Online & On-Campus**

NYC summer programs for students from 3rd grade to 12th grade - Portfolio building
in 3-credit immersive design, studio art, photography, illustration, and game design
Paris Program – Design & Mgmt, Explorations in Drawing & Painting, Fashion Design

**Pathway Summer Program Dept of Energy RENEW Initiative- HS/College Students**

Mentorship, hands-on engineering/technology - Brookhaven National Lab

**Purchase College - SUNY SummerTech - HS Students w/day camp & overnight options**

This tech camp offers Python, Java, animation, 3D modeling & individual instruction.

**Rensselaer Polytechnic University – Summer Architecture Program - Troy, NY**

2-week Program in July or August, building 3D models, drawings, image editing

**Rochester Institute of Technology - FREE - Stipend - Army Laboratory Research Program**

Dissect brains, conduct research, meet scientists, interactive lectures - age 16+

**Rockefeller University Summer Neuroscience Program - 2-Week, NYC Students**

Dissect a brain, research, meet scientists, interactive lectures - 16+ years old

**Rome Laboratory - Rome, NY - Air Force Research Labs - 8-12 Weeks**

Students participate in mentored ongoing research. Paid internship: comp sci,
physics, materials science, & aerospace. Workshops, seminars, presentations.

**Roswell Park Cancer Research Institute for HS Juniors - Poster Presentation**

Independent research, classroom instruction on cancer, seminars w/invited speakers
Cancer biophysics, genetics, pharmacology, cancer therapeutics, tumor immunology

**School of Creative & Performing Arts (SOCAPA) – New York (13-18-year-olds)**
2-, 3-week - Learn Filmmaking, Screenwriting, Dance, Music, Photography

**Sotheby's Summer Institute – Pre-College, Undergrad, Graduate, and Professional**
New York, London, and virtual programs; Intensives in painting & drawing, curating, luxury marketing, art crime/art law, fashion, and art business

**Spotify – Summer Internship with The Journal – New York (Remote Eligible)**
Research, writing, news stories, podcasts: Partnership w/Gimlet and WSJ

**Stony Brook University - Simons Summer Research Prog - FREE/Stipend HS Outreach**
Simons Fellows conclude the internship by writing a research abstract & poster. Weekly faculty talks; research workshops, tours, events, poster symposium.

**Stony Brook University - Garcia Center for Polymers at Engineered Interfaces**
7-Week Program for HS/college students (June-Aug); Apply (Jan-March) projects, possible recognition in national competitions & publication in refereed journals

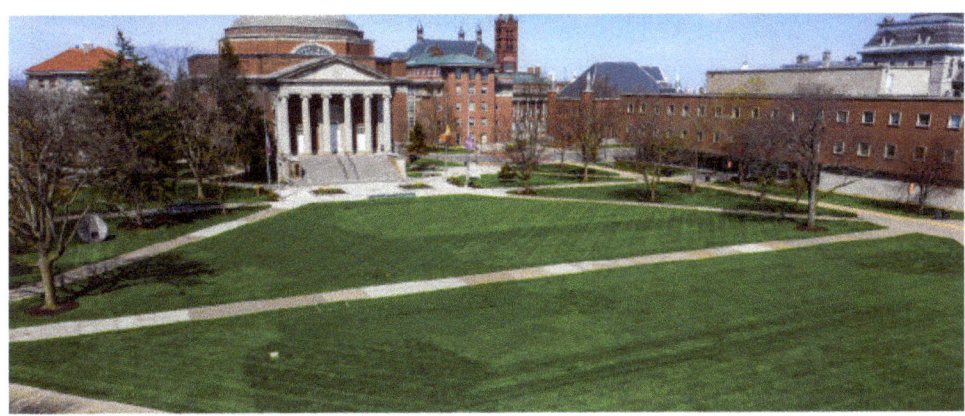

**Syracuse University - Neuroscience: Introduction to the Brain - HS Students**
This 2-week program provides a foundation to study the nervous system's structure, function, and disorders, including lectures, reading, and lab exercises.

**Syracuse University – 2-, 3-, 6-week On-Campus & Online Programs for HS Students**
3-D studio art; sculpture; architecture; design studies; writing immersion

**University at Buffalo School of Pharmacy and Pharmaceutical Sciences (SPPS)**
**Pharmacy Summer Institute (PSI) - 3-days - Buffalo, NY - HS/College Students**
Hands-on experiences, exposure to research, career pathways

**University of Rochester - Laboratory for Laser Energetics - 16 Rising Seniors Selected**
Attend weekly seminars on LLE research, write reports, present research results

**Wave Hill Forest Project - 7-week Environmental Proj - HS NYC Resident (16+ yrs old)**
Paid Summer Internship/Fieldwork in ecological restoration & urban ecology. Build/maintain wooded trails, remove invasive plant species, fix eroded slopes.

## North Carolina

### Bank of America Student Leaders Program - 10+ NC Cities - HS Students - 8 Wks

Paid internships with nonprofits. Work experience & leadership development. Week long all-expense-paid Student Leaders Summit in Washington, DC in July. Submit application essays, recommendations, and resume in January.

### Corning Summer Internships for College Students – NW Charlotte, NC

Advanced optics, Gorilla Glass, emerging innovations, life sciences, pharmaceuticals.  Internships offered in engineering, science, & business

### Cyberpatriot - Air Force Assn National Youth Cyber Education Program - 1 Week

HS Students - Multiple camp locations include Central Piedmont CC & Wayne CC

### Duke University Summer Program in Psychology & Neuroscience for HS Students

4-Week Hands-on research program in psychology & neuroscience labs.

### Duke University Summer Workshop in Math (SWiM) - Free - 1-Week Program

Focused on advancing female participation in math, SWiM participants attend 2 math courses, afternoon lectures by professors and social activities.

### GenCyber – 5-day Nat Security Agency-Sponsored Cybersecurity Camp for HS Students - NC Central University – Taught by Cyber Industry Professionals

Engaging & Dynamic - Role-playing, visual aids, activities, discussions: Computer networking, systems security, cyber operations, defense, AI, virtual reality

### National Institute of Health – 8-week Paid Internship – Research Triangle Park

Biomedical research internship for students 17 years or older by June. HS-SIP for high school juniors & seniors June to August hands-on research.

### North Carolina State University - Residential Engineering Camp for HS Students

11th & 12th graders - Three 1-wk sessions. Topics include: Aerospace, biomedical, civil, chemical, computer science, industrial/systems, materials science, & textile engineering, AI, robotics, bioenergy, agriculture, sustainability, paper science.

### Science & Engineering Apprenticeship Program (SEAP) – US Navy – Cherry Point

8-weeks, 300 openings, 30 research labs nationwide, $4,000-$4,500 salary. HS students must be 16+ years old. Apply starting in August for following summer.

### University of North Carolina Summer Science Program - HS Students 5-6 Wks

Biochemistry and molecular biology research - highly competitive, hands-on, collaborative; mentors; student teams; analysis, scientific writing, presentations

### Wake Forest University - Highly Selective Cancer, Bioscience, and Sports Medicine

These in-person and virtual programs offer HS students hands-on experience with medicine. Passionate students will find this first-hand experience inspiring.

## North Dakota

### GenCyber – 5-day Nat Security Agency-Sponsored Cybersecurity Camp for HS Students - Bismark State College – Taught by Cyber Industry Professionals

Engaging & Dynamic - Role-playing, visual aids, activities, discussions: Computer networking, systems security, cyber operations, defense, AI, virtual reality

## Ohio

### Bank of America Student Leaders Program - 4+ OH Cities - HS Students - 8 Wks

Paid internships with nonprofits. Work experience & leadership development. Week long all-expense-paid Student Leaders Summit in Washington, DC in July. Submit application essays, recommendations, and resume in January.

### Cyberpatriot - Air Force Assn National Youth Cyber Education Program - 1 Week

HS Students - Camp locations include the National Museum of the U.S. Air Force

### Science and Engineering Apprenticeship Program (SEAP) – US Navy – Dayton

8-weeks, 300 openings, 30 research labs nationwide, $4,000-$4,500 salary. HS students must be 16+ years old. Apply starting in August for following summer.

### Wright-Patterson AF Base - Dayton, OH - Air Force Research Labs - 8-12 Weeks

Students participate in mentored ongoing research. Paid internship: comp sci, physics, materials science, & aerospace. Workshops, seminars, presentations.

## Oklahoma

### Bank of America Student Leaders Program - 5+ OK Cities - HS Students - 8 Wks

Paid internships with nonprofits. Work experience & leadership development. Week long all-expense-paid Student Leaders Summit in Washington, DC in July. Submit application essays, recommendations, and resume in January.

### GenCyber – 5-day Nat Security Agency-Sponsored Cybersecurity Camp for HS Students - Rose State College – Taught by Cyber Industry Professionals

Engaging & Dynamic - Role-playing, visual aids, activities, discussions: Computer networking, systems security, cyber operations, defense, AI, virtual reality

### University of Oklahoma Architecture Summer Academy - HS Students - 1 week

Residential Program: Architecture, interior design, construction science design in action: creativity, innovation, & sustainability shaping the built environment

## Oregon

### Bank of America Student Leaders Program - 4+ OR Cities - HS Students - 8 Wks

Paid internships with nonprofits. Work experience & leadership development. Week long all-expense-paid Student Leaders Summit in Washington, DC in July. Submit application essays, recommendations, and resume in January.

GenCyber – 5-day Nat Security Agency-Sponsored Cybersecurity Camp for HS Students - Chemeketa CC, Oregon State, Portland CC – Taught by Cyber Industry

Engaging & Dynamic - Role-playing, visual aids, activities, discussions: Computer networking, systems security, cyber operations, defense, AI, virtual reality

## Pennsylvania

Bank of America Student Leaders Program - 10+ PA Cities - HS Students - 8 Wks

Paid internships with nonprofits. Work experience & leadership development. Week long all-expense-paid Student Leaders Summit in Washington, DC in July. Submit application essays, recommendations, and resume in January.

Carnegie Mellon University - Art, Math, Science, and Game Design Programs

**National HS Game Academy - 6-Week Game Design Program** - Design video games from ideation, development, & pitch, to final product.
**AI Scholars Program** - FREE - 4-Week Program for HS Students - AI, seminars, discussions, research, projects, and engagement with tech companies
**Pre-College Residential Art Program:** 3-, 4-, 6-week (July-August) Intensive Studio Studies Portfolio development in Drawing, Sculpture, Animation and Concept Studio Art Chestnut Hill College Global Solutions Lab
**Summer Academy for Math & Science (SAMS)**-Free Hands-on STEM program for underrepresented students, explore science w/projects & class instruction.

Cyberpatriot - Air Force Assn National Youth Cyber Education Program - 1 Week

HS Students - Multiple locations include Univ. of Pittsburgh, Gannon University, Community College of Beaver County, & Pittsburgh Technical College

Drexel University Westphal College of Media Arts & Design – Discovering Architecture

2-week Residential Program – HS Students – Intensive Studio Architecture Program Visit prominent architectural, multi-disciplinary design offices; meet architects

GenCyber – 5-day Nat Security Agency-Sponsored Cybersecurity Camp for HS Students - Indiana U. of Pennsylvania – Taught by Cyber Industry Professionals

Engaging & Dynamic - Role-playing, visual aids, activities, discussions: Computer networking, systems security, cyber operations, defense, AI, virtual reality

Gettysburg College - Camp Psych - 1-Week HS Student Program

In-person summer camp in psychology gives an insider's view of the field.

Great Books Summer Program - Haverford College - Grades 6-8 and 9-12

Great Books & Big Ideas, Writer's Workshops, and Literary Travel Programs Read, Write, & Discuss Big Ideas in Literature and Philosophy with scholars

Interactive Global Simulation, Electrifying Africa, & UN Sustainable Growth

1-week – HS Students – Intensive collaborative team solutions to big problems

Lehigh University - IGEI (4 Weeks) and SEI (2 Weeks) - HS Programs for 11th & 12th

**Iacocca Global Entrepreneurship Intensive(IGEI)** - HS Entrepreneurship Program Sustainable design, global citizenship, design challenges, business hackathons, teams

**Summer Engineering Institute (SEI)** - Intensive classroom study, discussions, team projects, problem-solving, integrated technology

### Maywood University Pre-College Summer Workshop School of Architecture
2-week (July) Residential Program – HS Students – Design/Build Your Future

### Pennsylvania State University Architecture & Landscape Architecture Summer Camp
1-week (July) – HS Students – Architecture, graphics, design, built environment

### Pennsylvania State University Summer Discovery Program in Engineering & STEM, Also Engineering Ahead (Free 4-Week Program for Minorities)
Students are introduced to engineering disciplines, design, and research.

### Science and Engineering Apprenticeship Program (SEAP) – US Navy – Philadelphia
8-weeks, 300 openings, 30 research labs nationwide, $4,000-$4,500 salary. HS students must be 16+ years old. Apply starting in August for following summer.

### Temple University Tyler School of Art and Architecture Pre-College Program
2-week (July-August) Residential Program – HS Students – Studio Architecture

### University of Pennsylvania HS Students Science, Engineering, Research, Comp Sci
**TREES Program** - Tuition Free - 2 weeks - Environmental Science Research at the UPenn Ctr of Excellence in Environmental Toxicology, independent research
**Summer Coding Academy** - 3 weeks - HTML, Cascading Style Sheets, JavaScript, and webpage creation
**Engineering Summer Academy at Penn (ESAP)** - Rigorous on-campus program: biotech, computer graphics, computer science, nanotechnology, & robotics.

### University of Pittsburgh Medical Center - FREE - Hillman Cancer Center Academy
Immersive 7-week mentored medical research program for high school students (15+ yrs). Research in biology, medicine, and computer science.

### Wistar Institute High School Fellowship in Biomedical Research - Philadelphia
4-week - cancer biology, genetics, vaccine development, infectious diseases, and bioinformatics. Work in state-of-the-art training lab; literature review.

## Rhode Island

### Bank of America Student Leaders Program - 5+ RI Cities - HS Students - 8 Wks
Paid internships with nonprofits. Work experience & leadership development. Week long all-expense-paid Student Leaders Summit in Washington, DC in July. Submit application essays, recommendations, and resume in January.

### Brown University – 1-4 Weeks – Art Themed Courses & the Environmental Leadership Lab (Climate Change 2-week hand's on program for HS Students
Creative writing, music, studio art, art history, & environment/sustainability

### Cyberpatriot - Air Force Assn National Youth Cyber Education Program - 1 Week
HS Students - Multiple camp locations include the Comm College of Rhode Island

GenCyber – 5-day Nat Security Agency-Sponsored Cybersecurity Camp for HS Students - Rhode Island College – Taught by Cyber Industry Professionals
Engaging & Dynamic - Role-playing, visual aids, activities, discussions: Computer networking, systems security, cyber operations, defense, AI, virtual reality

Rhode Island School of Design Pre-College School of Design – Providence, RI
6-week (June-July) Residential Program – High school students – Foundational Art & Design Studies. Figure drawing, projects, trips, & exhibitions.

Roger Williams University High School Summer Academy in Architecture
4-week (July-August) Residential Program – Grades 11 & 12 – Explore Studio Architecture - Seminars, fieldwork, studio, portfolio development

## South Carolina

Bank of America Student Leaders Program - 7+ SC Cities - HS Students - 8 Wks
Paid internships with nonprofits. Work experience & leadership development. Weeklong all-expense-paid Student Leaders Summit in Washington, DC in July. Submit application essays, recommendations, and resume in January.

Clemson University Pre-College School of Architecture Program
1-week (July-August) Residential Program – Grades 7-12 - Engineering design, mechanical/civil engineering, intelligent vehicles, materials engineering

Cyberpatriot - Air Force Assn National Youth Cyber Education Program - 1 Week
HS Students - Multiple camp locations, including USC Upstate & USC Aiken

GenCyber – 5-day Nat Security Agency-Sponsored Cybersecurity Camp for HS Students - The Citadel – Taught by Cyber Industry Professionals
Engaging & Dynamic - Role-playing, visual aids, activities, discussions: Computer networking, systems security, cyber operations, defense, AI, virtual reality

Mentorship for Environmental Scholars (MES) Program - 10 Wk Paid - HS/College
Savannah River Site Dept of Energy - Aiken, SC - Environmental Science & STEM

Science and Engineering Apprenticeship Program – US Navy – Charleston
8-weeks, 300 openings, 30 research labs nationwide, $4,000-$4,500 salary. HS students must be 16+ years old. Apply starting in August for following summer.

University of South Carolina HS Summer Computer Tech & Engineering Programs
**Carolina Master Scholars Adventure Series** - 1 Week Hands-on design thinking in VEX Robotics, digital content creation, and green engineering
**Partners for Minorities in Eng & Comp Sci (PMECS)** 9th-12th AI, Cyber, Coding

## South Dakota

GenCyber – 5-day Nat Security Agency-Sponsored Cybersecurity Camp for HS Students - Dakota State Univ. – Taught by Cyber Industry Professionals
Engaging & Dynamic - Role-playing, visual aids, activities, discussions: Computer networking, systems security, cyber operations, defense, AI, virtual reality

## Tennessee

**Arnold Air Force Base - Tullahoma, TN - Air Force Research Labs - 8-12 Weeks**

Students participate in mentored ongoing research. Paid internship: comp sci, physics, materials science, & aerospace. Workshops, seminars, presentations.

**Bank of America Student Leaders Program - 8+ TN Cities - HS Students - 8 Wks**

Paid internships with nonprofits. Work experience & leadership development. Week long all-expense-paid Student Leaders Summit in Washington, DC in July. Submit application essays, recommendations, and resume in January.

**Mentorship for Environmental Scholars (MES) Program - 10 Wk Paid - HS/College**

Oak Ridge Nat Lab Dept of Energy Site - Research in Environmental Science/STEM

**University of Memphis Discovering Architecture + Design - 1-day – HS Students**

Design programs on architecture, interior design, and the built environment.

**University of Tennessee, Knoxville College of Architecture + Design**

1-week UT Summer Design Camp (July) Residential – HS Students
Immersive architecture, graphic design, and professional practice program

**Vanderbilt Summer Academy – Nashville, TN – 3-Week Program**

" Digital Storytelling", "Writing Fantasy Fiction", "Math & Music", "Writing Short Stories"

**Vanderbilt Research Experience for High School Students (REHSS) - 6-Week Intensive**

Only for specific Nashville STEM HS - 40 hrs/wk, weekly workshops, final symposium

## Texas

**AFWERX Air Force Innovation - Austin, TX - Air Force Research Labs - 8-12 Weeks**

Students participate in mentored ongoing research teams. Paid intern: comp sci, physics, materials science, & aerospace. Workshops, seminars, presentations.

**Aggie STEM Summer Camps -  Texas A&M - Grades 6-8 & 9-12 - 1 & 2 Week**

STEM topics include robotics, rockets, coding, and engineering design principles. Students also meet professors & tour STEM labs on the TAMU campus.

**Bank of America Student Leaders Program - 10+ TX Cities - HS Students - 8 Wks**

Paid internships with nonprofits. Work experience & leadership development. Week long all-expense-paid Student Leaders Summit in Washington, DC in July. Submit application essays, recommendations, and resume in January

**Baylor Engineering & Computing Summer Academy (BECSA) - 10th - 12th**

Focus on rolling, electrical, calculating energy, energy in flight & harvesting energy

**Baylor University - CASPER HS Scholars Program - EE/Aerospace - 11th & 12th**

Astrophysics, gravitation, condensed matter, plasmas & beam physics

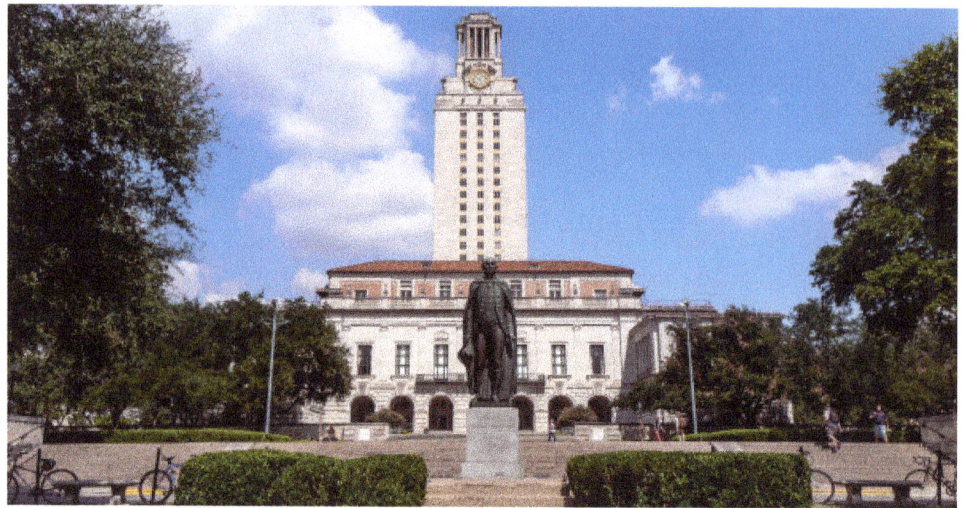

### Boeing Summer Internship – HS & College– Lewisville and San Antonio
Hands-on industry experience - Aviation and engineering Internships

### Corning Summer Internships for College Students – Keller, TX
Advanced optics, Gorilla Glass, emerging innovations, life sciences, and pharmaceuticals Internships offered in engineering, science, and business.

### Cyberpatriot - Air Force Assn National Youth Cyber Education Program - 1 Week
HS Students - Locations include Angelo State U. South Texas College, UTEP, Baylor Collaborative, Texas Women's University, St. Philip's College Texas State

### GenCyber – 5-day Nat Security Agency-Sponsored Cybersecurity Camp for HS Students - San Antonio College, Texas A&M – Taught by Cyber Industry Prof.
Engaging & Dynamic - Role-playing, visual aids, activities, discussions: Computer networking, systems security, cyber operations, defense, AI, virtual reality

### Jacobs Engineering Internship – Summer Internship (College) - Dallas
Civil, electrical, environmental, geotechnical, & transportation engineering; sustainability, cybersecurity, mobility, and R&D with worldwide projects.

### National Security Agency (NSA) – Paid Computer Internship – San Antonio
Students must be at least a junior in high school with interest in business, engineering, or computer science. Apply between September 1 and October 31.

### Rice University Summer Scholars Programs - Middle & High School Students
**Aerospace Academy** - 12 days - Hands-on in industry facilities w/NASA reps Immersion attend flight school w/flight prep simulation, launch a satellite.
**Creative Writing Camp** - Develop writing skills while living on campus.
**National Youth Leadership Forum: Medicine & Health Care** - 8 days hands-on HS students gain clinical training in medical diagnostics, surgery & first aid
**Pre-College Programs** - Economics, Entrepreneurship, Genome Engineering, Global Affairs, Law, Physiology, & Psychology

**Rice Center for Engineering Leadership (RCEL) Rice ELITE Tech** - Real world advanced engineering & technology - AI, IoT, machine learning, data science
**Rice U School Mathematics Project (RUSMP)** - Summer Math Camps
**Tapia Camps** - 1 Week on campus - STEM projects, presentations, field trips

## SpaceX – Summer Engineering/Co-op Program – Brownsville & McGregor

Paid Internship - Must be in an undergraduate in a STEM subject.

## Southern Methodist University - STEM Works, Kids Ahead, TEDXKids@SMU

**Introduction to Engineering** - 7th & 8th - Basic hands-on project approach
**Advanced Engineering** - 9th & 10th - Project-based engineering design
**Engineering Design Experience** - 11th & 12th - Civil, EE, Comp Sci, Mechanical

## Tesla Internships – More than $35/hr – FT Automotive Design/Engineering

Austin: Manufacturing Eng; Waco: People Analytics, Vehicle Service Research

## Texas Tech Anson L Clark Scholars Program – Research Areas: Advertising, Architecture, Art, Dance, Engineering, or Theatre - 7-week – Grades 11 & 12

Residential Program (must be 17 years old by start date) – No program fee.
Intensive research-based program; $500 meal card; $750 tax-free stipend.

## University of Houston & Wonderworks Pre-College Summer Discovery Program

**Hines College of Architecture & Design** – Intro to Architecture 6-week – HS Students – Design in hands-on studio, field trips, & portfolio workshop.
**UH Coding and AI Camp** - Hands-on programming with AI applications.

## University of Texas at Austin Summer Programs for HS Students

**Computer Science Summer Academy** - 1 Week - HS Students learn C++, project management, machine learning, artificial intelligence, & Python.
**My Introduction to Engineering (MITE)** - 5-day camp for 11th grade students to work on team-based engineering projects
**Digital Design** - 2-D Game Design, 3-D Game Design, 3-D Animation/Motion - School of Design & Creative Technologies - 1-week – HS Students – portfolio development
**STEM Enhancement in Earth Science (SEES)** - NASA, Texas Space Grant, Ctr for Space Research - Interpret NASA satellite remote sensing data while working w/ NASA scientists. Field investigation - HS Jr/Sr 16+ years old by July 1 - FREE

## Welch Summer Scholar Program (WSSP) - 5-Week - HS Jr/Sr from Texas

@UT Austin, UT Arlington, UT Dallas, University of Houston, & Texas Tech
Hands-on chemical research, mentorship, research paper, presentation, poster

# Utah

## Bank of America Student Leaders Program - 4+ UT Cities - HS Students - 8 Wks

Paid internships with nonprofits. Work experience & leadership development.
Week long all-expense-paid Student Leaders Summit in Washington, DC in July.
Submit application essays, recommendations, and resume in January.

**Cyberpatriot - Air Force Assn National Youth Cyber Education Program - 1 Week**
HS Students - Multiple camp locations, including Utah Valley University.

**Edwards Lifesciences Summer College Internship Program - Draper, Utah**
Currently enrolled in college - Interested in healthcare related programs
Proficient in engineering drafting software, writing, or business/leadership

**GenCyber – 5-day Nat Security Agency-Sponsored Cybersecurity Camp for HS Students - Brigham Young University – Taught by Cyber Industry Professionals**
Engaging & Dynamic - Role-playing, visual aids, activities, discussions: Computer networking, systems security, cyber operations, defense, AI, virtual reality

## Vermont

**Columbia Climate School in the Green Mountains - Green Mountains - HS Students**
2-week program on Climate and Sustainability - discussions, seminars, fieldwork, hands-on projects, critical thinking, & problem solving

**School of Creative & Performing Arts ( SOCAPA) – Burlington, VT (13-18-year-olds)**
2-week, 3-week - learn filmmaking, screenwriting, dance, music, photography

## Virginia

**Bank of America Student Leaders Program - 25+ VA Cities - HS Students - 8 Wks**
Paid internships with nonprofits. Work experience & leadership development. Week long all-expense-paid Student Leaders Summit in Washington, DC in July. Submit application essays, recommendations, and resume in January.

**Cyberpatriot - Air Force Assn National Youth Cyber Education Program - 1 Week**
HS Students - Locations, incl Mtn Gateway CC & Lynchburg Nat Guard Academy

**Defense Intelligence Agency Summer College Internship - Engineering/Technology**
10-14 Week Summer Internship Program Intelligence/Tech Apply in February
Arlington, Charlottesville, Quantico, Reston - College Jr/Sr or Grad Student

**Federal Bureau of Investigation -  Future Agents in Training - Teen Academy**
FBI classes on terrorism, cyber crime, public corruption, polygraph exams, evidence response, and SWAT. Meet w/special agents and intelligence analysts.

**GenCyber – 5-day Nat Security Agency-Sponsored Cybersecurity Camp for HS Students - Marymount Univ. & Virginia Tech - Taught by Cyber Industry Prof.**
Engaging & Dynamic - Role-playing, visual aids, activities, discussions: Computer networking, systems security, cyber operations, defense, AI, virtual reality

**NASA Langley Research Center Paid Internship Program (16+ years old) 8-10 weeks**
Aerospace program in public affairs, multimedia, statistics, aerial robotics, apace hardware design, testing, Mars surface habitat, & high temperature materials

**NASA's  Wallops Flight Facility Summer Internship - High School & College**
Research, mentorship, and experiential learning opportunities

### Northrop Grumman – Engineering Intern– Space Systems R & D Team

Graduating HS Seniors – Join an engineering team to design, develop and test space systems and satellites; R & D - land, sea, air, space, and cyberspace.

### Pentagon - Arlington, VA - Air Force Research Labs - 8-12 Weeks

Students participate in mentored ongoing research. Paid internship: comp sci, physics, materials science, & aerospace. Workshops, seminars, presentations.

### Science and Engineering Apprenticeship Program (SEAP) – US Navy Hampton Roads and Dahlgren

8-weeks, 300 openings, 30 research labs nationwide, $4,000-$4,500 salary. HS students must be 16+ years old. Apply starting in August for following summer.

### Virginia Commonwealth University (VCUArts) Pre-College - 3-Week

On-Campus Program  – 2D Portfolio devt, photography; Clay: More Than Just Mud, Sketchbook to Controller,  animation workshop, sculpture, jewelry & fashion design, stage combat, musical theatre, & Acting From Page to Stage

### Virginia Tech Inside Architecture + Design & Imagination Camp

1-week – HS Students – Hands-on design studio architecture program 1-week Electrical & computer engineering; drone, build, & fly program.

## Washington

### Bank of America Student Leaders Prog - Various WA Cities - HS Students - 8 Wks

Paid internships with nonprofits. Work experience & leadership development. Week long all-expense-paid Student Leaders Summit in Washington, DC in July. Submit application essays, recommendations, and resume in January.

### COPE Scholars Program – Healthcare Internship – 280 Hours Training Locations in Puyallup, Seattle, Spokane, and Tacoma

Health Scholars must be 18+. Students assist w/basic healthcare for medical or nursing school, etc. Certificate of Completion -  Keck Graduate Institute

### Cyberpatriot - Air Force Assn National Youth Cyber Education Program - 1 Week

HS Students - Multiple camp locations, including Marysville NUROTC.

### DigiPen Academy – K-12 Film, Music, Game Design  Summer in Redmond, WA

1-week and 2-week  programs, including Teen Art & Animation; Film Scoring Music & Sound Design; Video Game Development; Animation Masterclass

### Fred Hutchinson Cancer Research Center's Summer HS/College Internship Program

Seattle - 8-Week, FT, Paid Internship - Mentored research, seminars, workshops

### GenCyber – 5-day National Security Agency-Sponsored Cybersecurity Camp for HS Students - Eastern Washington University, Spokane Falls Community College, & Whatcom Community College – Taught by Cyber Industry Professionals

Engaging & Dynamic - Role-playing, visual aids, activities, discussions: Computer networking, systems security, cyber operations, defense, AI, virtual reality

### Microsoft Discovery Program - 4 Weeks - HS Students - Redmond, Washington

Work on real-world projects during the summer at Microsoft to gain business skills and mentorship. Students must live & attend high school within 50 miles of Redmond or Atlanta. Resume, application, & questions; apply in February.

### Mentorship for Environmental Scholars (MES) Program - 10 Wk Paid - HS/College

Hanford Dept of Energy Site Richland, WA Environmental Science/STEM Research

### NatureBridge Summer Programs - Olympic National Park - 1-2 weeks

Environmental science education, & hands-on fieldwork while backpacking for students in 7th - 12th grades. Connect to nature with trail building, habitat restoration, and wilderness exploration.

### Pacific Northwest National Laboratory - Summer STEM Programs for HS/College

**HS** - 10-Week Student Research Apprenticeship Prog & Young Women in Science
**College** - 10 Week Science Undergraduate Lab Internship, National Security Internship Program, Energy & Environment Internship Program

### Pathway Summer Program Dept of Energy RENEW Initiative- HS/College Students

Mentorship, hands-on engineering/technology - Pacific NW National Laboratory

### Seattle Children's Research Institute STEM Internships - Biomedical Research

* 4 Week Paid 10th Grade HS Research Training Program - Bio lab - July/Aug
* Yearlong HS Program - biomedical research in healthcare - Lab exp, guest lectures
* College - 9 & 12 Week Paid Summer Scholars & STAR Biomedical Research Prog

### University of Washington – Seattle, WA – Middle & HS STEM Students - 1 Week

Neurotechnology Young Scholars Program, DawgBytes Computer Science Camp, Engineering & Tech, Material Science Camp, & summer art classes

### Wilderness Awareness School's Summer Day Camps - 5-days for 6-12 year olds

Nature/environment activities; survival skills training in State Parks - St. Edward, Cougar Mountain, Seward, Tolt MacDonald, & Carnation Farms. Kids camps

### Youth Engaged in Sustainable Systems (YESS) - HS Student Summer Program

This hands-on paid internship includes natural resources, conservation, ecological restoration, & sustainable environmental practices. Replace invasive plant species to restore ecological environments. Highline & Riverview School Districts

## West Virginia

### NASA Independent Verification and Validation Facility, Fairmont, WV

Research, Mentorship, and Experiential Learning Opportunities
HS Students - Focus on robotics, programming, engineering, & STEM projects.

### National Youth Science Academy - FREE - Camp Pocahontas, WV - STEAM

Two delegates (high school juniors or seniors) are selected to attend from each state and D.C. attend for 3 weeks. Housing, meals, transportation, and supplies are provided at no cost. Washington, D.C. trip included.

West Virginia Governor's STEM Institute (GS0) - high-achieving 8th & 9th Graders
Hands-on computer science, cybersecurity, & AI program to advance science exp

## Wisconsin

Bank of America Student Leaders Prog - Various WI Cities - HS Students - 8 Wks
Paid internships with nonprofits. Work experience & leadership development.
Week long all-expense-paid Student Leaders Summit in Washington, DC in July.
Submit application essays, recommendations, and resume in January.

Cyberpatriot - Air Force Assn National Youth Cyber Education Program - 1 Week
HS Students - Camp locations include Marquette University

Experimental Aircraft Association - 1 Week Aviation Camps for students 12 - 18
**Young Eagles Camp** - 12-13-year-olds - Aeromodeling, Wing Construction, basic
flight, interactive computer simulator ground school, fly designed missions
**Basic Camp** - 14-15-year-olds Ground School, Tech Workshop, Models, Demos
**Advanced Camp** - Action-packed aviation ground instruction & flight experience

GenCyber – 5-day Nat Security Agency-Sponsored Cybersecurity Camp for HS
Students - U. of Wisconsin-Whitewater – Taught by Cyber Industry Professionals
Engaging & Dynamic - Role-playing, visual aids, activities, discussions: Computer
networking, systems security, cyber operations, defense, AI, virtual reality

University of Wisconsin - Madison - Engineering Summer Program - 11th & 12th
Free, 3-week residential program for students interested in engineering.
Mechanical engineering & electrical/computer engineering

University of Wisconsin Milwaukee School of Architecture & Urban Planning
1-week – HS Students – Online architectural design & interior design activities,
lectures, workshops, and interactive architectural concepts and design thinking.

## Wyoming

Sierra Club's Summer Outings - Gros Ventre Wilderness - Yellowstone Ecosystem
Trail restoration trip - 7 days - Forest Service personnel drive gear to the trailhead.
Hike the rugged landscape to scenic rivers while working on the trail.

### TAKE ADVANTAGE OF THIS TIME TO EXPLORE

During high school and college, explore your interests in summer programs,
skill-building camps, and internships. You never have the chance to consider
alternatives in quite the same way. Learn something new. There are hundreds of
career areas you may never have considered. Have some fun while you are at it!

"

Every expert was
once a beginner.

— Helen Hayes

## CHAPTER FOURTEEN
# STUDY SKILLS & TUTORING

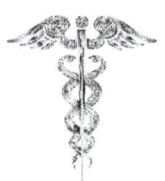

Learning comes in many forms. You need to determine the way you prefer to master the information you learn. "Teachers" also come in all forms: video, in-person, live-interactive, tutoring, study groups, friends, online courses, Google Classroom, handouts, books, library resources, visuals, test banks, etc.

Sometimes we get stuck thinking that we can learn in only one way. Yet, some of our biggest teaching moments are when we make a mistake. So, change your mindset since AI robots will soon be trained to be our teachers and we will use whatever resources are available to master whatever we need to learn.

Study skills are equally important. You have probably heard that some people are more auditory, visual, or kinesthetic. Do you prefer hearing, seeing, or touching the material you learn? You need to try out the where, when, and how that works best for you.

For example, research says that only ten percent of students complete their reading assignments. If sitting down to read a textbook does not work, get your books in an audio format. Listen to them in the car if it is not distracting or when you take a walk, run on a treadmill, or lift weights.

Many schools and almost all colleges offer free tutoring. A good tutor can save hours of valuable time. If they are a master of the subject, they can explain material in multiple ways, including any method, order, or format your teacher prefers that you to submit your work. I no longer tutor chemistry, physics, or mathematics, but when I did, I discovered the multitude of teachers' unique ways of presenting material, including their idiosyncrasies. I either showed students easier methods or adjusted they way I explained concepts to their teacher. Note: A tutor can be immeasurably valuable in saving students both time and stress.

There are numerous other avenues to learn subject matter and many of them are free. Here are a few suggestions to study for the SAT/ACT, classes, or possibly information you feel would be helpful like computer programming, machine learning, writing research papers, or data science.

## Khan Academy

* 100% free nonprofit platform.
* Geared toward K–12 and early college students.
* Excellent for AP courses, MCAT/SAT/ACT prep, and math/science topics.
* Accessible and friendly for all learning levels.

## MITx

* Part of the edX platform, created by MIT and Harvard.
* Offers college-level courses in physics, biology, computer science, and more.
* Many courses are free to audit, with optional paid certificates.
* Focuses on rigorous academic material often aligned with real MIT classes.

## Coursera

* Partners with top universities (like Stanford, Yale, and Johns Hopkins).
* Offers both free and paid courses, specializations, and full degrees.
* Great for pre-med, public health, AI, psychology, and humanities courses.
* Provides certificates and credentials; often recognized by employers.

## Other Platforms:

**Brilliant.org** – Interactive STEM learning, great for problem-solving skills.
**edX** – The broader platform hosting MITx, HarvardX, etc.
**FutureLearn** – UK-based, university-taught courses with a global focus.
**Harvard Online** – Free and paid courses from Harvard (via edX or directly).
**Open Yale Courses** – Free recorded lectures from Yale professors.
**Saylor Academy** – 100% free college-level courses with certificates.
**Stanford Online** – Offers free and professional-level courses.
**Udemy** – Offers affordable, practical skill-based courses (but less academic).

With free or low cost resources, you do not need expensive books, classes, training, or tutors. There are numerous resources for you to obtain the knowledge you need. Some students supplement their learning in online classes, community college, service experiences abroad, specialized programming, reading materials, and videos. Learning ways to study that are best for you takes practice.

Making lists and organizing information varies widely from person to person. Some people keep lists on their phone, some say what they need to remember into an audio recording device. While still others prefer Google Docs, planner pads, or simply handwritten notes.

# STUDY SKILLS CHECKLIST

- ☐ **Active Listening in Class** – Engage and take meaningful notes during lectures.
- ☐ **Active Recall** – Test yourself on the material rather than just rereading.
- ☐ **Concept Mapping** – Draw diagrams that show relationships among ideas.
- ☐ **Daily Review** – Spend 10–15 minutes each day reviewing notes or key concepts.
- ☐ **Dual Coding** – Combine words and visuals (e.g., diagrams with explanations).
- ☐ **Environment** – Ensure lighting, quiet, minimal distractions, and good posture.
- ☐ **Feynman Technique** – Teach the concept in simple terms as if explaining it to someone who knows nothing about the subject.
- ☐ **Flashcards** – Create physical or digital "index" cards for key terms, formulas, or concepts (Anki, Brainscape, Cram, Quizlet, or StudyBlue).
- ☐ **Goal Setting** – Set "SMART" (Specific, Measurable, Achievable, Relevant, and Time-bound) study goals.
- ☐ **Group Study** – Study with peers to explain concepts and test each other.
- ☐ **Inquisitive Interrogation** – Ask "why?" to deepen understanding of facts.
- ☐ **Limit Multitasking** – Focus on one task at a time for better concentration.
- ☐ **Mind Mapping** – Create visual maps of key ideas and their connections.
- ☐ **Mnemonics & Acronyms** – Use memory aids to remember lists or concepts (e.g., PEMDAS).
- ☐ **Note-Taking Systems** – Use methods like the Charting Method, Cornell Notes, Mapping Method, Outline Format, or Sentence Method to stay organized.
- ☐ **Pomodoro Technique** – Study for 25 minutes, then take a 5-minute break; repeat.
- ☐ **Positive Reinforcement** – Reward yourself after meeting study goals.
- ☐ **Practice Problems** – Solve math/science problems or case studies to apply knowledge.
- ☐ **Prioritization (Eisenhower Matrix)** – Focus on urgent and important tasks first.
- ☐ **Self-Quizzing** – Generate your own test questions and answer them regularly.
- ☐ **Spaced Repetition** – Review content at increasing intervals to cement long-term memory.
- ☐ **SQ3R Method** – Survey, Question, Read, Recite, Review (for reading comprehension).
- ☐ **Summarization** – Write concise summaries of what you learned.
- ☐ **Teach Others** – Reinforce your learning by teaching it to someone else.
- ☐ **Time Blocking** – Schedule specific time slots for subjects or tasks.

This is a good start. Some will work for you! I highly recommend getting ahead during breaks. Not to ruin your summer, but your break times are excellent times to prepare. The summer before I started Organic Chemistry, I made posters, models, and nomenclature notecards. When school started, I stuck models of the major molecules to my ceiling, put posters of the reactions and concepts to be memorized on my wall, and flipped through my flashcards. Just a thought. That worked for me. What works for you may be different.

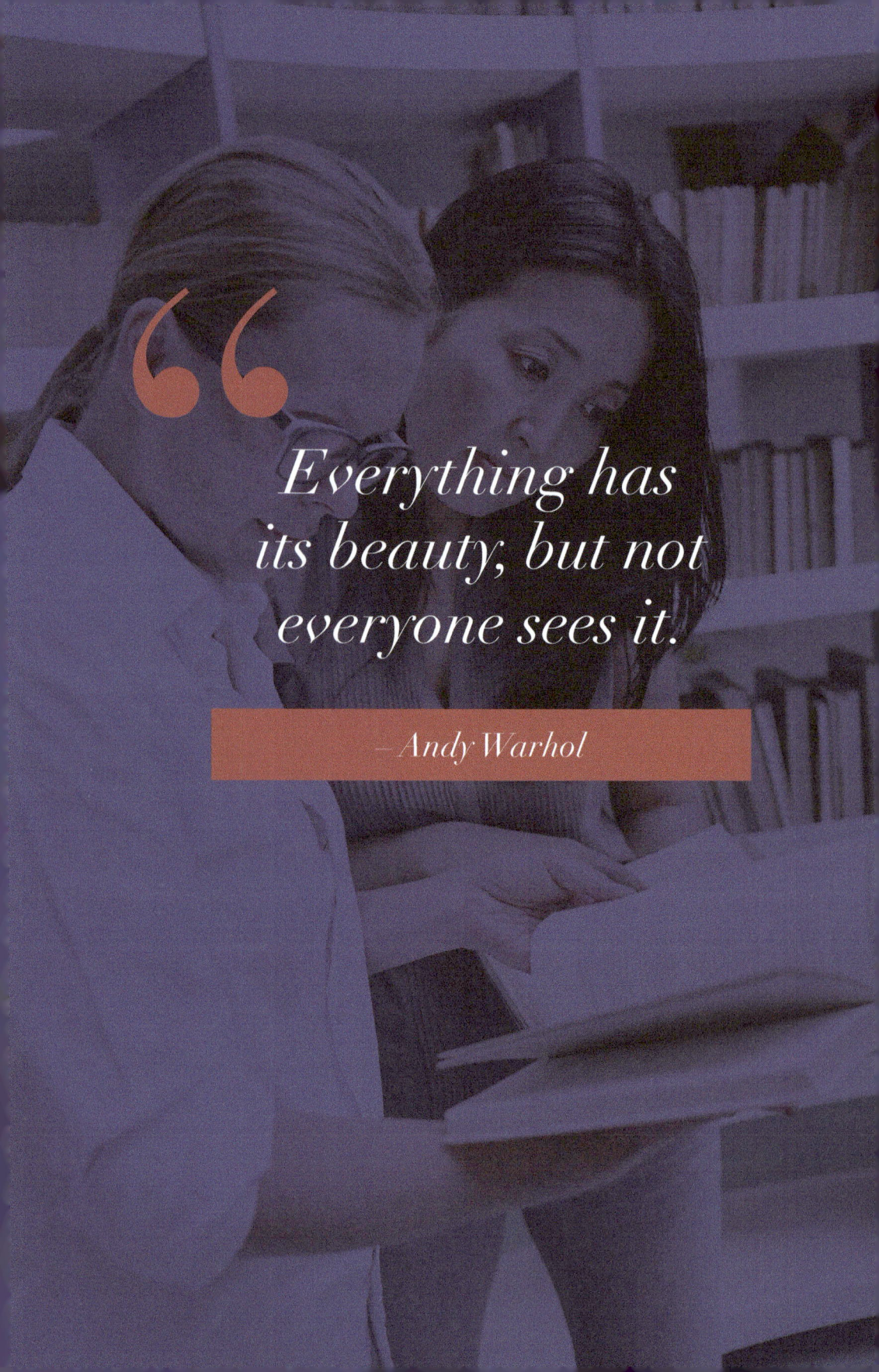

"

*Everything has its beauty, but not everyone sees it.*

– *Andy Warhol*

## CHAPTER FIFTEEN

# DESIRED QUALITIES

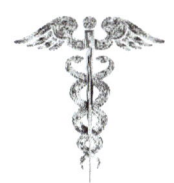

### BECOMING A PHYSICIAN:
### QUALITIES THAT SHAPE A FUTURE DOCTOR

I f you are dreaming of one day becoming a doctor or are working hard to be admitted to a competitive BS/MD or BS/DO program, this chapter is a reminder that you already hold the seeds of what it takes. Yes, academics are essential. Yes, test scores and coursework matter. Yet, at the heart of every excellent physician lies something deeper: character. Medical schools, and especially direct medical programs, are not looking for perfection, they are looking for promise. They want students who do not just study medicine, but who embody the humanistic values needed in medicine.

Medicine demands the mastery of science, yet what underlies diagnosis and treatment is a calling to serve. The intense study requires intellectual rigor and emotional intelligence, technical skill and empathetic compassion. The best physicians are problem-solvers and peacemakers, listeners and leaders. The journey begins early, both in the classroom and in how you live. It is how you treat others and the kind of responsibility you consistently embrace.

BS/MD programs are designed to identify students who show the maturity, dedication, and heart to become doctors. These programs are highly competitive, not just because they offer a streamlined path to medical school, but because they seek students who will uphold the integrity of medicine.

Admissions committees ask, "Can we trust this student to wear the white coat one day with humility and honor?"

These inward and outward qualities are epitomized by the student who helps their classmates understand biology, not for extra credit or payment, but out of a genuine desire to see others succeed. Or the athlete who rises before daybreak to train and studies late into the night, demonstrating discipline as a core part of their identity. Or the student who volunteers at the local hospital, remaining focused not on logging hours and checking their watch for the moment their time is fulfilled, but on completing every task with care and purpose. Or the teen who works to support their family, cares for a sick relative, or checks in on a friend who is in pain. These individuals know strength, resilience, and illness are not abstract concepts, but a lived, daily reality.

Unsurprisingly, these individuals are also those who step out of the box to help and sometimes fail, learning and growing stronger with each experience. Medicine requires resilience. Not everything goes as planned. The road to becoming a doctor will test your mind, your patience, and your spirit. But those who endure with grace, forgiveness, and wisdom make the most trusted, inspiring healers.

## CORE QUALITIES OF A FUTURE PHYSICIAN

Whether you are applying to a direct med program now or planning for medical school later, the following traits will help shape your path. They are not traits you are born with but rather habits, attitudes, and choices you develop every day.

**Adaptability** – Calmly navigating change, stress, and the unknown.

**Communication** – Listening actively and speaking clearly.

**Compassion** – Showing genuine care for the well-being of others.

**Creativity** – Thinking outside the box to solve problems.

**Critical Thinking** – Analyzing evidence and making thoughtful decisions.

**Cultural Sensitivity** – Respecting differences in background and beliefs.

**Curiosity** – A hunger to ask why, explore how, and go deeper.

**Emotional Maturity** – Staying composed and kind, even under stress.

**Empathy** – Putting yourself in others' shoes, especially patients'.

**Ethical Judgment** – Choosing integrity over convenience when no one is watching.

**Global Awareness** – Understanding health in a diverse, interconnected world.

**Gratitude** – Showing appreciation for the mentors, teachers, and patients who shaped you.

**Grit** – Doing hard things, again and again, because the goal matters.

**Humility** – Understanding your limits and always being open to learning.

**Initiative** – Taking action without being told, starting meaningful projects.

**Integrity** – Being honest, accountable, and trustworthy.

**Leadership** – Inspiring others through service, not status.

**Observation** – Noticing subtle details others might miss.

**Passion** – A deep, authentic drive to be part of something bigger than yourself.

**Reflection** – Looking back on the past in order to improve.

**Resilience** – Bouncing back from setbacks and using them to grow.

**Self-Discipline** – The ability to stay focused and committed over time.

**Service Orientation** – Wanting to help, not for praise, but for purpose.

**Teamwork** – Collaborating respectfully and effectively with others.

**Time Management** – Prioritizing and organizing, while managing demanding responsibilities.

## FINAL THOUGHTS

There is no one perfect path to medical school. But there are common threads among those who get there. They lead with heart and act with purpose. Whether you are conducting research, helping your siblings with homework, leading a club, or comforting a friend, every moment is a chance to grow into the person you are meant to become.

I am reminded about the child who asks, "Are we 'there' yet?" Mull that over a bit. Where is there? If you mean medical school, then residency will be next. When you get to residency, "there" will be your practice, your family, your home, your future. We are here, today, living life to the best of our ability. Our persistent efforts encompass the best we can do because there will always be another "there". Live vivaciously today and be the very best version of you.

Be proud of the steps you take. Stay curious. Keep serving. Be kind. And remember that the journey to becoming a doctor is not just about where you are headed, but about who you are becoming.

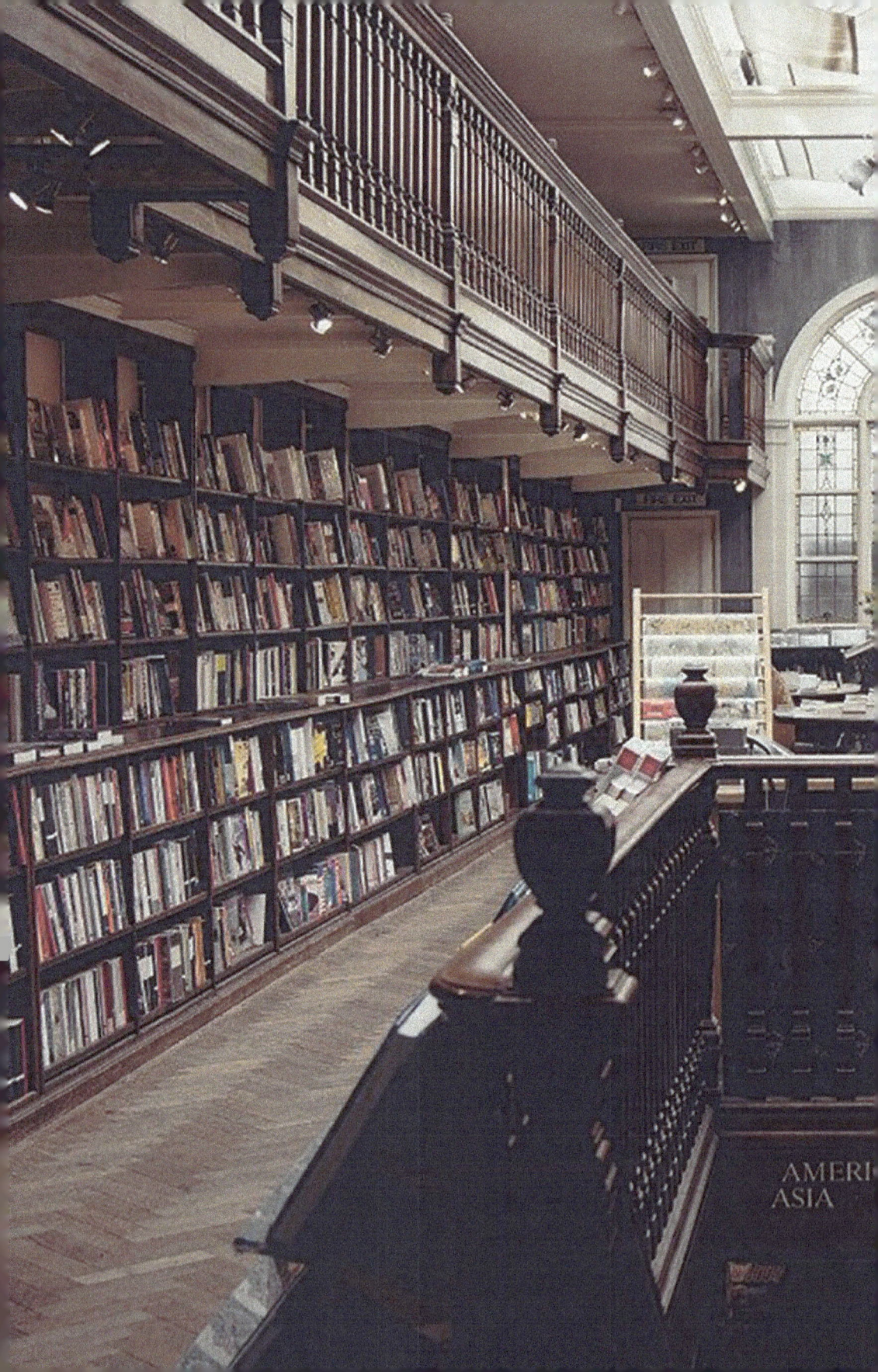

# PART THREE

# TIMELINES, CALENDARS, AND CHECKLISTS

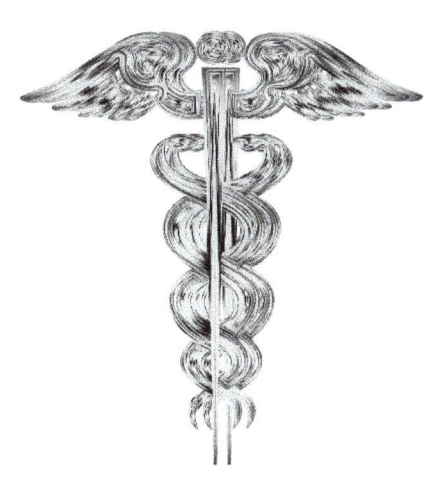

# "

The natural healing force within each of us is the greatest force in getting well.

– *Hippocrates*

# CHAPTER SIXTEEN

# PLANNING AHEAD 8TH – 10TH GRADE

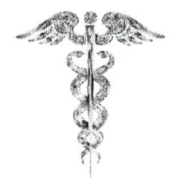

## BECOMING A DOCTOR STARTS NOW

If you dream of becoming a doctor, by reading this book you are already on the right path, even in middle or early high school. You do not have to wait for college to start thinking like a future physician. In fact, many students who pursue BS/MD, BS/DO, or BS/DDS programs or gain early admission to medical/dental school begin building the right habits and mindsets now. This chapter is for you and your family.

The pathway to medicine or dentistry is not just about test scores or science classes, you must also embody curiosity, compassion, and commitment. When you volunteer to help others, lead a school project, study late to understand how the heart works, or take time to listen to someone who is hurting, you are already becoming the kind of person medicine needs.

You may not wear a white coat yet, but you can already act with the heart of a healer. Each step, as you join a science club, visit a local hospital, read about diseases, or watch a medical documentary plants a seed. Then, as you nourish that seed with learning, discipline, and service, you grow into someone capable of changing lives.

Parents play a powerful role in this journey with encouragement, structure, and faith. Each action helps build confidence and drive. Ask questions. Explore opportunities. Reflect together. Becoming a doctor may be a goal, but it is also a process of growth, resilience, and purpose.

So, start now. Whether you are choosing classes or looking for volunteer roles, remember that every moment matters. With vision, preparation, and heart, you can turn today's decisions into tomorrow's dream career.

## BS/MD, BS/DO, BS/DDS, AND PRE-MED PREPARATION CHECKLIST

Here is a checklist to stay on track for your future.

- ☐ Maintain strong academic performance (especially in math and science).
- ☐ Enroll in honors, AP, or IB coursework when available.
- ☐ Develop strong study and time management habits.
- ☐ Participate in science fairs, math competitions, or STEM enrichment programs.
- ☐ Shadow a healthcare professional (doctor, nurse, PA, dentist, vet, ).
- ☐ Join school clubs such as Science Olympiad, HOSA, or Red Cross Club.
- ☐ Engage in meaningful community service or volunteer work.
- ☐ Start a project or service initiative in your community.
- ☐ Build leadership skills by taking on roles in clubs or team activities.
- ☐ Pursue summer programs focused on medicine or science (e.g., medical camps, pre-college STEM programs).
- ☐ Read books and watch documentaries related to health and medicine.
- ☐ Begin keeping a journal of volunteer, academic, and extracurricular experiences.
- ☐ Develop strong communication skills through writing or public speaking.
- ☐ Build relationships with teachers and mentors who may later write letters of recommendation.
- ☐ Stay informed about current events in healthcare and medical research.
- ☐ Learn about BS/MD, BS/DO, and BS/DDS programs and keep a running list of potential colleges.
- ☐ Attend college fairs, webinars, or campus visits with a medical/dental focus.
- ☐ Take care of your mental and physical health through balanced nutrition, rest, and exercise.
- ☐ Discuss goals regularly as a family and create action steps each semester.
- ☐ Explore anatomy, biology, or health sciences through online platforms like or MITx, Coursera, and Khan Academy.

The key at this point is to develop the key skills that will take you all the way to the finish line. This first means to learn ways to maintain balance and not feel overwhelmed. Gain a rhythm in your life where you enjoy what you do, pursue your interests, study because you love learning, and find fascination in the world around you.

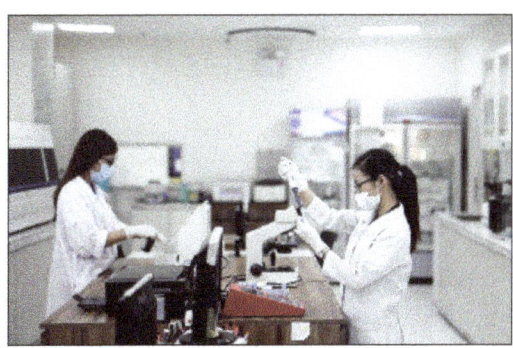

Challenging yourself academically should not be a chore or drudgery, but a way to explore your curiosities. Find ways to reduce the pressure you might feel to perform at the highest level and forgive yourself if you make a mistake. Everyone makes mistakes and we grow and learn from them. Wisdom is an outcome of life's lessons, both good and bad.

So here are some tips as you get started:

1. Balance your school, extracurricular, and personal life.

2. Form study groups with people who are academically motivated.

3. Set realistic goals. Hold yourself to the highest standards, but be kind to yourself in case you miss the mark at some point.

4. Break down larger tasks into smaller steps and cheer on your victories.

5. Take breaks. Stand up and stretch. Take a walk. Take a short nap. Meditate.

6. Figure out ways that work for you to recharge and gain a fresh perspective.

7. Ask for help if you are overwhelmed or confused. Ask a parent, friend, teacher, or counselor if you need help. You gain no points pulling your hair out if you are stuck academically or interpersonally. Someone will offer a pearl of advice.

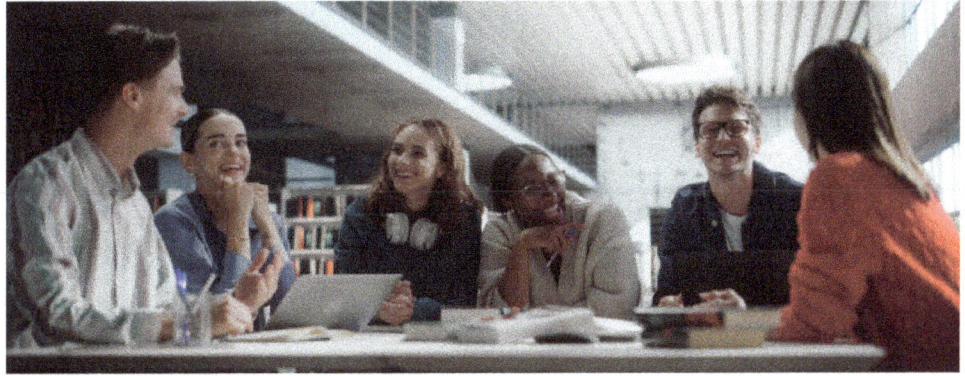

# "

*Wherever the art of medicine is loved, there is also a love of humanity.*

— *Hippocrates*

AMERICA · AFRICA
ASIA · AUSTRALASIA

CHAPTER SEVENTEEN

# JUNIOR YEAR RAMP UP

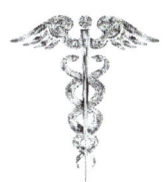

Eleventh grade is a critical year for students aspiring to become a doctor. This moment is when challenging courses meet demanding activities and passion meets focus. Your interest in science, healthcare, and service becomes a roadmap to your future. Whether your goal is a BS/MD, BS/DO, BS/DDS or traditional pre-med track, now is when your momentum builds. Colleges will look closely at your academic trajectory, leadership roles, service record, and ability to articulate why medicine/dentistry matters to you.

Sharpen your story. Do not just participate, lead. Do not just volunteer, reflect. Ask bigger questions the kind of physician/dentist you envision yourself to be, and then begin to build upon that vision through your choices, actions, and relationships. Research opportunities, summer programs, and internships will shape your understanding of healthcare's complexity and humanity. Your job now is to learn, lead, and listen.

Parental support continues to be vital. Parents can encourage curiosity, consistency, and compassion, helping to balance ambition with health and reflection. Although medical/dental school is still years away, the qualities that define a great physician/dentist are already forming.

Your counselor is also an important puzzle piece in your future since your counselor, whether they are supportive or not, will need to write one of your letters of recommendation. Get to know them. Ask their advice. They are a partner and guide in your journey.

# CHECKLIST FOR 11TH GRADE

- ☐ Take the PSAT seriously and use results to prep for SAT/ACT.

- ☐ Register and prep for SAT or ACT (consider taking both).

- ☐ Maintain high grades in AP/IB/honors science and math courses.

- ☐ Seek shadowing opportunities in clinics, hospitals, or private practices.

- ☐ Pursue a summer program in medicine, research, or STEM (e.g., NIH, RMP, HSHSP, RISE, RSI, SEEP, etc.; see the lists provided).

- ☐ Expand your leadership. Become a president, captain, or founder of a meaningful activity.

- ☐ Volunteer consistently in healthcare or community service environments.

- ☐ Participate in science fairs, Olympiads, or research-based projects.

- ☐ Build relationships with teachers for future letters of recommendation.

- ☐ Update your résumé and log experiences (shadowing, service, jobs, awards).

- ☐ Explore colleges with BS/MD, BS/DO, and BS/DDS programs. Review their admission criteria.

- ☐ Write reflections of your experiences. What did you learn? What moved you? Penning your thoughts in the moment may be valuable later.

- ☐ Start outlining a personal statement or story of why medicine or dentistry.

- ☐ Ask a trusted mentor to help you shape your academic and service narrative.

- ☐ Attend local health lectures, medical webinars, or pre-med info nights.

- ☐ Take dual enrollment courses at a college if possible.

- ☐ Read medical memoirs or follow physician-scientists online.

- ☐ Discuss goals with your family and set clear priorities for summer.

- ☐ Practice time management and balance academics with sleep and mental health.

- ☐ Continue to be curious, courageous, and compassionate.

Unfortunately, at this point, you have probably met people who cheat in a multitude of ways. You have undoubtedly witnessed academic, athletic, leadership, or personal events that seemed profoundly unfair. You may have even poured a great deal of energy and frustration into cruelty, bullying, adversity, inequity, prejudice, injustice, drugs, alcohol, and possibly even disease, injury, or death.

Whether or not you believe in a higher power, the Serenity Prayer is helpful for reflection.

*God, grant me the serenity to accept the things I cannot change, the courage to change the things I can, and the wisdom to know the difference.*

Remember, you cannot change others. You can only change yourself.

Here is one more quote to help you through the inconsistencies, inequities, and tragedies you might face in life. This one, by Charles Swindoll, is on attitude, emphasizing the profound impact our mindset has on life's outcomes.

*The longer I live, the more I realize the impact of attitude on life.*
*Attitude, to me, is more important than facts.*
*It is more important than the past, than education, than money, than circumstances, than failures, than successes, than what other people think or say or do.*
*It is more important than appearance, giftedness, or skill.*
*It will make or break a company...a church...a home.*
*The remarkable thing is we have a choice every day regarding the attitude we will embrace for that day.*
*We cannot change our past.*
*We cannot change the fact that people will act in a certain way.*
*We cannot change the inevitable.*
*The only thing we can do is play on the one string we have, and that is our attitude.*
*I am convinced that life is 10% what happens to me and 90% how I react to it. And so it is with you. You are in charge of your attitude.*

This is your junior year, a year of remarkable growth and tons of questions as people ask you what you plan to do with the rest of your life. You may feel the pressure to decide and the uncertainty of whether you can keep up the pace, often with no sleep and tons of questions about right and wrong, good and evil, virtue and immorality surrounding you. Seek wisdom from morally-wise mentors. They will guide you through the thicket of uncertainty until you gain your bearings.

" "

*Don't be afraid...*
*Science is light...*
*and it is through*
*science that we*
*will find a way*
*out of this.*

*– Luiz Henrique Mandetta*
*Brazil's former Health Minister*

## CHAPTER EIGHTEEN
# SENIOR YEAR SERIOUSNESS

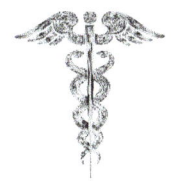

### YEAR FOR APPLICATIONS & DECISIONS

Twelfth grade is the year when everything you have prepared for comes into focus. The application season is here. Your story, character, and choices are ready to speak for you. Whether you are applying to BS/MD, BS/DO, BS/DDS, or traditional pre-med college programs, this is the time to showcase, your knowledge, passions,and what you have become.

You are more than a transcript. You are a leader, a volunteer, a thinker, and a future physician. Own your journey. Be proud of the moments you grew through service, struggled with integrity, or found strength in supporting others. Colleges and medical/dental programs want students with heart and substance, people who are ready to succeed and ready to care.

Your parents' presence, patience, and perspectives are invaluable. This year is filled with conversations, questions, deadlines, essays, decisions, and emotions. Trust that the foundation you have helped build will carry into this next chapter of your life's book of wisdom. Together, continue nurturing the qualities that medicine will one day require: resilience, reflection, and hope.

This is the breakthrough year where you are challenged throughout the fall as you apply to schools and balance academics. Then, in the spring, you must decide the college you will attend. The safety of somewhere close to home meets the adventure of moving away to a place where you may not know anyone and desire to start anew. It is a time when your self-driven motivation kicks into gear.

## CHECKLIST FOR MED-SCHOOL BOUND 12TH GRADERS

- ☐ Finalize college list (BS/MD, BS/DO, BS/DDS and traditional pre-med programs).
- ☐ Make a Google Doc for essays and Google Sheet for your college list.
- ☐ Determine the deadlines for EA, ED, REA, or RD applications and decide how you will submit each of your applications.
- ☐ Check to see if the direct med program requires an honors program application.
- ☐ Request letters of recommendation from science and humanities teachers.
- ☐ Complete Common App and school-specific applications early.
- ☐ Locate and fill out the separate applications for BS/MD, BS/DO, and BS/DDS programs along with their essays and additional requirements.
- ☐ Write/revise personal statement and BS/MD, BS/DO, and BS/DDS essays.
- ☐ Submit SAT/ACT scores (or confirm test-optional policies).
- ☐ Ensure transcripts and school reports are submitted by counselors.
- ☐ If you have taken college courses outside of school, send those transcripts from the school's registrar's office.
- ☐ Prepare for BS/MD, BS/DO, and/or BS/DDS interviews.
- ☐ Research MMI (multiple mini interviews) and ethical scenarios.
- ☐ Continue volunteering, shadowing, or clinical work throughout your senior year.
- ☐ Keep your grades strong. Colleges see your first semester grades.
- ☐ Participate in relevant extracurriculars and stay committed to your roles.
- ☐ Log hours and details of shadowing, research, and service experiences.
- ☐ Update your résumé with senior year accomplishments.
- ☐ Look into gap year or summer pre-med programs to gain additional experience or if you are unsure of your next steps.
- ☐ Be proactive about financial aid. Submit FAFSA, CSS Profile, and scholarship applications early.
- ☐ Practice mock interviews with a mentor, counselor, or parent.
- ☐ Ask a healthcare professional for a reference if applicable.
- ☐ Keep exploring healthcare, medicine, biotechnology, and other scientific topics in journals, books, podcasts, or documentaries.
- ☐ Stay connected to mentors and thank those who help your along your journey. A thank you note showing gratitude goes a long way.
- ☐ Celebrate your growth and find peace in doing your best.
- ☐ Believe that your kindness, grit, and purpose will guide you forward.

## INTEGRITY: THE FOUNDATION OF TRUST

Amid the decisions about your future and reality that you may leave the nest on your own, you need to believe that you have learned enough lessons to fly. Your parents also face challenges as they ask themselves, "Did I teach my children enough so they can rise with humility and face challenges with grace?"

The most important part of this juncture is your attitude and behaviors as you face each new and unexpected life event. You will ask yourself questions every day throughout college as you make decisions. If you are focused on your future and not the novelties and pleasures of the present, you will keep heading in the right direction, even when those around you take part in activities you know are wrong.

Use your senior year to cultivate integrity. This means doing the right thing, even when no one is watching. Be honest in your applications, authentic in your essays, and respectful to peers, teachers, and mentors. In medicine, trust is sacred. The character you build now will follow you in every patient interaction and every clinical decision you make in the future.

As you begin your journey toward a BS/MD, BS/DO, BS/DDS, or along the pre-med/pre-dent path, remember, the road is long, but it is navigable. If other people can do it, why can't you? Construct timelines to give yourself structure. Use calendars to manage your time. Lean on checklists to take action. And, finally, let focus, organization, responsibility, vision, positivity, and integrity be your constant guides.

Medicine is more than a career, it is a calling. Your journey starts now, one step at a time.

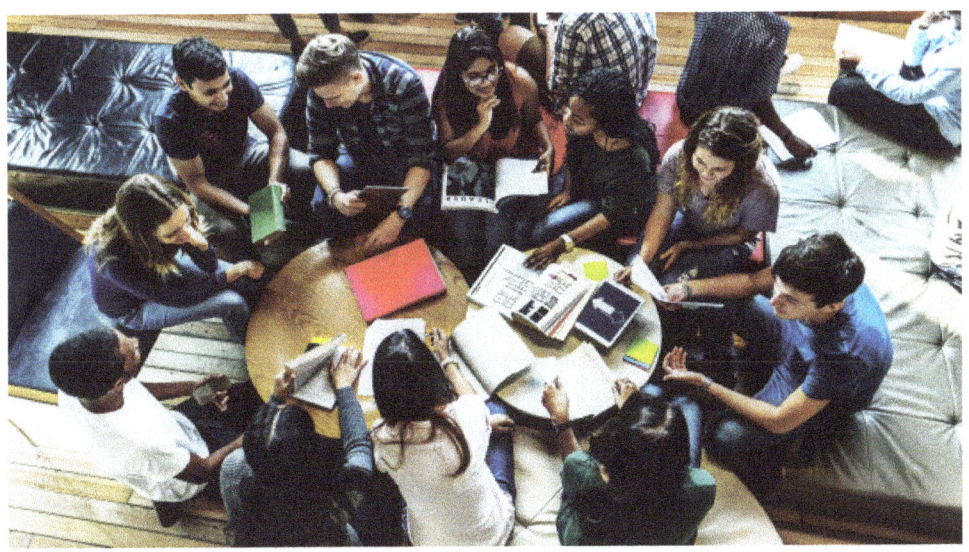

"

*Have the courage to follow your heart and intuition. They somehow know what you truly want to become.*

– Steve Jobs

# CHAPTER NINETEEN
# COLLEGE PREP CALENDAR

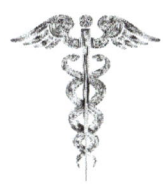

Probably the most important factors you can control in the admissions process are your personal statements, additional supplement essays, and optional questions. When an essay is compelling, reviewers can give the applicant a second look, even when they may have been put on the "probably not" pile. Passion, empathy, humility, and resilience resonates with admissions officers.

First rule of thumb is to be authentic. Tell your story. Since everyone's story is different, look back at pivotal moments in your life. Tell those short stories that impacted your decision to pursue medicine. Capture the reader's attention with the clarity and detail that elucidate the events in your life and reveal the humanity and compassion you have for others. Who inspired you along the way? When were you touched by the healing power of medicine?

Be respectful, vulnerable, and thoughtful. What experiences show your best qualities, core values, and character? Connect anecdotes seamlessly so the flow is easy for readers to follow. Do not be afraid to share a moment where you questioned your decisions, wondered if you were headed along the right path, or worried about how you might approach a patient with news about cancer or the possibility of death. Humility is endearing.

The most off-putting essays to read are the ones that are blatantly boastful. Most students do not write this way intentionally and fail to realize how arrogant they sound. Initially, they seek to describe the pride they have their successes and tell those in admissions they are a winner. However, what comes across is not the leadership, growth, and self-awareness they intended.

Difficult decisions, tough choices, challenges, and hopelessness are part of life and demonstrate your cognizance that medicine does not always have a positive outcome. Moreover, you may not always turn out to be the story's hero. What sacrifices did you make? What did you prioritize? What is important to you? Reveal your true self, the humility of the experience, and your commitment to medicine.

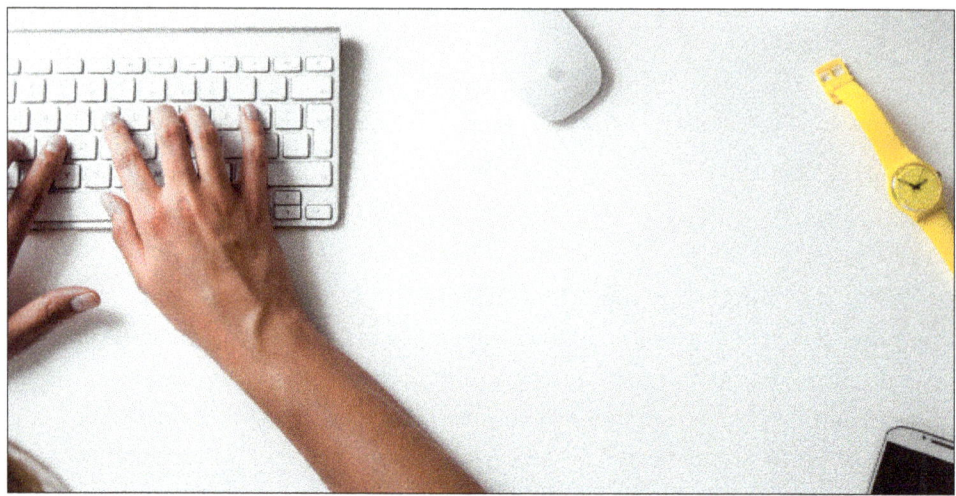

Those tidbits of advice may seem wise and encouraging. However, when you are ready to incorporate them into your essay, sit back and ask, "How can I turn the story of my life into a compelling, interesting, and clarifying personal statement?" How will your story be seen as one that is as thoughtful and moving as someone else's story?

Here is my advice. Write down five pivotal or transformational moments in your life. What did you learn from each? Write down the five experiences that impacted your pursuit of medicine. These could be personal experiences or those with family members or through your volunteer service. Again, what stuck out as being meaningful to you? Finally, since this is a personal statement, name five attributes you believe define you. Why are these important to you and your pursuit of medicine? This exercise will help you hone your story into episodes so you can select from those that resonate the most with you and show the fullness of your character.

Rarely will you submit only one essay. Typically your Common App or Coalition App personal statement will not be about medicine, but about a life experience that shows resilience, an epiphany, or heartfelt moment. However, you will also have supplement essays, like your "Why Medicine" essay (or two or three), diversity essay, and/or why do you want to attend that school. Some programs will ask short answer questions from 50 to 350 words. Do not tell the same stories in each essay.

Consider ways to describe yourself by separating and elaborating upon the experiences on your life's canvas. Your personal statement might describe your identity, heritage, challenges, or lessons from your upbringing. Your 'Why Medicine" essay might present swatches of science, research, experimentation, nursing home volunteerism, and shadowing. Most importantly, help the committee understand your personality, how you came to want to be a physician, and a glimpse how this knowledge will translate into your future in medicine.

You can do this. You just have to take some time and think through the five moments, five medical experiences, and five attributes. If you are worried about how your writing will sound, record your voice telling short versions of your stories and then transcribe them. Humans are natural storytellers. That is how we record, recall, and relay events.

Some students come to me and say they cannot make their essay profound. They express grave concern that their life is "vanilla," they do not have a tear-jerking event, or their stories are not tragic. Nevertheless, they are able to tell their friends or family members incidents they find intriguing or experiences they felt were profound. Try telling your story to someone else. People are often better at telling their stories verbally because they do not worry so much about the grammar. Write these down. You can edit your "personal statement" later.

When you write your personal statement, bring the reader into your world. Describe how your life purpose came to be and how you evolved in the person you are today. Reveal qualities in your character that show up in your life. Cherry-pick life events that show the reader who you are and what you are committed to becoming. Each event in your life story is a critical piece that fits together like a jigsaw puzzle. There is a reason you made certain decisions. You are here today applying to BS/MD, BS/DO, or BS/DDS programs because you are committed to pursuing medicine. Nobody has your story. Show the committee who you are.

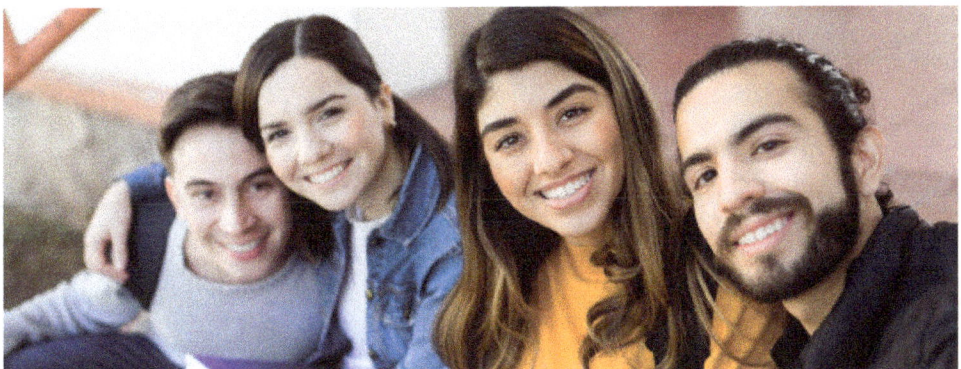

> " Nothing we do is more important than hiring and developing people. At the end of the day, you bet on people, not on strategies.

Former COO of General Electric

CHAPTER TWENTY

# COLLEGE ADMISSION CHECKLIST

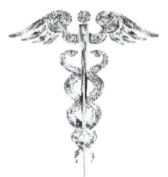

## THE IMPORTANCE OF A COLLEGE PLANNING CHECKLIST

### *Planning, Organization, Evaluation*

Your college planning checklist is an essential tool to navigate the complex path toward higher education, especially at highly competitive colleges and programs. With opportunities, deadlines, and decisions along the way, a structured checklist with choices at each intersection ensures that nothing critical is overlooked and provides peace of mind during an often stressful process.

From middle school through high school, you will encounter a series of academic, extracurricular, and personal milestones that shape your college readiness. A checklist will help you break the process into manageable steps, while staying on track year by year. Whether you are selecting rigorous courses, preparing for standardized tests, exploring careers, or visiting campuses, having a written plan turns intention into action.

Additionally, a checklist promotes early and consistent engagement. For example, middle school students can begin developing study habits and exploring interests, while high school freshmen can start building resumes and identifying passions. By junior and senior year, when the workload intensifies and application deadlines come into focus, students who have followed a checklist are much better prepared and more confident in the strides they took toward their goals.

A checklist also encourages parental involvement and advisor support, making it easier for families to communicate with school counselors, track financial aid, and register for key milestones like the PSAT, SAT, ACT, or FAFSA.

Ultimately, a college planning checklist offers organization and empowerment, transforming a daunting journey into a clear roadmap while helping you stay proactive, intentional, and goal-driven throughout your education.

## COLLEGE PLANNING CHECKLIST BY GRADE LEVEL

### Middle School

- ☐ Develop study habits and time management.
- ☐ Read to build vocabulary and comprehension.
- ☐ Explore interests through clubs and activities.
- ☐ Research careers.
- ☐ Talk to your school counselor about long-term goals.
- ☐ Build positive relationships with teachers.
- ☐ Use a planner to track homework and activities.
- ☐ Participate in community service.
- ☐ Attend a summer camp to build interpersonal skills; explore interests.
- ☐ Practice budgeting/saving to learn the value of money.
- ☐ Visit a local college campus to get inspired.

### 9th Grade

- ☐ Meet with your school counselor to map a 4-year plan.
- ☐ Take challenging courses (honors, AP, IB if possible).
- ☐ Join clubs, sports, or arts programs.
- ☐ Start a resume or activity tracker (with hours spent).
- ☐ Explore college websites.
- ☐ Attend local college and career fairs.
- ☐ Read books outside of class.
- ☐ Volunteer or get involved in the community.
- ☐ Build dependability with attendance and grades.
- ☐ Take a career interest survey.
- ☐ Research summer programs that challenge you to learn something new.
- ☐ For the go-getter, take a community college class.

### 10th Grade

- ☐ Continue Honors, AP, IB, & accelerated coursework.
- ☐ Take the PSAT for practice.
- ☐ Ask teachers and mentors for feedback on strengths.
- ☐ Consider STEM, art, or writing contests or competitions.
- ☐ Shadow a professional in a career interest.
- ☐ Apply for and attend a summer program and/or take a community college class.
- ☐ Actively participate in clubs, sports, and activities.

- ☐ Find ways to serve your community.
- ☐ Update your resume with new achievements.
- ☐ Start thinking about possible majors.
- ☐ Create a list of 10–15 potential colleges.
- ☐ Begin learning about financial aid and scholarships.

## 11th Grade

- ☐ Take the PSAT/NMSQT (qualifying for National Merit).
- ☐ Register and prepare for the SAT, ACT, TOEFL.
- ☐ Visit college campuses (virtual or in person).
- ☐ Talk to current college students or alumni.
- ☐ Attend college planning nights at school.
- ☐ Begin drafting a personal statement or essay ideas.
- ☐ Ask teachers for letters of recommendation early.
- ☐ Determine if your teacher and/or counselor has a special form to obtain a recommendation and fill out that form.
- ☐ Narrow your college list based on preferences.
- ☐ Research admission requirements and deadlines.
- ☐ Consider research labs, writing, creative supplements.
- ☐ Look for opportunities to mentor or lead.
- ☐ Create an activity list w/descriptions, dates, responsibilities, & leadership.
- ☐ Revise your resume for summer opportunities.
- ☐ Apply for summer programs, take a college class, language immersion, study abroad, medical mission trip.
- ☐ Conduct an eco project, publish a poem/short story.
- ☐ Investigate financial aid: FAFSA, CSS Profile, & scholarships.
- ☐ Create Common App account and begin filling it out.

## 12th Grade

- ☐ Finalize your college list (reach, match, safety).
- ☐ Create a Google Doc or Sheet of your college list.
- ☐ Consider ED, EA, REA, RD and make a timeline.
- ☐ Plan for science, art, music, theatre, film portfolio (if possible).
- ☐ Outline personal statements and supplement essays.
- ☐ Start a UC, CSU, ApplyTexas, MIT, Coalition, and/or Common App as necessary.
- ☐ Fill in your college applications.
- ☐ Proofread and submit essays.
- ☐ Interview, attach video introduction, resume, & website.
- ☐ Send official transcripts and test scores (if required).
- ☐ Apply for scholarships (local and national).
- ☐ Complete the FAFSA and other financial aid forms.
- ☐ Monitor application portals for updates.
- ☐ Keep up your grades; tackle something new.
- ☐ Visit colleges to which you were admitted; attend open houses.
- ☐ Compare financial aid packages.
- ☐ Make your final college decision and submit your deposit.
- ☐ Consider housing, roommates, and your academic plan.

> ## "
> *We all have dreams. But in order to make dreams come into reality, it takes an awful lot of determination, self-discipline, and effort.*

– *Jesse Owens*

## CHAPTER TWENTY-ONE

# WORDS OF ADVICE

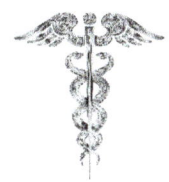

### ADVICE FOR YOUR PRE-MED JOURNEY

The path to medical school begins long before college. For students aiming for BS/MD, BS/DO, BS/DDS, or pre-med tracks, the journey demands stellar grades, test scores, and thoughtful planning. Discipline and an unwavering sense of purpose lie at the heart of this journey.

Be the master of your timeline, calendar, and checklists. These essential tools will transform ambition into action. But beyond organization, you must embrace values like focus, responsibility, organization, vision, integrity, and a positive attitude. Together, these form the compass that guides you toward becoming a physician.

### TIMELINES, CALENDARS, AND CHECKLISTS MATTER

Medical/dental school admissions are among the most competitive in the world. These programs raise the bar even higher by compressing the timeline and expecting maturity beyond your years. To meet these challenges, you must treat high school not just as a phase of academic development, but as a launchpad. This is where timelines, calendars, and checklists matter most.

A timeline helps you visualize the bigger picture. Start by marking key milestones: when to take the PSAT, SAT/ACT, AP/IB exams, and when to apply for summer research or volunteer opportunities. Add college application deadlines, FAFSA submission dates, and scholarship cutoff dates. Work backward from key events to pace yourself and avoid last-minute scrambling.

A calendar breaks down your plan into months and weeks. Use digital tools like Google Sheets/Calendar or apps like Notion or Trello to set reminders for studying, submitting forms, meeting with counselors, or attending college fairs. Color coding helps you separate academic, extracurricular, and personal tasks, and builds habits of daily time management.

| App | Best For | Key Features |
|---|---|---|
| Google Calendar | Seamless scheduling, integration, & reminders | Syncs across devices, recurring events, color-coding, reminders |
| Microsoft To Do | Simple task management w/MS integration | Daily planners, reminders, subtasks, Microsoft 365 sync |
| Notion | All-in-one planning, notes, and databases | Customizable pages, databases, collaborative tools, habit trackers |
| Todoist | Task and deadline tracking w/reminders | Natural language input, recurring tasks, labels, productivity goals |
| Trello | Visual project and assignment tracking | Kanban boards, checklists, calendar view, project organization |

Finally, checklists turn goals into action. Want to shadow a doctor? Add the following steps: research physicians, draft an email, follow up, schedule a time. By checking off each task, you build momentum. Seeing tangible progress on the path to your dreams is truly satisfying.

## THE POWER OF FOCUS

Pre-med students often juggle a heavy course load, test prep, extracurriculars, and leadership roles. Amid this whirlwind, focus becomes your superpower. Choose deep engagement over constant multitasking. Turn off distractions during study time and give your full attention to your tasks. "Be Here Now," wherever here is, instead of checking in elsewhere and thinking about other responsibilities.

Focus also means clarity of purpose. Remind yourself regularly why you want to pursue medicine. Whether you are driven by the memory of a loved one's illness, a fascination with biology, or the desire to improve access to healthcare, anchoring yourself in your "why" will give you the stamina to persist when the journey gets hard.

## ORGANIZATION BUILDS CONFIDENCE

To become a successful pre-med applicant, you must practice organization. Just as muscles need training, life management is a developed skill. Keep track of your classes, grades, test scores, volunteer hours, awards, and recommendations, so you do not scramble when application season arrives. More importantly, organization builds confidence. When you know what you have accomplished, you are better prepared to advocate for yourself, write compelling essays, and face interviews with poise.

## TAKE RESPONSIBILITY

Responsibility is not just about completing your homework or arriving on time. It is about owning your journey. In high school, this means seeking out opportunities, following through on commitments, and showing up even when it is inconvenient. Pre-med students need to cultivate an internal drive, because no one else is going to carry your dream for you. Your family will not set alarms or reminders when you move into your dorm. The more responsibility you take, the more trustworthy you become not just to teachers and mentors, but to yourself.

## VISION FUELS THE LONG GAME

Committing to BS/MD, BS/DO, BS/DDS or pre-med/pre-dent is not a sprint; heading to and through medical/dental school is a marathon. You must be able to visualize not just where you want to be next year, but five, ten, even fifteen years from now. Vision provides a forward-thinking mindset that helps you prioritize long-term rewards over short-term convenience. That may mean choosing summer research or clinical internship over a trip with friends. It may mean sacrificing sleep for a hospital shift or a last-minute test review. When you have vision, sacrifices feel purposeful, not burdensome.

## EXUDE A POSITIVE ATTITUDE

No path to medical/dental school is free from setbacks. You might get rejected from a summer program, underperform on an exam, or feel overwhelmed by pressure. This is where your positive attitude becomes essential. Positivity does not mean pretending everything is fine. It means believing that tough moments are opportunities for growth. Resilience is a key, allowing you to bounce back, reframe failure, and keep moving forward with humility and hope. Doctors face setbacks all the time. Learning to keep a steady, optimistic mindset starts now.

Finally, you will hit speed bumps. You may get bruised. Your wounds will heal. Pick yourself up and renew your spirit. Life is long and you will survive whatever challenges you face.

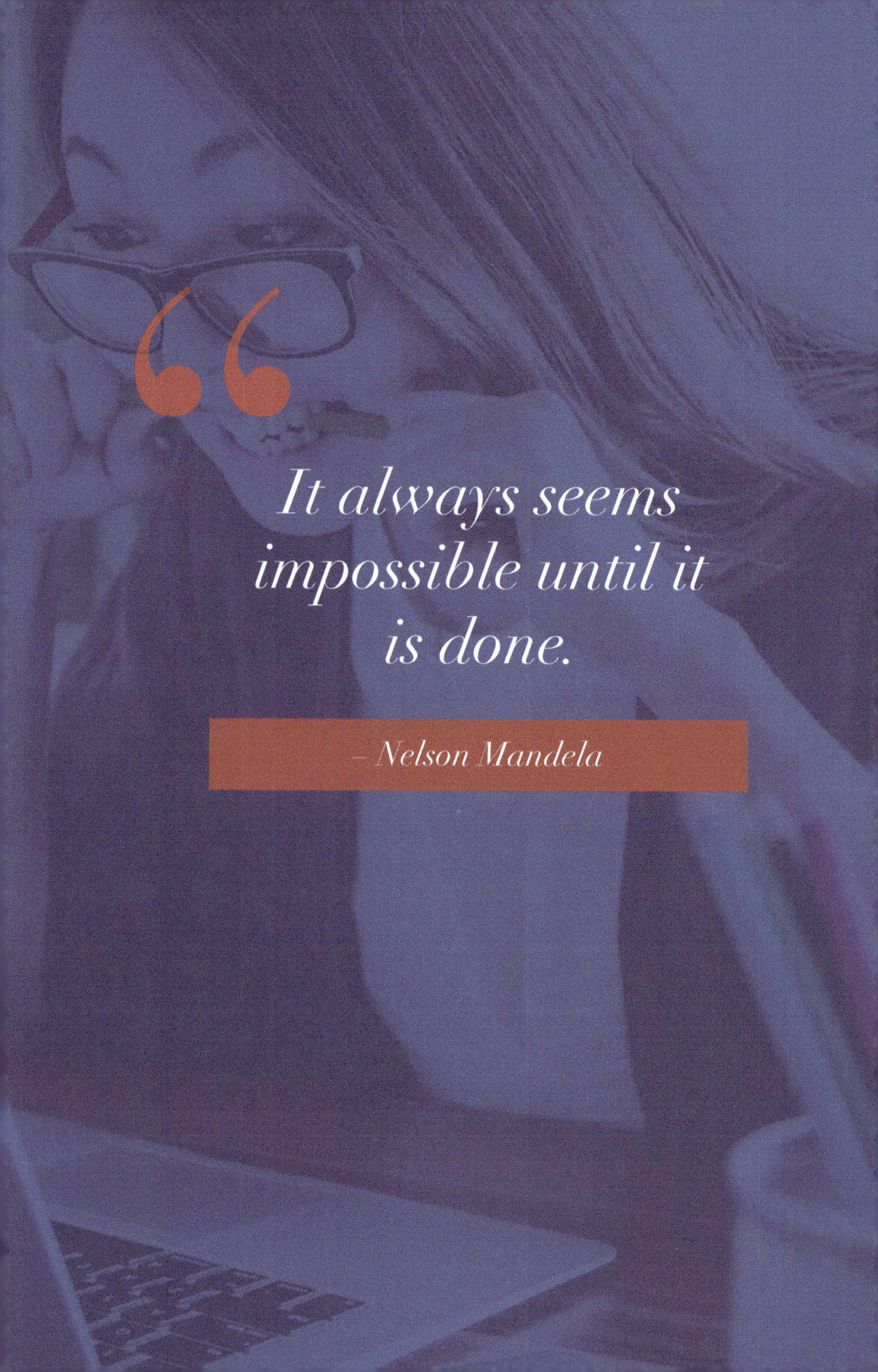

"

*It always seems impossible until it is done.*

*– Nelson Mandela*

CHAPTER TWENTY-TWO

# NOTE TO PARENTS

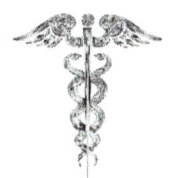

## PARENT'S ROLE IN NAVIGATING THE PRE-MED PATH

Watching a teenager choose the path toward medicine, especially competitive BS/MD, BS/DO, or BS/DDS programs, evokes a mix of pride, excitement, and concern. The road is a ambitious, marked by rigorous academics, high-pressure testing, and long-term commitment. As your teenager prepares for this journey, your role is to lead and guide, not for them but beside them. By helping them establish clear timelines, calendars, and checklists, and by modeling and encouraging values like vision, focus, responsibility, organization, integrity, and a positive attitude, you can help lay the foundation for success both in college admissions and in life.

## SUPPORTING STRUCTURE

College admission, particularly for BS/MD or pre-med hopefuls, is not a one-year sprint; it is a six to ten year orchestration of academic performance, extracurricular engagement, test prep, and self-discovery. Moments may feel overwhelming for you and for them with the sheer number of moving parts.

Encourage your child to track their own timelines as you cheer on their major milestones. Offer an outline to help them create their own roadmap. In college, they will need to do this alone and you will not be there. Remember the wisdom: "Give someone a fish and they will eat for today; teach them to fish and they will eat for a lifetime." This adage holds true for time management and pre-med tracking too. The sophomore PSAT determines where they stand and their weaknesses in timed testing. The junior-year PSAT, which is also the National Merit Scholar Qualifying Exam, is a bellwether sign. Make sure they prepare for and take the SAT/ACT by the end of their junior year.

Summer research or healthcare internships are valuable, though they require applications, and attention to deadlines. Summer is good for getting ahead in math and science. Also consider community service, medical experiences, and leadership opportunities. After junior year AP testing, begin preparing applications, resumes, and essays. The application process for BS/MD, BS/DO, and BS/DDS programs is extensive. Many programs require numerous essays. Some have multi-step application processes. Visual timelines help students see the big picture and relieve the stress of last-minute requirements or unexpected challenges.

Next, guide them in using calendars. These tools shift students from reactive to proactive. Whether it is a physical planner or digital app, calendars keep track of deadlines, study plans, shadowing hours, and interview dates. Review the calendar together weekly, not to micromanage, but to offer accountability and support.

Finally, checklists help transform goals into tasks. If your teenager is applying for a summer STEM program, support them in outlining steps: researching programs, gathering recommendation letters, writing essays, and submitting forms. Small wins will keep them motivated and ensure nothing falls through the cracks.

## CULTIVATING FOCUS IN A DISTRACTED WORLD

High school today is saturated with social media distractions, academic pressure, extracurricular overload, and uncertainty about the future. One of the most powerful gifts a parent can offer is helping their child develop focus. This does not mean demanding perfection or eliminating every outside interest. It means guiding your teenager to make intentional choices about how they spend their time and energy.

Help them recognize what matters most at each stage. For a future physician, this might mean prioritizing chemistry homework over binge-watching a television show, even one on medicine, or choosing a research internship over video game challenges. These decisions build long-term focus and self-discipline, essential habits for success in medicine.

## MODELING AND ENCOURAGING ORGANIZATION

Organization should be modeled. Create an environment at home that supports organized living. For example, you might set aside quiet study spaces, visible family calendars, and routines that reinforce time management.

Ask questions that encourage strategic thinking and be supportive: "What proactive step can you accomplish this weekend?" and "What can I do to help?" These questions help shift the mindset from procrastination and last-minute completion to thoughtful preparation. "Never put off to tomorrow what you can do today!"

## TEACHING RESPONSIBILITY, NOT CONTROL

One challenge for parents is balancing support with independence. The college admissions process is your teenager's journey, not yours. However, that does not mean you should take a passive role. Encourage task ownership like requesting transcripts, scheduling interviews, or researching schools. Resist the urge to do everything for them. If you do, you are likely to get a call during their freshman year that they forgot a project, did poorly on a test, or did not complete an assignment.

Instead, position yourself as a mentor and sounding board. If your teenager forgets a deadline or struggles with a grade, help them reflect on what went wrong and how to improve. Instill responsibility rather than blame. Learning from setbacks is just as important as succeeding and far more instructive in the long run.

## DEFINE A VISION

Teenagers often struggle to connect present effort with future goals. Help your child visualize their future as a doctor not just in terms of prestige or income, but as a life of service, resilience, and intellectual growth. Ask reflective questions like, "What kind of doctor do you want to be?" or "What do you hope your future patients say about you?" These conversations help them build a purpose-driven mindset, which fuels their motivation through difficult moments.

## FOSTER A POSITIVE, RESILIENT ATTITUDE

Students face rejection, burnout, and comparison. Parents play a crucial role in helping teenagers build resilience, reframing disappointments as growth. Celebrate effort, not just outcomes. Attitude influences how teenagers handle pressure for the rest of their academic journey. Most importantly, keep the tone at home hopeful and encouraging. A student who feels emotionally safe and supported is more likely to take academic risks and stay committed through the toughest challenges.

## BUILDING INTEGRITY FROM THE INSIDE OUT

Finally, integrity is the bedrock of any medical career. From high school essays to patient care, honesty, humility, and ethics must define each choice. Reinforce the idea that their worth is not tied to achievements or accolades, but to character. Discourage shortcuts, plagiarism, or resume padding. Frankly, when caught, these lead to serious downfalls. Instead, praise authenticity, kindness, and accountability.

In the admissions process, integrity shines through in an essay's tone, sincerity in an interview, or a follow-up email. Help teenagers realize that integrity mirrors their identity as they seek to become a competent, deeply compassionate doctor.

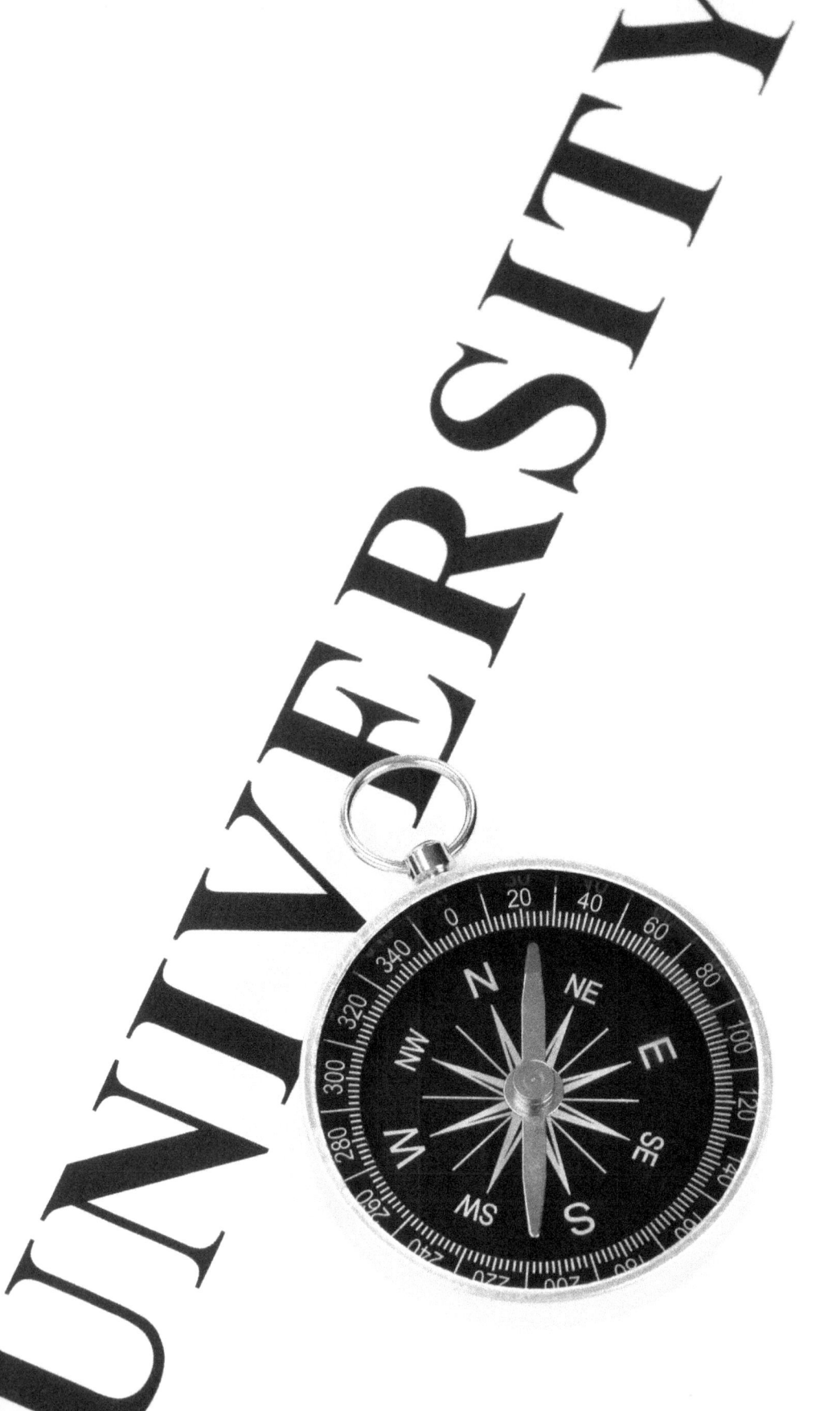

# PART 4

# WHICH PROGRAMS ARE BEST FOR YOU?

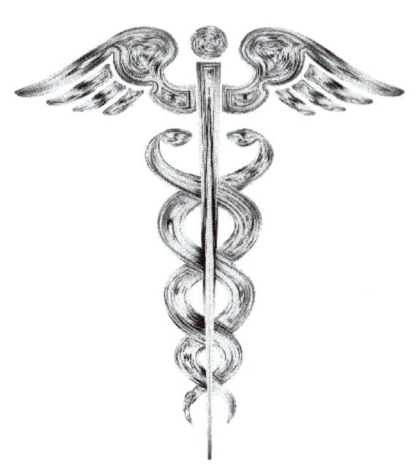

> **Between stimulus and response there is a space. In that space is our power to choose our response. In our response lies our growth and our freedom.**

—Viktor E. Frankl

## CHAPTER TWENTY-THREE

# RESEARCHING SCHOOLS

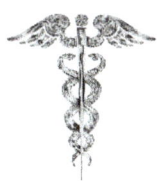

Researching BS/MD, BS/DO, and BS/DDS programs requires planning, attention to detail, and a deep understanding of your personal and academic goals. These programs are designed to fast-track highly motivated students into a medical career, so it is essential to be thorough and strategic in your approach. Below are practical tips to help you navigate this complex process.

Consider traditional 8-year program and accelerated options. Think about the school's location, size, affiliated medical/dental school, campus culture, and proximity to hospitals. Determine whether you will apply to the MD, DO, and/or DDS pathway. What are their philosophical and clinical differences?

Use official sources for current information. Search AAMC, AACOM, ADA or university websites for resources. Look for admissions requirements, GPA and test score ranges, program length, MCAT/DAT expectations, and any in-state residency preferences. Also research guaranteed vs. conditional medical school acceptance like secured entry and academic thresholds.

Stay organized. Include columns for program name, location, deadlines, GPA/test score requirements, MCAT policy, interview process, program length, and notes on unique features such as early clinical exposure, research, required summer programs, and residency matches. Compare programs side-by-side.

Look for insights beyond official materials. Use forums such as Student Doctor Network or College Confidential to read about student experiences, but be cautious and verify claims with official sources. Attend virtual information sessions and/or campus events. Reach out to program advisors, current students, or recent alumni with thoughtful questions. Visit the campus if possible to get a sense of the environment.

In your research, collect and organize information. If you use a Google Doc, make tabs: Notes, Deadlines, Major, Requirements, Personal Statement, Resume, Essays, Transcripts, Abstract/Art Supplement, Honors Program, Recommenders/Requests, Interview Questions, Financial Aid, Scholarships, Portal Logins, College Specific Info, Date Submitted/Portal Checks, Deferral/Waitlist Updates, and Additional Information. For the Google Sheet, you might make columns for the following. You choose what works for you!

| COLLEGE OR UNIVERSITY | Due Date | EA, RD, REA | Request Info Done | SAT Scores Sent? | Recs Assigned | Arts Supp? | Research Abstract or Supplement | HONORS PROGRAM | Interviews | Major | Scholarships | FAFSA, CSS PROFILE & SUBMIT DATES |
|---|---|---|---|---|---|---|---|---|---|---|---|---|
| | | | | | | | | | | | | |

Some people insist the best universities are those with large lecture halls. However, some students work better in small, project-based environments with hands-on activities and field trips to labs, research centers, and events.

Every student is different. You need to find a school that fits you. Large, fiercely competitive schools can be motivational or they can leave you with a pit in your stomach and a sense of failure. If graduate school is your goal, you may want to attend a university where you can get research opportunities, master your classes, and get involved. Thus, the best university is the one where you will thrive. Fortunately, there are many colleges and variables to consider.

Here is the big picture data for U.S. college student enrollment:

* 19.25 million college students
* 2,691 4-year colleges
* 1,496 2-year colleges
* 5.2 million attend private colleges
* 13.7 million attend public colleges

In another interesting statistic, undergraduate enrollment dropped more than 8% from fall 2019 to fall 2022, representing nearly 2,000,000 loss of students during the pandemic. However, in 2024, enrollment grew 1.2% with greatest increase in community colleges. Test-optional admissions opened the door to students without test scores or those who test poorly. Thus, more students applied to the top schools. Beware, though, some colleges are moving back to requiring tests.

*The secret of getting ahead is getting started.*
*The secret of getting started is breaking your complex, overwhelming tasks into small manageable tasks, and then starting on the first one.*

**– Mark Twain**

## CONSIDER MORE THAN JUST RANKINGS

Rankings can help you start your search. However, they miss important factors that determine whether the school is a good fit for your circumstances. Here are a few variables to consider:

| | |
|---|---|
| Ability to Enroll in Required | Internships |
| Classes Acceptance Rates | Intramural Sports |
| Access to Professors | Majors |
| Book Costs | Research Opportunities |
| Competitiveness | Safety |
| Diversity | Scholarship Money |
| Dorm Life | School Spirit |
| Financial Aid | Security |
| Graduate School Acceptance | Size of Lower Division Classes |
| Housing Availability | Social Life |
| Inclusiveness | Study Abroad |

Note: Colleges with 400 students in first and second year classes often say their "average class size" is somewhere around 25. Do not be deceived by statistics that deviate from reality. Also, almost every school offers study abroad, though in many cases the study abroad programs are under another school's or program's umbrella and rarely include students or professors from your university.

Ask students at a school you are interested in attending if they are able to register for the classes they need, get support for internships or summer programs, and have access to professors and not just graduate school assistants who, frankly, have a full load of their own classes.

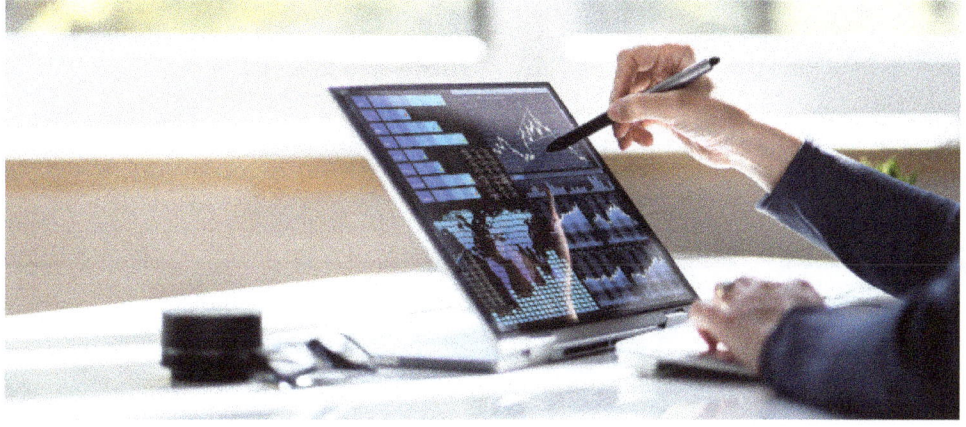

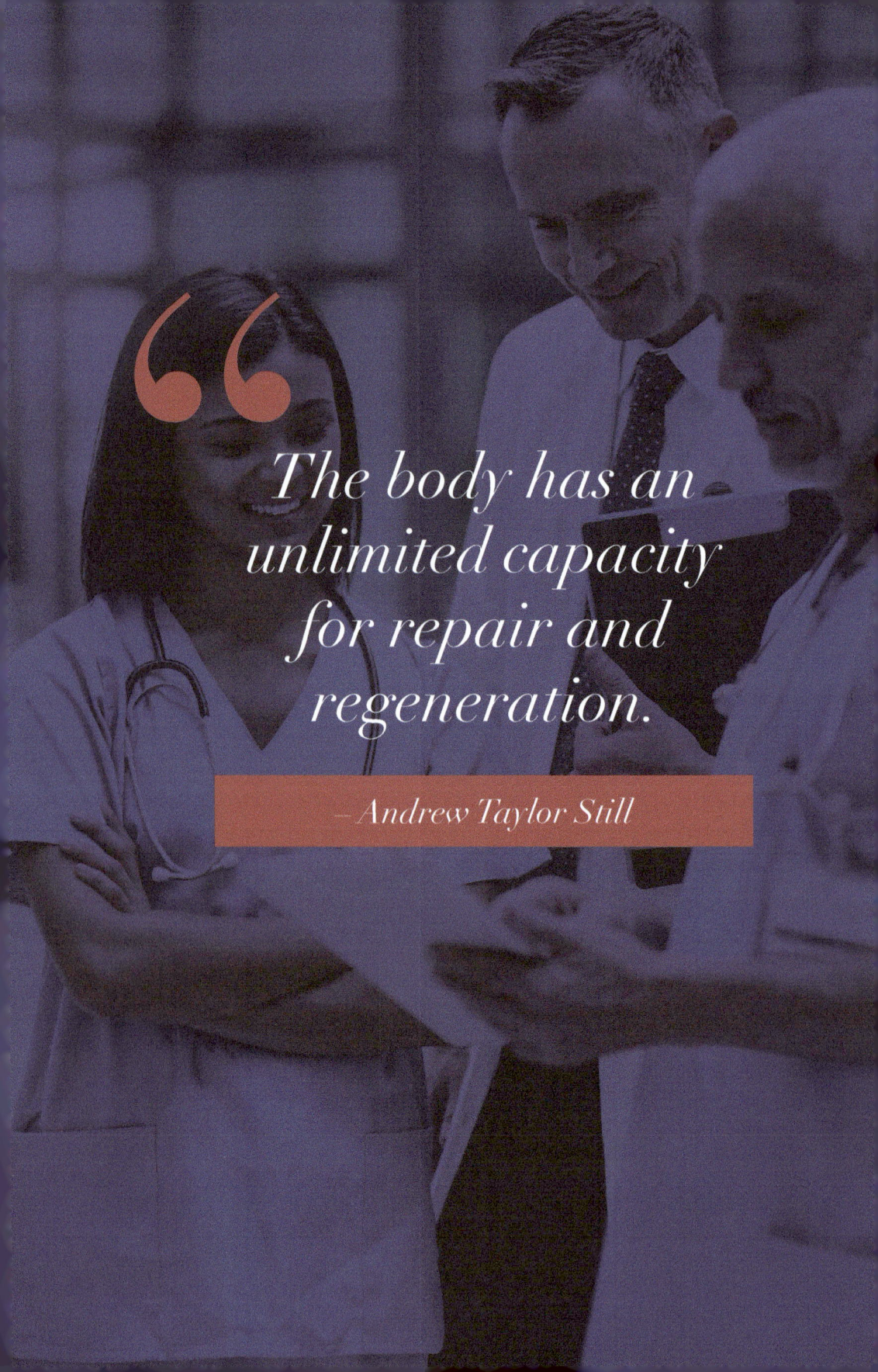

"

*The body has an unlimited capacity for repair and regeneration.*

—Andrew Taylor Still

# CHAPTER TWENTY-FOUR

# ALLOPATHIC VS. OSTEOPATHIC MEDICINE

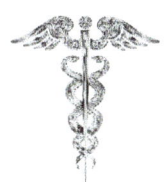

Allopathic and osteopathic medicine are the two schools of medical practice in the United States. The two systems diagnose, care, and prevent diseases, approaching medicine from different perspectives and with specific philosophies. Their approaches are found in the methods of education, treatment, and provision of medical care. Within the past decade, allopathic medicine has adopted more osteopathic whole person approaches while osteopathic medicine has increased its training in medicines and surgery. This 'coming together' has also given greater credibility to DOs and increased the numbers of DOs in specialized residency programs.

## EDUCATIONAL PATHWAYS

Both allopathic and osteopathic physicians receive similar types medical training. Education for both include undergraduate education, medical school, and residency. Students study anatomy, physiology, biochemistry, and pharmacology, followed by clinical rotations in various medical subspecialties. However, osteopathic medical students undergo additional training in Osteopathic Manipulative Treatment (OMT). OMT uses hands-on methods to diagnose, treat, and prevent illness or injury. OMT

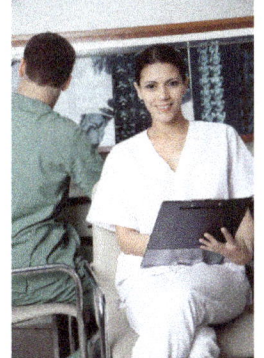

ensures the body's proper structure and function. Thus, osteopathic medical education combines allopathic medicine with unique skills to determine the body dysfunction.

**Here are a few interesting statistics to note. For the class of 2028,**

* 23,156 students started an MD program
* 9,644 first-year students enrolled in D.O. schools

In the 2024 National Resident Matching Program Main Residency Match, match rates for U.S. MD and DO seniors varied across specialties. Here's a breakdown of a few match rates:

## Dermatology

* MD: ~ 80%
* DO: ~ 70.7%

## General Surgery

* MD: ~ 68%
* DO: ~ 68%

## Neurology

* MD: ~ 53.1%
* DO: ~ 16.4%

## Orthopaedic Surgery

* MD: ~ 73%
* DO: ~ 48%

## Otolaryngology

* MD: ~ 80%
* DO: ~ 70.7%

## Plastic Surgery

* MD: ~ 80%
* DO: ~ 70.7%

## TREATMENT APPROACHES

One of the key differences between allopathic and osteopathic forms of medicine is the method of treatment. Allopathic medicine may be defined most precisely as the application of drugs, surgery, and other standard orthodox therapies to conditions and their symptoms. Treatment depends on results of scientific studies and control trials to inform decisions. Whereas osteopathic medicine offers a holistic approach, focusing on how the body can heal itself. DOs employ OMT alongside conventional methods to boost the body's natural disease-fighting ability. Specifically, OMT may be optimal for musculoskeletal issues, such as back pain, issues with the joints, and even headaches. Recent research shows that patients who received OMT experienced less pain and had better functionality as an adjunct to more conventional forms of therapy.

## HEALTHCARE PHILOSOPHIES

Another area of difference is in the philosophical underpinnings of allopathic and osteopathic medicine. Allopathic medicine might be framed as a more reductionistic approach, one that looks at specific symptoms or illnesses and applies a defined intervention or treatment. Studies show that this approach is useful in the management of acute conditions, infections, and emergencies. Osteopathic medicine explores the human body is a whole, believing that the human body is the interconnection of systems. With a more preventive approach, DOs focus on patient education, preventive care, and lifestyle modification. DO's holistic approach considers the root cause instead of just the symptoms of the illness.

## SIMILARITIES IN PRACTICE

Despite the subtle differences in medical practice, allopathic and osteopathic physicians have several similarities. MDs and DOs are both full-fledged physicians with the same licensing ability to prescribe medication and surgery. They can pursue any medical specialty and often hold positions alongside MDs in a hospital or clinic. These distinctions between MDs and DOs have blurred over time. Many DOs incorporate allopathic treatments into their practice, while many MDs use similar holistic methods as DOs. The integration of these two medical traditions have resulted in a more unity-driven healthcare system where the main aim is to serve the patient to the best of the ability available.

## DIFFERENCES IN PRACTICE

An MD is more likely to prescribe medicine for lymphatic flow disorders, which is sometimes effective. A DO is more likely to use lymphatic pump treatment (LPT), a manual technique aimed at encouraging lymph flow in the lymphatic system. This technique is used in treatments such as fractures, abscesses or localized infections, bacterial infections, and elevated body temperature.

In an *International Journal of Osteopathic Medicine*, LPT has shown promise in treating pneumonia. Antibiotics prescribed by MDs are generally effective, although some bacterial strains have been shown to be resistant. By using LPT, the flow through the lymphatic system can be enhanced to rid the body of pathogens.

Another difference might be seen in orthopedics and neurology in areas like:

* Muscle Spasms
* Cramping
* Stiffness
* Chronic Muscle Pain
* Limited Range of Motion
* Shoulder Pain
* Scoliosis
* Sciatica
* Fractures
* Injuries
* Dislocations
* Joint instability
* Strains
* Osteoporosis
* Whiplash injury
* Vertebrobasilar insufficiency
* Some surgeries
* Unsymmetrical Legs, Hips, or Arms

# SHADOWING

Shadowing an MD and/or DO is central to understanding the differences between allopathic and osteopathic medicine. These physicians could be your doctor, family friend, or professional medical contact. While you may seek medical experiences to demonstrate to BS/MD and BS/DO programs your commitment, you also need to understand medical practices. Witness the day-to-day physician-patient experience and immerse yourself in the whole of the healthcare process. Ask the doctors questions. Observe. You are likely to be asked in your interviews to tell about a situation that left an impression upon you.

The specialty does not matter. You might start with a doctor who you know well and then, either ask that doctor or a family friend if they know of another person you might shadow. Diverse experiences are helpful as well since a sample of one rarely provides a wide-ranging perspective.

Shadowing a doctor is not a ticket to gain admissions into a program, but it is an excellent way to know whether you want to pursue the long haul to and through medical school. While you may choose to shadow a doctor in a specific area of your interest, you might want to shadow a second doctor in another area to gain a broader understanding of the field. First, the life of a general 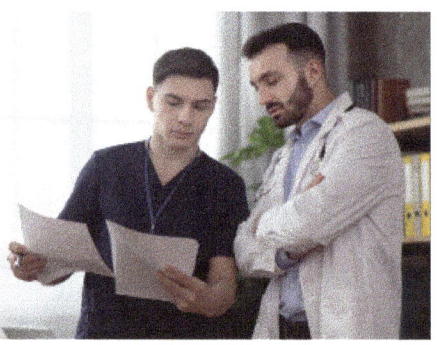 practitioner can be very different from the day-to-day experience of a pathologist or surgeon. Second, while the idea of medical discovery is fascinating, there is a great deal more to helping patients. Seek practical insights into a physician's concerns, commitment, responsibility, and ethical practices.

You will interview at some point. During that interview, you can point to the understanding you gained from your shadowing experiences. Ask yourself these questions.

1. What experiences left an impression on you?
2. What did you learn from the doctors you shadowed?
3. What challenges and opportunities do you believe physicians face?
4. What specific formative experiences led you to be sure medicine is your future?

## INTEGRATION IN HEALTHCARE

The integration of allopathic and osteopathic medicine has been made possible by the creation of one single accreditation system for graduate medical education in the United States. This system is managed by the Accreditation Council for Graduate Medical Education, which aims to maintain the highest standards in allopathic and osteopathic medicine. MDs and DOs are trained under stringent conditions and their knowledge and skills are comparable.

## PUBLIC PERCEPTION AND MISCONCEPTIONS

Due to the differences in approaches and misconceptions, the public often view allopathic and osteopathic medical treatments differently, though most hospitals have both. First, the development of osteopathic medicine was seen, historically, as less scientific than allopathic training. However, perceptions have changed with the increasing integration of osteopathic medicine into the mainstream healthcare system and with the greater unification of training. Today, MDs and DOs often have equal qualifications in providing medical services. Despite this fact, past distinctions cloud perception, particularly in the legitimacy and effectiveness of adding OMT. Further information campaigns are necessary to counteract these misconceptions and clearly explain the evidence-based standards in osteopathic practice.

## CONCLUSION

Thus, it is appropriate to say that allopathic and osteopathic medicine complement one another. Although they are different in their treatment approaches and philosophies, both strive for the best medical care of their patients. With these similarities in their training processes, some parallel practices, there is an increase in allopathic-osteopathic comparisons. Further collaborations between allopathic and osteopathic physicians will push patient care to the next level in ever-changing and always improving medical care.

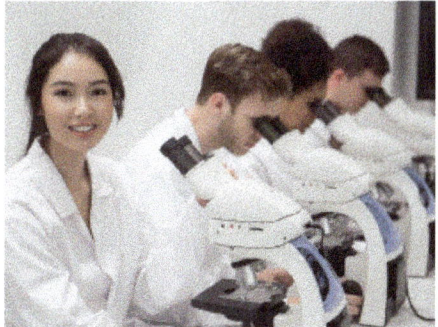

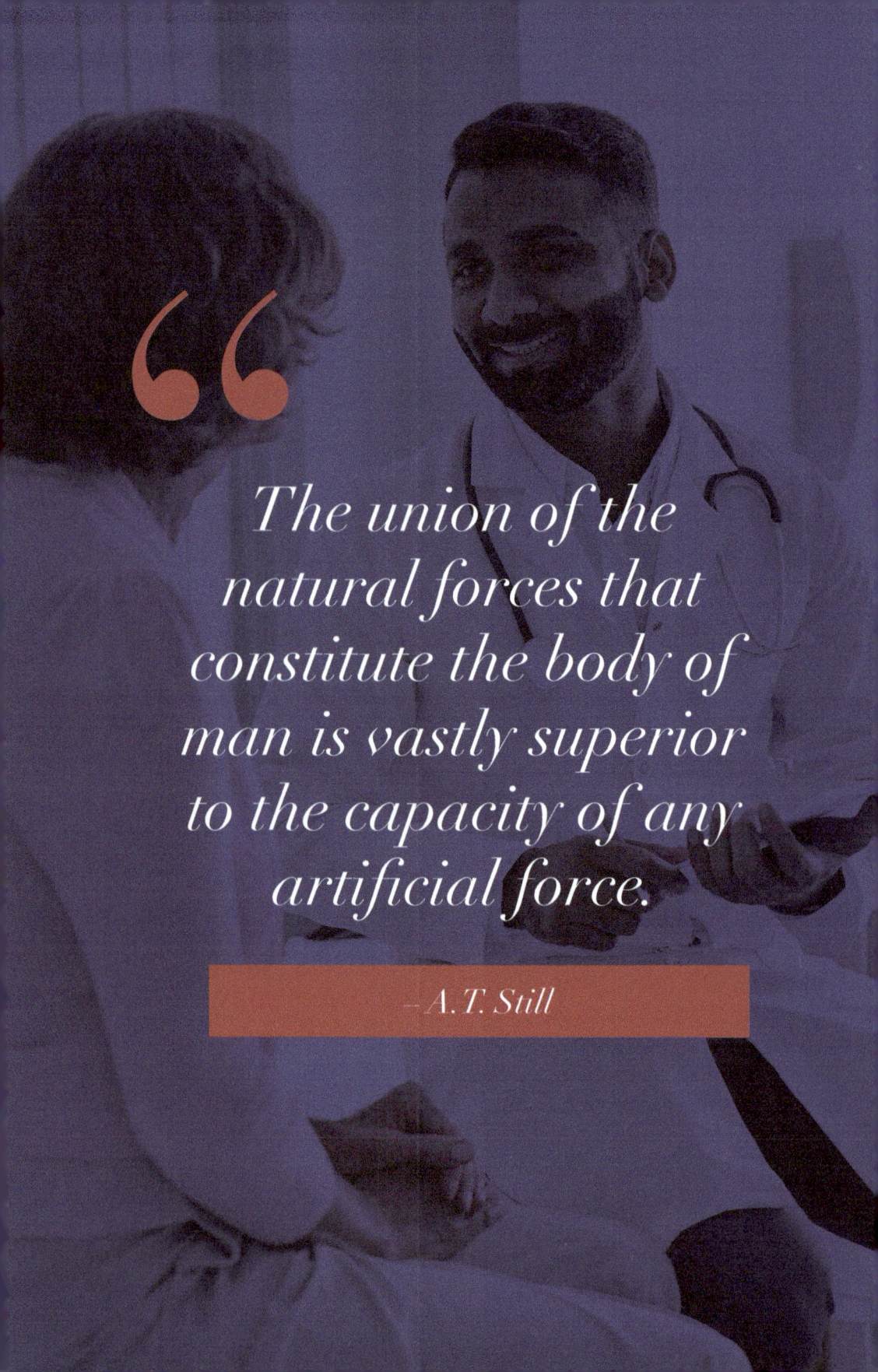

"

*The union of the natural forces that constitute the body of man is vastly superior to the capacity of any artificial force.*

*–A.T. Still*

# CHAPTER TWENTY-FIVE

# BS/MD, BS/DO, DIRECT MED, EARLY ACCEPTANCE

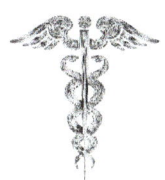

Navigating the pathway to becoming a physician is long, often spanning over a decade of education and training. However, for students with a clear and early commitment to the medical profession, alternative pathways such as BS/MD, BS/DO, Direct Med, and Early Acceptance offer streamlined routes. These programs provide significant advantages, thought they also come with their own set of challenges and considerations. This chapter delves into the nuances of these programs, highlighting their differences, opportunities, and the competitive landscape, with a focus on developments from fall 2024 (class of 2028) admissions.

## UNDERSTANDING PROGRAM TYPES

**BS/MD and BS/DO Programs:** These programs allow students to secure admission to both undergraduate and medical school simultaneously. Spanning 6-8 years, they offer a seamless transition from undergraduate studies to medical education, often with conditions such as GPA requirements, minimum MCAT score, and successful interview.

**Accelerated Programs:** As a subset of BS/MD and BS/DO programs, the accelerated options are designed to shorten the duration of medical education, sometimes to as few as six years. These are intensive, requiring students to undertake a rigorous curriculum with little room for academic exploration outside the medical track. Many also require summer coursework and training.

**Direct Med Programs:** Similar to BS/MD programs, Direct Med programs offer high school seniors a direct path to medical school. The terms are often used interchangeably, but some institutions may differentiate based on specific program structures or requirements.

**Early Assurance Programs (EAPs):** These programs allow undergraduate students, typically in their sophomore or junior years, to apply for early admission to medical school. Unlike BS/MD programs, EAPs accept students further along in their academic studies after having completed tough lower division requirements. These often provide more flexibility in undergraduate course selection.

## OPPORTUNITIES AND ADVANTAGES

**Streamlined Admission Process:** A significant benefit of these programs is the reduction uncertainty associated with the traditional medical school application process. For instance, many BS/MD programs waive the MCAT requirement or set a lower threshold score, allowing students to focus more on their studies and less on standardized test preparation.

**Time and Financial Savings:** Accelerated programs, by design, reduce the total time spent, allowing students to enter the medical profession sooner. This not only saves time but also reduces the financial burden associated with prolonged education, often requiring gap years, intensive test preparation, and post-baccalaureate expenses.

**Early Commitment to Medicine:** These programs are ideal for students who are certain about their desire to pursue a career in medicine. Early commitment provides a clear and focused path, enabling students to engage deeply with medical studies from the outset.

## ADMISSION CHALLENGES AND COMPETITIVENESS

While these programs offer numerous advantages, gaining admission is highly competitive. For example, Brown University's Program in Liberal Medical Education (PLME) had an acceptance rate of 2.3% for the class of 2024, with 3,516 applicants vying for 82 spots. Similarly, the Sophie Davis BS/MD program at CUNY School of Medicine reported an acceptance rate of 2.5%.

Applicants are expected to demonstrate exceptional academic performance, with average SAT scores often exceeding 1,500 and GPAs near 4.0. Beyond academics, successful candidates typically have substantial clinical exposure, research experience, and a demonstrated commitment to community service.

Embarking on a medical career is a significant commitment, and for aspiring physicians, the journey begins well before medical school. Several specialized programs offer streamlined pathways to a medical degree, each with its unique structure, benefits, and challenges. Understanding the nuances of BS/MD, BS/DO Accelerated, Direct Med, and Early Assurance programs is crucial for students aiming to secure a spot in medical school early in their academic careers.

## BS/MD AND BS/DO PROGRAMS

### *Direct Route from High School*

**Definition and Structure:**

BS/MD and BS/DO programs are combined undergraduate and medical school programs that allow students to gain admission straight out of high school. Typically spanning 6 to 8 years, these programs integrate undergraduate education with medical training, culminating in an MD or DO degree.

**Opportunities:**

*   **Guaranteed Medical School Admission:** Students bypass the traditional medical school application process, provided they meet program requirements.

*   **Integrated Curriculum:** A cohesive educational experience, aligning undergraduate and medical studies.

*   **Time Efficiency:** Some programs offer accelerated timelines, reducing the total number of years of study.

**Admission Challenges:**

Admission to BS/MD and BS/DO programs is highly competitive.

## ACCELERATED PROGRAMS

### *Fast-Tracking Medical Education*

**Definition and Structure:**

Accelerated medical programs condense the traditional education timeline, allowing students to complete both undergraduate and medical degrees in a shorter period, often 6 to 7 years.

**Opportunities:**

*   **Reduced Time and Cost:** Students enter the field of medicine sooner and incur fewer educational expenses.

*   **Intensive Learning Environment:** These rigorous curricula foster discipline and resilience.

The demanding nature of accelerated programs requires students to manage a challenging set of STEM courses with limited breaks. For example, the Penn State-Jefferson Accelerated Premedical-Medical Program requires students to complete undergraduate studies in three years before transitioning to medical school. UMKC's six year program requires students to spent their summers taking courses and working in their clinical environments.

# DIRECT MED PROGRAMS

*Securing a Medical Future*

## Definition and Structure:

Direct Med programs, like BS/MD and BS/DO programs, offer high school students a direct path to medical school, often with conditional acceptance based on undergraduate performance.

## Opportunities:

*   **Early Acceptance:** Students secure spot in medical school, reducing the stress of future applications.

*   **Focused Academic Path:** Curricula are designed to thoroughly prepare students for medical education.

## Admission Challenges:

Direct Med programs are selective, with stringent requirements. For instance, the University of Missouri-Kansas City's BA/MD program requires applicants to have a very high GPA.

# EARLY ASSURANCE PROGRAMS (EAPS)

*Commitment During College*

## Definition and Structure:

EAPs allow undergraduate students to apply to medical school during their sophomore or junior years, securing a place before completing their bachelor's degree.

## Opportunities:

*   **Reduced Application Stress:** Students avoid the traditional medical school application process. Some EAPs do not require students to complete the AMCAS.

*   **Flexibility:** Some programs waive the MCAT requirement, allowing students to focus on their studies while gaining clinical and research experience.

## Admission Challenges:

EAPs are competitive and often limited to students from specific institutions. For example, Tufts University's Early Assurance Program offers admission to selected Tufts undergraduates without an MCAT score, emphasizing strong academic performance and a commitment to medicine.

## COMPARATIVE ANALYSIS

### *Choosing the Right Path*

| PROGRAM | ENTRY POINT | TIME | MCAT REQ | ADMISSION TIMING | CONSIDERATIONS |
|---------|-------------|------|----------|------------------|----------------|
| BS/MD, BS/DO | HS | 6-8 yrs | Varies | HS Senior | Highly competitive; commitment required |
| Accelerated | HS | 6-7 yrs | Often Required | HS Senior | Intense academics; faster entry |
| Direct Med | HS | 6-8 yrs | Varies | HS Senior | Conditional acceptance; structured path |
| Early Assurance | College Soph/Jr | 8 yrs | Sometimes Waived | College Students | Secure spot early; check requirements |

Each pathway to medical school offers unique advantages and challenges. BS/MD, BS/DO and Direct Med programs provide early assurance and a structured route, ideal for students certain about a future as an MD or DO. Accelerated programs appeal to those eager to enter the medical field swiftly, while Early Assurance programs offer flexibility for college students who solidify their medical aspirations during undergraduate studies. Prospective applicants should assess their readiness, academic credentials, and long-term goals to choose the path that aligns best with their aspirations.

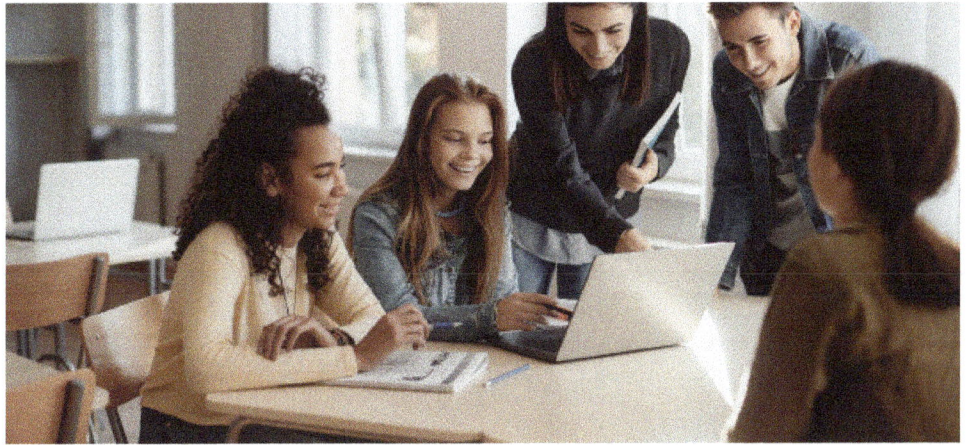

Do your best. One day, you will be someone's hero.

— Unknown

# CHAPTER TWENTY-SIX

# CURRICULUM, CATALOG, & REQUIREMENTS

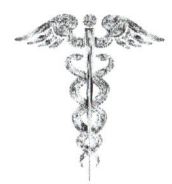

### DEMYSTIFYING THE PATH

*How to Investigate BS/MD, BS/DO, BS/DDS, & Pre-Med Curricula*

For highly academic high school students pondering a future in medicine, one key decision is whether to apply to BS/MD, BS/DO, BS/DDS or pre-med programs. While these programs share common goals, the curriculum, structure, expectations, and responsibilities can vary significantly.

Understanding these differences is essential. First, students need to determine whether the programs are the right fit and, second, they need to decide whether they will succeed once enrolled. This chapter will walk you through how to research and compare programs by exploring their academic catalogs, curricular structures, expectations, and long-term commitments.

### WHY INVESTIGATE CURRICULA AND CATALOGS?

Before you commit to either a BS/MD, BS/DO, BS/DDS or traditional pre-med pathway, it is essential to move beyond promotional brochures and deeply examine the curriculum, course structure, student body, and medical admission requirements. These components reveal how each school educates, shapes, and decides who will be its future physicians.

For BS/MD, BS/DO, and BS/DDS programs, the undergraduate courses are often closely integrated with medical school preparation, and some even begin medical coursework in the third or fourth year. Conversely, pre-med tracks at traditional four-year colleges may offer more flexibility but require students to self-navigate the prerequisites and application process for medical school.

By exploring each program's curriculum and academic catalog, you can answer key questions like:
* How rigid or flexible is the schedule?
* Are there research or clinical hour requirements?
* Is the MCAT/DAT required for matriculation into medical/dental school?
* What GPA must be maintained for acceptance?
* Are study abroad, electives, or non-STEM minors permitted?

## Step 1: Locate the University Catalog and Program Page

Nearly every university publishes an academic catalog on its official website. These are the year-by-year requirements, much like a contract. For BS/MD, BS/DO, BS/DDS, or early assurance programs, look for a dedicated program page often located under the university's college of science, health sciences, or honors college section.

**Key search terms include:**
* "BS/MD curriculum xxxuniversity.edu"
* "Pre-med academic requirements xxxuniversity.edu"
* "Undergraduate catalog xxxuniversity.edu"

**Download or bookmark the following:**
* Curriculum guides
* Course descriptions
* Pre-medical advisory tracks
* Program handbooks
* GPA/MCAT requirements
* Medical/dental school transition policies

## Step 2: Compare BS/MD, BS/DO, BS/DDS & Pre-Med Requirements

To evaluate a school's offerings, compare core components across programs. Focus on:

**1. Coursework**
* BS/MD, BS/DO, and BS/DDS programs often prescribe a strict course sequence in biology, chemistry, physics, and humanities.
* Pre-med/pre-dent students usually follow a standard track including:
  o General Biology w/lab
  o General Chemistry w/lab
  o Organic Chemistry w/lab
  o Physics w/lab

- o    Biochemistry
- o    English/writing-intensive courses
- o    Calculus and/or statistics

Check to see if AP credits, dual enrollment, or community college classes fulfill requirements and whether summer courses are accepted.

## 2. MCAT/DAT Policy

- *    Some BS/MD, BS/DO programs waive the MCAT entirely (e.g., Brown PLME, UMKC).
- *    Others require a minimum MCAT/DAT score for advancement.

In contrast, traditional pre-med/pre-dent students will nearly always need to take the MCAT/DAT and prepare extensively outside of class.

## 3. GPA and Progress Requirements

- *    Many BS/MD, BS/DO, and BS/DDS programs require a minimum GPA, often around 3.5 overall and 3.6 in science courses.
- *    Falling below the minimum may risk dismissal from the medical/dental track or revocation of conditional admission.

For pre-med/pre-dent students, the burden of maintaining a strong GPA is no less important, but there is usually more flexibility in course pacing and academic support.

## 4. Clinical, Volunteer, and Research Hours

- *    BS/MD, BS/DO, and BS/DDS programs often embed clinical exposure.
- *    Some mandate a specific number of volunteer, research, or clinical hours.
- *    Research experience may be a formal part of the program or required before transitioning to medical/dental school.

Pre-med/pre-dent students must actively seek out these opportunities independently, and their competitiveness for medical/dental school will heavily depend on these experiences.

## Step 3: Review Sample Schedules and Course Plans

Most schools publish sample four-year plans or advising guides for BS/MD, BS/DO, BS/DDS, and pre-med students. These documents include:

- *    Semester-by-semester workload
- *    Prerequisite completion requirements
- *    Summer opportunities (shadowing, research, study abroad)
- *    How medical/dental school courses are integrated into their programs

For example, the Sophie Davis BS/MD Program at CUNY School of Medicine incorporates medical coursework as early as year three, while other programs (e.g., the University of Connecticut's Special Program in Medicine) maintain a split between undergraduate and graduate years.

## Step 4: Investigate Unique Offerings, Minors, and Interdisciplinary Options

Does the school allow or require students in the BS/MD, BS/DO, or BS/DDS track to pursue double majors, minors, or honors programs? What about studying public health, medical humanities, or bioethics?

Programs like Case Western's Pre-Professional Scholars Program or Brown's PLME allow for greater academic freedom and are designed to foster well-rounded physicians, not just science majors.

Students with strong interests in psychology, literature, or sociology may want to prioritize programs that allow interdisciplinary exploration without jeopardizing their medical/dental school seat.

## Step 5: Look for Enrichment, Advising, and Support Resources

A critical part of your success in either path will be the advising and mentorship network. Investigate:
* Are pre-med/pre-dent advisors full-time, specialized staff?
* Is there a formal committee letter process for pre-med/pre-dent students?
* Does the BS/MD, BS/DO, or BS/DDS program offer medical/dental school mentors or peer advising?

Also look for structured enrichment programs such as:
* Summer research fellowships
* MCAT prep courses (included or discounted)
* Medical ethics seminars
* Clinical immersion programs
* Medical journal clubs
* Going on rounds with physicians
* Biotechnology workshops, medical imaging practice, or human simulators
* Auxiliary certificates like AED, CPR, EMT, phlebotomy, medical assisting

These can greatly influence your readiness and sense of belonging in the field of medicine.

# WHAT'S THE RIGHT FIT?

Ultimately, choosing between a BS/MD, BS/DO, or BS/DDS program and a pre-med/pre-dent route comes down to learning style, career certainty, and academic goals. Some students thrive in the structure and security of BS/MD, BS/DO or BS/DDS programs, while others benefit from the flexibility, interest exploration, and social environment of a traditional path.

By closely reading each school's curriculum and catalog, you can plan your schedule and map out the next seven to ten years of your life. Make sure your choice aligns with your ambition and your academic/personal needs. Being a physician starts with being a thoughtful and informed student.

# SAMPLE CATALOG PAGE

University of South Florida BS/MD Program (straight from their catalog page)

**7-YEAR B.S./M.D. PROGRAM ELIGIBILITY**
*As you review the information below, feel free to reach out to Carter Harbert, coordinator of health pathway programs, with additional questions at harbert@usf. edu.

To be eligible for this program incoming students must meet the following criteria, without exception:

4.0 weighted HS grade point average (GPA), as calculated by USF Undergraduate Admissions, and

SAT (Critical Reading and Math sections) score of 1500 or ACT score of 34 (we super-score all attempts for both tests, scores must be finalized and received by USF no later than June 1 of the entering year), and

Receive acceptance to both USF and the Judy Genshaft Honors College

**ENTERING THE 7-YEAR B.S./M.D. PROGRAM**
There is no formal application for the 7-Year B.S./M.D. Program.

Students interested in following the 7-Year B.S./M.D. track must reach initial eligibility requirements (above) and declare a major in biomedical sciences when applying to the university.

Those students will be directly assigned to work with the program coordinator during summer orientation and confirmed as participating in the program at that time as well as registered for the appropriate first-semester courses.

View a detailed and annotated course sequence for the 7-Year B.S./M.D. program here.

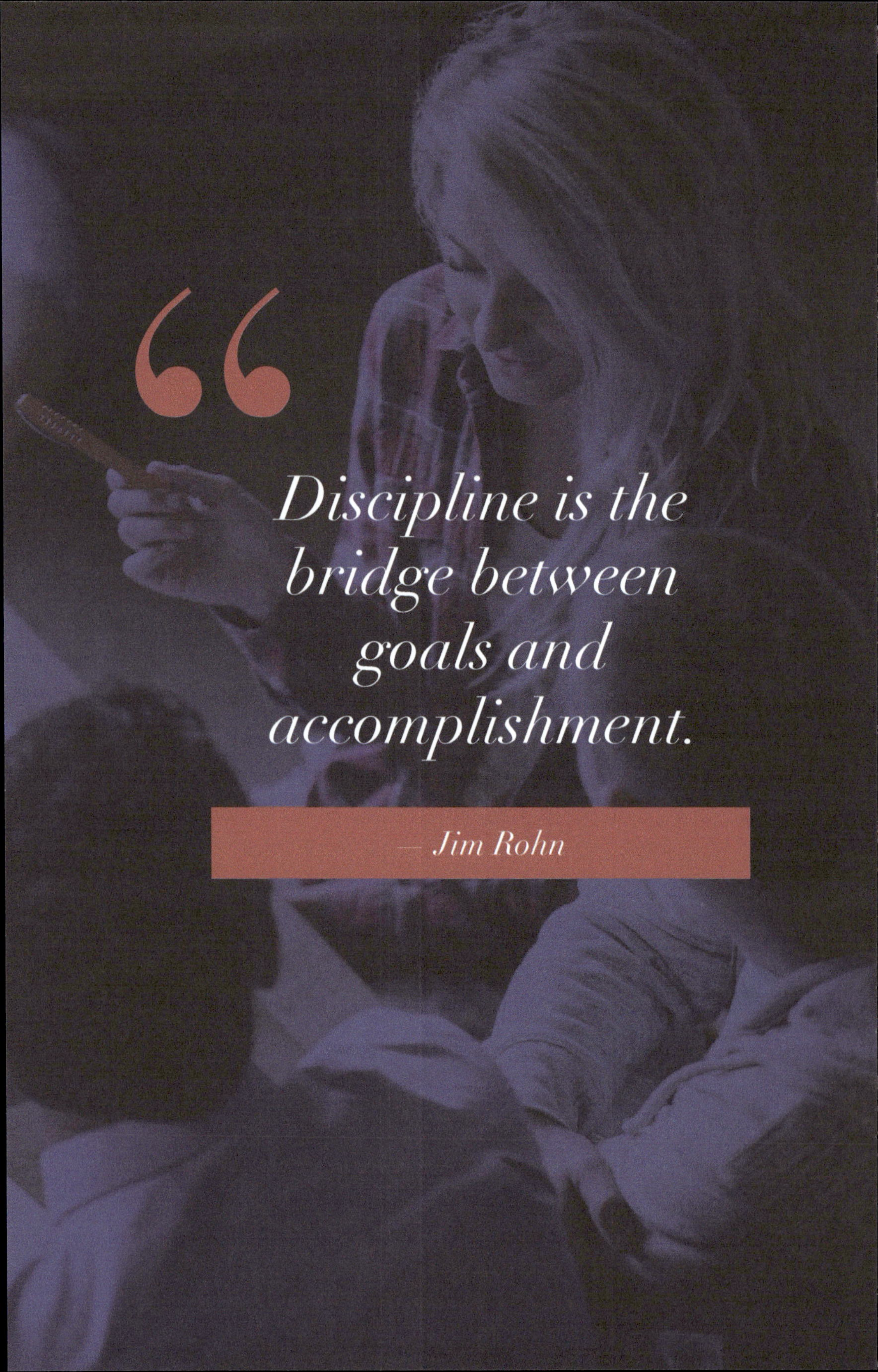

" "

*Discipline is the bridge between goals and accomplishment.*

— *Jim Rohn*

# CHAPTER TWENTY-SEVEN

# SUPPORT SERVICES

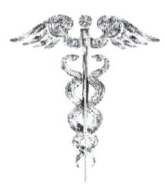

Success in a BS/MD, BS/DO, BS/DDS, Direct Med, or Accelerated program is fundamentally based on academic ability, but students must also be able to sustain their effort. Often, support, direction, or guidance are invaluable. These programs are rigorous, compressed, and emotionally demanding. Whether a student has a documented disability, needs additional tutoring, or simply feels overwhelmed by the workload, the quality of support services can make a critical difference. This chapter explores the types of support available, how to investigate them, and what families should look for to ensure their student is supported throughout their pre-medical and medical journey.

## UNDERSTANDING THE SCOPE OF SUPPORT SERVICES

Support services in BS/MD and accelerated medical programs can generally be grouped into the following categories:

1. **Academic Support**
   o  Peer and professional tutoring
   o  Study skills workshops
   o  Structured advising and academic coaching
   o  Time management and exam preparation resources

2. **Disability Accommodations**
   o  Extended testing time
   o  Note-taking assistance
   o  Accessible classroom environments

o   Individual learning accommodations under the Americans with Disabilities Act

3. **Mental Health and Wellness Services**
   o   Counseling centers
   o   Stress management workshops
   o   Crisis support and group therapy

4. **Career and Professional Mentoring**
   o   Medical school integration support
   o   Shadowing and research opportunities
   o   Interview prep and resume building

## How to Investigate Support Services

To evaluate a program's support structure, students and families should:
- Visit the university's Office of Student Affairs or Student Services website.
- Look up the university's Disability Services Office or ADA Compliance Office.
- Search "[university name] + academic support for pre-med" or "student success center."
- Contact the BS/MD, BS/DO, or BS/DDS program and ask:

   o   "What accommodations are available for students with documented learning or medical conditions?"
   o   "Do BS/MD, BS/DO, BS/DDS students have access to tutors or medical school faculty early on?"
   o   "Is there a dedicated advisor for program participants?"
   o   "Are support resources integrated with the medical school?"

## Four Program Examples

To illustrate how support systems vary and how to find them, here are four specific BS/MD or Direct Med programs and their services:

### 1. CUNY School of Medicine (Sophie Davis BS/MD Program) – *New York, NY*

The CUNY School of Medicine, which houses the Sophie Davis BS/MD program, is deeply focused on serving underserved communities. This extends to its student support.

- **Disability Services:** The CUNY Office of Accessibility provides individualized accommodation plans, testing accommodations, note-taking, and assistive technology.
   o   Website: www.ccny.cuny.edu/accessability

- **Academic Support:** Tutoring is available through the City College Academic Resource Center.

- **Wellness Services:** The Counseling Center at CCNY provides therapy and support groups with easy access for medical and pre-medical students.

*How to Investigate:* Search the CCNY and CUNY School of Medicine websites for "student services" and "academic success." Email the Sophie Davis coordinator to ask how these services integrate into the BS/MD curriculum.

## 2. University of Missouri-Kansas City BA/MD Program – *Kansas City, MO*

UMKC offers a six-year BA/MD program that is academically intense but supported by a well-established advising and support infrastructure.

- **Disability Services:** The UMKC Office of Services for Students with Disabilities coordinates all ADA accommodations including exam modifications and classroom adjustments.
  - o   Website: www.umkc.edu/disability-services
- **Academic Support:** The School of Medicine Academic Enrichment Office provides tutoring, peer-led group review sessions, and study skills workshops.
- **Advising Model:** Each student is assigned a docent team, which includes a physician mentor, academic advisor, and peer mentors.

*How to Investigate:* Visit the School of Medicine's Enrichment and Advising sections. Ask about the frequency of advising meetings and how early students begin clinical work with mentors.

## 3. Nova Southeastern University (BS/DO Dual Admission Program) – *Fort Lauderdale, FL*

Nova's Dual Admission DO program prepares students for osteopathic medicine while providing a supportive undergraduate-to-medical school bridge.

- **Disability Services:** NSU's Office of Student Disability Services coordinates ADA compliance and provides accommodation plans, testing services, and emotional support animal registration.
  - o   Website: www.nova.edu/disabilityservices
- **Tutoring and Academic Support:** The Tutoring and Testing Center offers one-on-one sessions, supplemental instruction, and writing assistance for science-heavy courses.
- **Health and Wellness:** NSU's Center for Student Counseling and Well-being offers medical school-specific counseling services, wellness events, and a 24/7 crisis hotline.

*How to Investigate:* Use the NSU undergraduate and DO school websites. Call the Office of Undergraduate Admissions to request a checklist of support resources available to Dual Admission students.

## 4. Case Western Reserve University (Pre-Professional Scholars Program - PPSP) – *Cleveland, OH*

Though technically a pre-med program with conditional acceptance into Case Western Reserve School of Medicine, PPSP is highly flexible and deeply supported.

- **Academic Support:** Case Western offers a Student Success Initiative with peer tutoring, academic coaching, and a science-focused study group program.
- **Disability Services:** The Office of Disability Resources provides comprehensive accommodations including assistive technology and alternative format textbooks.
  - Website: students.case.edu
- **Career Support:** The Pre-Professional Health Office works with PPSP students throughout undergrad, helping to prepare for research, clinical experiences, and the transition to med school.

*How to Investigate:* Explore Case Western's Office of Student Advancement and Disability Resources sites. Use the search tool for "PPSP advising" and "academic coaching."

## WHAT SHOULD STUDENTS ASK OR LOOK FOR?

Here are questions every family should ask during program info sessions or visits:

1. Is there a dedicated advisor for BS/MD, BS/DO, BS/DDS, EAP, or Direct Med students?
2. Are tutoring services built into the program or are they optional? Is there a fee?
3. How do students access mental health services during high-stress years (e.g., MCAT prep or medical school transition)?
4. Does the program support academic accommodations without stigma or additional barriers?

Look for support that is proactive, not reactive. The best programs anticipate student challenges and integrate resources into the program structure.

Finally, BS/MD, BS/DO, BS/DDS, EAPs, and accelerated medical programs are rigorous. However, no student should walk that path alone. From tutoring to disability accommodations, from mental health counseling to personalized advising, support services exist to help students thrive. By knowing what to look for and how to ask, families can ensure that their student applicant has a scaffold of support to carry them all the way to their white coat ceremony.

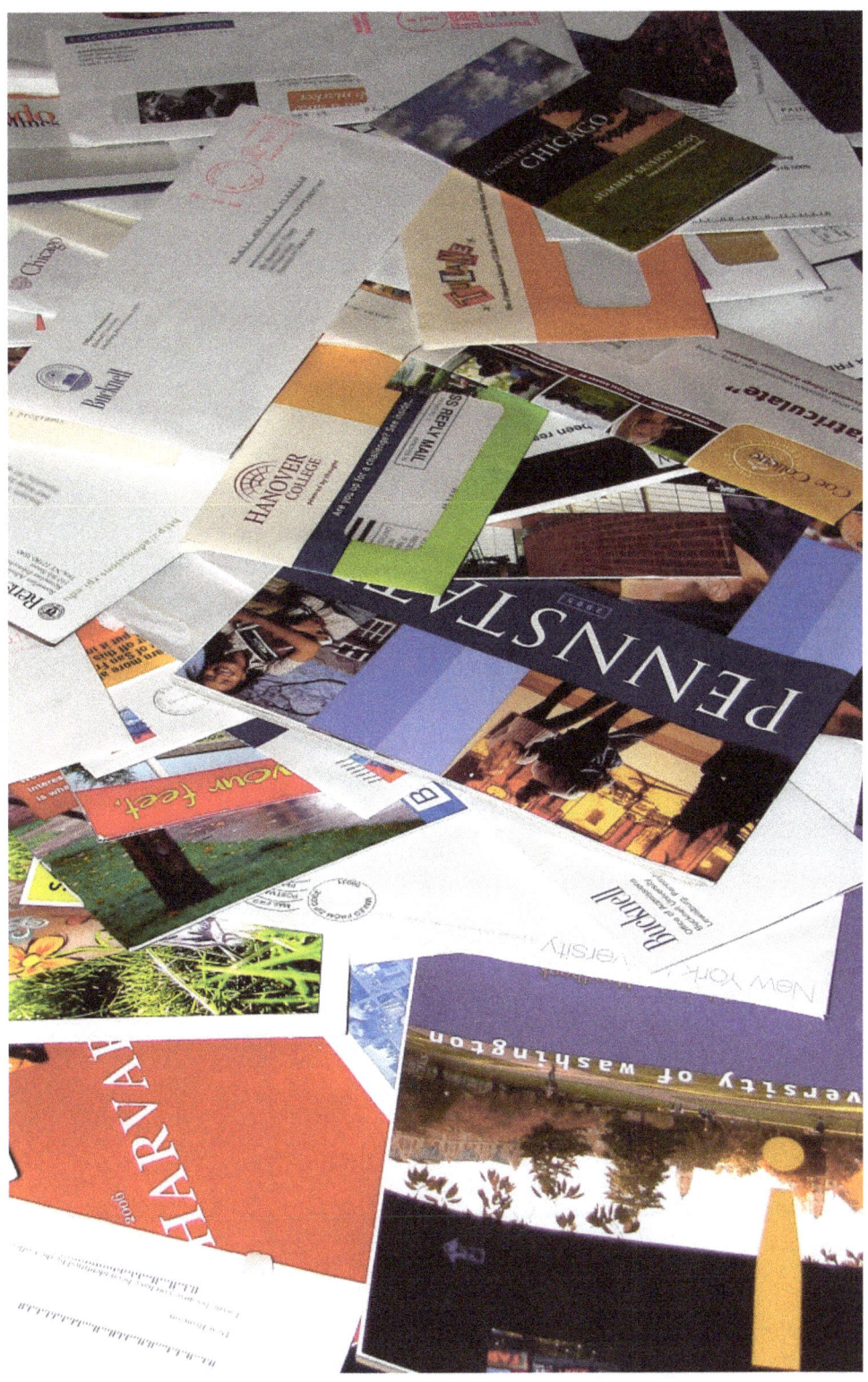

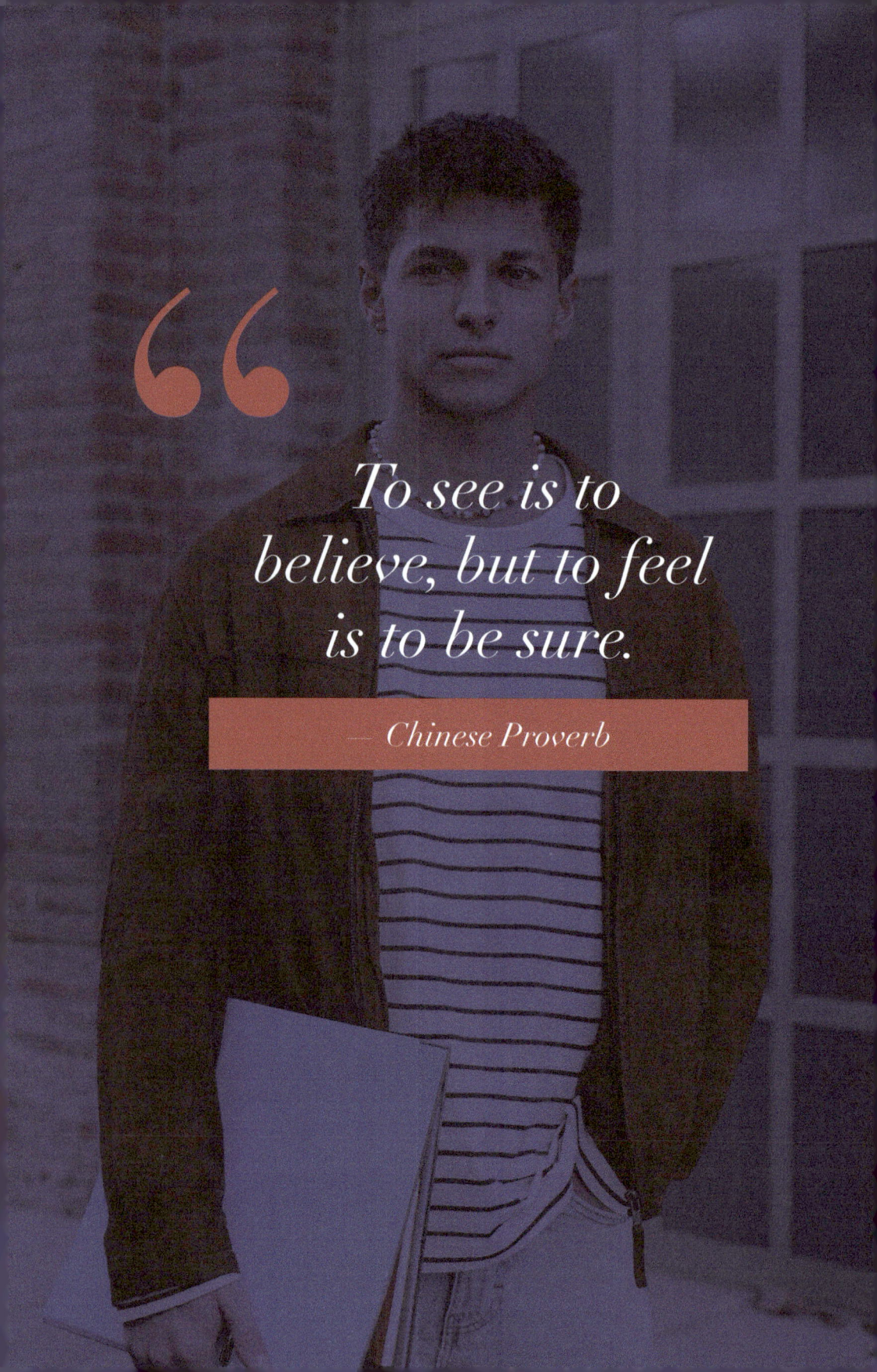

"

To see is to believe, but to feel is to be sure.

— Chinese Proverb

CHAPTER TWENTY-EIGHT

# COLLEGE VISITS

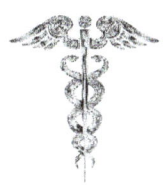

Visiting college campuses provides the best window to view your future college experience. While guidebooks and websites are helpful, there is no substitute for sensing the energy of the campus environment, academic rigor, student body, housing/dining, school spirit, and extracurricular activities. The following guidelines can help you to determine college characteristics that fit what you want in a school. What school will give you the best possible opportunity to learn, live, and love your college experience? What research opportunities, activities, and facilities will springboard your life in order for you to obtain your career and personal goals?

*   **Plan Your Trip in Advance**

    What colleges do you want to visit? Which additional universities might you visit if you had extra time? If there are formal tours, determine when they are available. Schedule a personal interview if possible. Take the tour before you interview so you can listen to the tour guide, ask questions, and become more are familiar with the programs and possibilities that are most interesting to you. Occasionally, the regional representative responsible for your area is in town and available. If so, definitely talk to him or her.

*   **Tours and Information Sessions**

    Tours and informational sessions usually last between 1-2 hours. Investigate residence halls, classroom buildings, the library, dining facilities, student center, and activities. Consider the atmosphere, environment, campus safety, transportation possibilities, and surrounding area. Look into classrooms. Sit in on a lecture if you have the time. Talk to several students and at least one faculty member. Eat a meal in the campus cafeteria or food court – not necessarily just to taste the food, but to get a sense of the campus culture. Remember, you are observing your prospective classmates. Maybe some will talk to you about their experience.

* **Write Down Campus Details, Information, and Contacts Along the Way**
There is so much more to determining if a particular college is the right place for you than the organized events provided by the admissions office. Don't forget that the college plans these activities with the goal of having every prospective student fall in love with their campus. Play the role of an investigator. Look behind the scenes and beyond what they want you to see. However, don't settle for only the positive information about the school.

* **Strike Up Conversations with Students**
  - What do they love about their school?
  - What majors are popular?
  - What clubs are the most active?
  - What do students do when they aren't studying?
  - What is your least favorite aspect of your experience?
  - What are two things you wish you could change?
  - Is it hard to get classes?
  - How much contact do you have with faculty?
  - How are your professors?
  - What is the typical class size?
  - Is the environment competitive?
  - Do most students remain on campus on weekends?

* **Pick Up and Read a Copy of the Student Newspaper**
Student newspapers often provide valuable insights into the campus culture. Articles provide a sense of school spirit, activities, political leanings, protests, controversies, and information about professors, internships, trips, the administration, dorm life, fun events, and local vendors.

* **Investigate the College's Record of Safety**
Remember, you are going to live there for four years. You want to know if the area and dormitories are safe, particularly walking back from class, library, or computer center late at night. Is there a safety program, shuttle service, buddy walking program, access to emergency phones, and good lighting?

| Activity/Program/ Sports/Admissions | Location on Campus | Name/Contact | E-mail |
|---|---|---|---|
| Admissions Office | | | |
| Computer Facilities/Labs | | | |
| Athletic Department and Facilities | | | |
| Department Offices/Professors | | | |
| Research Laboratories | | | |
| Business School - Investment Center | | | |
| Lecture Halls and Classrooms | | | |
| Visit a Class | | | |
| Music/Art/Theatre/ Dance/Cheerleading | | | |
| Dormitories | | | |
| Dining Halls | | | |
| Newspaper/Radio/ Television Center | | | |
| Tutoring Center | | | |
| Library | | | |
| Student Activities Center & Bookstore | | | |
| Career/Internship Center | | | |
| Financial Aid/ Scholarship Office | | | |
| Special/Disability Services Offices | | | |
| Bookstore | | | |

> An investment in knowledge always pays the best interest.

— *Benjamin Franklin*

# CHAPTER TWENTY-NINE

# COLLEGE EVENTS, FAIRS, & REPRESENTATIVES

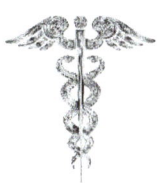

Many colleges around the United States have regional representatives who serve and support admissions and outreach operations. These dedicated and outgoing spokespeople are hired because of their knowledge and affiliations with the school, though not all are graduates of the college or university. At meetings held on your campus, local events, and national college fairs, you will find that these representatives are eager to talk about the benefits, opportunities, and unique aspects of their programs.

Take advantage of admissions representative visits to your school. These representatives frequently travel from school to school throughout the country. Each fall, representatives hold gatherings at schools throughout the region. Your college counseling office will have a list of the representatives that are coming. Many times, they also post the visiting colleges', dates, and admissions officer's names on the school's website and either physical or digital bulletin board. If not, ask your counselor where they post these visits.

Attend these information sessions if you can. They may reveal majors, clubs, or faculty that intrigue you. They may provide information about their financial aid and scholarship process. These visits often happen at different times of the day. Sadly, they are occasionally scheduled during a challenging AP class.

It would be convenient if admissions officers visit your school during lunch time when you are not in class. However, that is often not the case. Sometimes you cannot go because you have a test at the same time. If you can find a moment between classes to meet with them, introduce yourself and get their name and contact information so you can ask any questions you have.

These Regional Admissions Officers know the high schools in your region and are familiar with the curriculum and reputation of your school. They may also know the strength of your courses, the numbers of students who have applied in the past, and those who succeeded and failed when they matriculated.

While one aspect of their job is recruitment, they are primarily interested in proving information about their school. Frequently, another key role is serving as the first readers of your application. This is important for you because if you make a good impression, they may look twice in their review. These people are often friendly, approachable, and more than willing to answer questions.

## NATIONAL COLLEGE FAIRS

The NACAC National College Fairs provide invaluable opportunities for students exploring BS/MD, BS/DO, and BS/DDS programs. These fairs provide direct access to admissions representatives from a wide array of colleges and universities, allowing prospective applicants to gather detailed information about combined medical/ dental programs, application requirements, and institutional cultures. Engaging with representatives can offer insights into program specifics, such as curriculum structure, clinical opportunities, and support services, which are crucial for making informed decisions about your educational path.

NACAC hosts National College Fairs in cities across the United States. For instance, in the spring of 2025, fairs were scheduled in locations including Atlantic City, Baton Rouge, Birmingham, Chicago, Cincinnati, Dallas/Fort Worth, Denver, Fort Lauderdale, Honolulu, Houston, Jacksonville, Kansas City, Long Island, Los Angeles, Milwaukee, Minneapolis, Nashville, New Orleans, Philadelphia, Portland, Seattle, and Spokane. There may be one this year near you!

With geographically diverse colleges attending, these events are instrumental in connecting students with potential colleges and programs. The NACAC College Fairs collectively reach over 100,000 students annually and feature participation from more than 360 colleges and universities.

While there is no college fair exclusively dedicated to BS/MD, BS/DO, or BS/DDS programs, certain events focus on STEM fields often include institutions offering combined medical/dental programs. For example, the NACAC STEM College and Career Fairs provide platforms to explore these and related opportunities. The June 2025 STEM College and Career Fair was held at Colorado School of Mines. These specialized fairs provide students with opportunities to explore STEM-focused programs and careers by connecting with colleges and professionals in these fields.

Additionally, virtual events, like the AAMC Virtual Medical School Fair, enable students to connect with medical school admissions officers nationwide with sessions that can be particularly beneficial for those interested in direct medical pathways.

To stay informed about upcoming fairs and events, check the NACAC College Fairs website and the AAMC Virtual Medical School Fair page. These platforms provide updated schedules, registration details, and resources to help you make the most of these opportunities.

## LOCAL COLLEGE FAIRS

Similarly, local fairs held at nearby high schools feature dozens of colleges. They are smaller but equally valuable, maybe more valuable since the tables may feel more approachable and the representatives tend to know the local schools better.

Come for the second hour. People tend to go to these events early and leave around halfway through. At the beginning, the tables are full of students and parents. However, often the second half is quieter. Toward the end, the parking lots empty and many people are gone. Also, parents tend to want to return home early.

Get each representative's business card and follow up after the event. Write the name of the event and date on the business card. Surprisingly, many schools will ask if you ever interacted with a representative from that university. The application will also ask for the name of the person you met and when you went to that event.

I promise you, you will forget the name of the representative, the location, and the date months later when you are asked for that information. If you tend to lose the business cards, put the information of each college contact on a Google Sheet or Google Doc. If you can, take a few notes so you can refer to any pearls of wisdom.

Before you go, prepare by pulling together a few questions you want to ask. These events move swiftly. Some tables are literally surrounded by students and parents hungry to attend the most popular schools. You may not be able to ask questions at those tables. You could wait for a half hour, but the events are typically only two hours. I would just move on to a table where there are fewer people and the representatives are more than excited to speak to you about their school.

Whatever college fairs you attend, you will meet lots of people quickly. These are efficient ways to meet the representatives who are likely to read your application at some point and make a decision about you. Make a good impression. Follow up if you have questions. Get excited. College life and a new experience is just around the corner.

"

*Striving for success without hard work is like trying to harvest when you haven't planted.*

— David Bly

# CHAPTER THIRTY

# NARROWING YOUR LIST

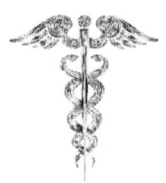

Embarking on a medical/dental career is both exciting and daunting. With numerous options, each with unique structures, requirements, and opportunities, it is crucial to approach the selection process methodically. This chapter provides a roadmap to make informed decisions.

### 1. Clarify Your Medical Career Goals

Reflect on your long-term quest to filter programs that align with your goals.

- ☐ **Specialization Interests:** Are you inclined towards primary care, surgery, research, or a specialty like oncology or dermatology?

- ☐ **Flexibility vs. Structure:** Do you prefer a rigid, fast-tracked program or one that allows for exploration?

- ☐ **Geographical Preferences:** Are there specific regions or cities where you prefer to study and eventually practice?

### 2. Understand Program Types, Structures, and Duration

Since each program has its pros and cons and caters to different student needs, determine whether you want an accelerated program that demands a higher workload in a shorter time or one that has more flexibility.

- ☐ BS/MD, BS/DO, BS/DDS programs: 7-8 years with traditional pacing.

- ☐ Early Acceptance/Direct Med Programs: Provides a direct pathway from high school to medical school, often with conditional acceptance.

- ☐ Accelerated Programs: Condenses the traditional timeline, allowing students to complete both degrees in a shorter span, sometimes as brief as 6 years: extremely rare and very intense, including summers.

### 3. Accreditation and Program Validity

Check if the program is still active and is accredited by a regional accrediting body like the LCME (MD) or COCA (DO). Since well-known and very popular programs (e.g., Northwestern HPME, USC, Rice/Baylor, Florida, BU Seven-Year Program) have been discontinued, confirming availability for the current year is essential.

### 4. MCAT and GPA Requirements

Some programs waive the MCAT entirely (e.g., Brown PLME), while others require a minimum score (e.g., 510) to progress. All programs have GPA thresholds.

### 5. Clinical and Research Opportunities

Programs integrated with teaching hospitals or research institutions provide better preparation for medical school. Look for guaranteed or preferred access to shadowing, labs, and internships.

### 6. Support Services and Flexibility

- ☐ Accessibility services for students with disabilities
- ☐ Peer tutoring or academic coaching
- ☐ Ability to pursue minors, study abroad, or extracurricular interests

### 7. Consider Geographic and Cultural Fit

- ☐ Size and vibe of the institution
- ☐ Proximity to home or urban/rural settings
- ☐ Campus diversity and student satisfaction

### 8. Evaluate Admissions Requirements

- ☐ **GPA and Test Scores:** Top programs often require unweighted GPAs above 3.8 and SAT/ACT scores in the 95th percentile or higher.
- ☐ **Extracurriculars:** Clinical experience, research, leadership roles, and community service can bolster applications.
- ☐ **Exceed Expectations:** Meet or exceed these criteria before applying.

### 9. Assess Program Rigor and Support Systems

- ☐ **Curriculum Intensity:** Accelerated programs might have fewer breaks and a denser curriculum.
- ☐ **Clinical Exposure:** Early and diverse clinical experiences can enhance learning and residency applications.

### 10. Financial Considerations

- ☐ **Tuition and Fees:** Compare costs. Determine "hidden" program fees.
- ☐ **Scholarships and Financial Aid:** Some programs offer merit-based scholarships or need-based aid.
- ☐ **Cost of Living:** Factor in living expenses in different cities or states.

**11. Research Residency Placement and Outcomes**

- ☐ **Residency Match Rates:** High match rates indicate strong programs.
- ☐ **Specialty Placements:** If you have a desired specialty, see how many graduates enter that field.
- ☐ **Alumni Networks:** Strong networks can aid in mentorship and job placements.

**12. Visit Campuses, First-Hand Experience, & Information Sessions**

- ☐ **Campus Visits:** Observe facilities, interact with current students, and gauge the environment.
- ☐ **Virtual Sessions:** Many programs offer online webinars and Q&A sessions.
- ☐ **Admissions Interviews:** Use these opportunities to ask detailed questions about the program.

## CASE STUDY

### George Washington University offers a Seven-Year BA/MD Program

#### Overview

The Seven-Year BA/MD is a joint degree program between GWU's Columbian College of Arts and Sciences and the School of Medicine and Health Sciences. This accelerated program is designed for high-achieving high school seniors.

#### Analyze the key features:

- ☐ **Accelerated Timeline:** Three years of undergraduate study followed by four years of medical school.
- ☐ **MCAT Waiver:** Students are not required to take the MCAT.
- ☐ **Early Clinical Exposure:** Engage in clinical work early in the program.
- ☐ **Mentorship:** Guidance from the Dean of MD Admissions and access to medical faculty.

Participants in the BA/MD must demonstrate academic excellence, leadership, community service, and a strong commitment to a career in medicine.

#### Competitiveness

Admission to GWU's BA/MD program is highly selective, admitting a small cohort each year, with acceptance rates typically ranging from 2% to 4%. Thus, the chances are small, but the payoff is high. Applicants are expected to have SAT or ACT scores in the 90th percentile or higher. Most have scores of over 1500.

GWU's program is among the more selective BS/MD programs in the United States. While not as competitive as programs like Brown University's PLME, which has an acceptance rate of approximately 2.3%, GWU's program is still considered highly competitive due to its low acceptance rate and rigorous admission standards.

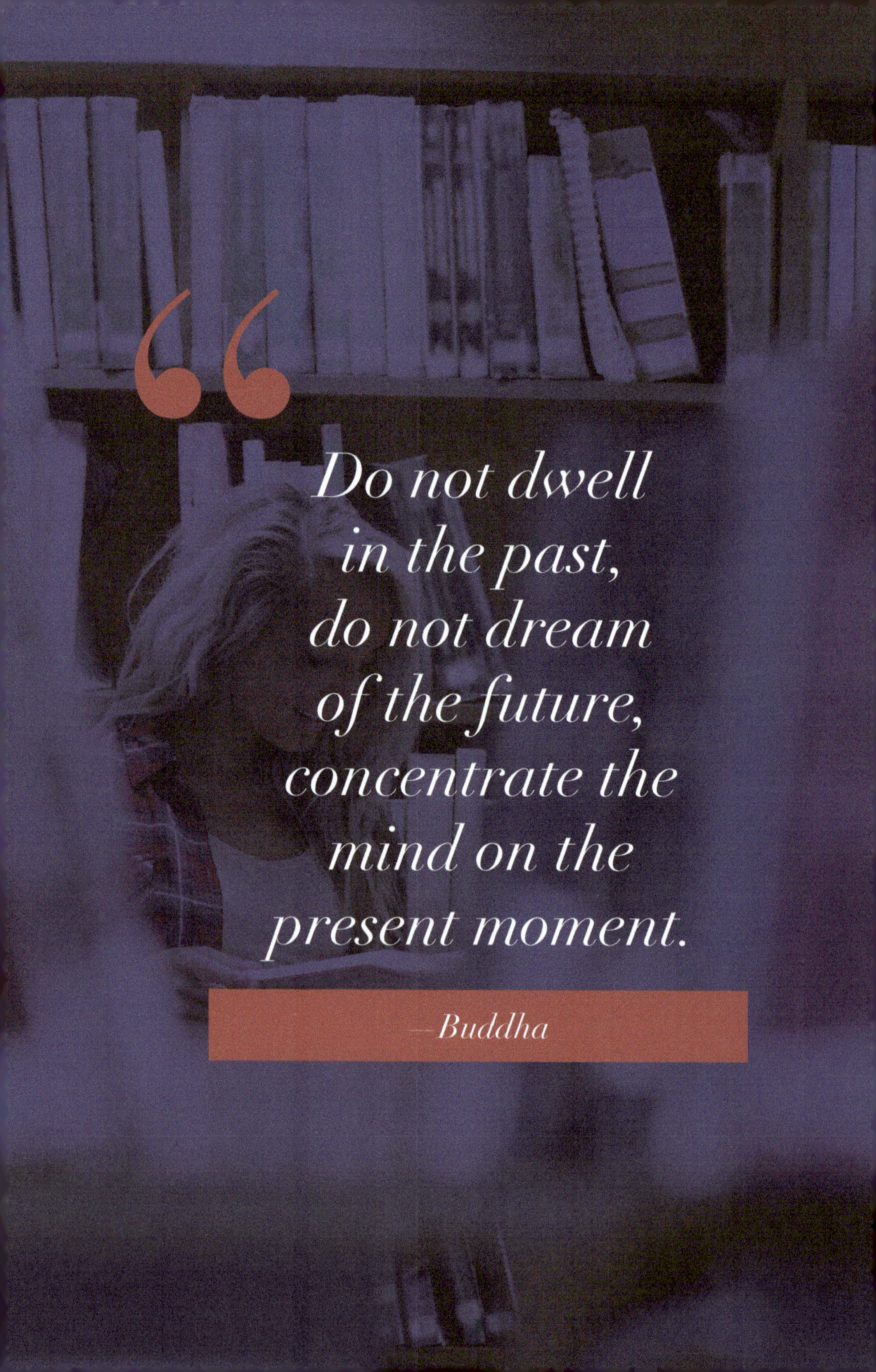

"

Do not dwell
in the past,
do not dream
of the future,
concentrate the
mind on the
present moment.

—*Buddha*

# CHAPTER THIRTY-ONE

# WHERE TO APPLY?

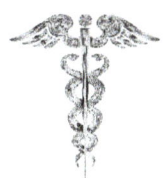

T he choice of where to apply is yours. In fact, many students start down the path toward a BS/MD, BS/DO, or BS/DDS and reconsider. This turnaround is often because of the student's time commitments. Frankly, if you are an athlete, musician, artist, school leader, researcher, hospital volunteer, and an academic powerhouse in tough classes, you have no time. And, to do a good job in your essays and interviews, the application process requires time...lots of time.

This is exactly why you must start planning by jumping on opportunities, creating a calendar, and researching schools early. Prepare your applications or at least organize your approach possibly in the summer after your sophomore year or during your junior year. The decisions are tough. Many students wonder whether they should shoot for their dream schools or put significant effort into a direct med program. Only you can answer this question.

By now, you have read enough of this book to know there are significant benefits to these direct med programs. However, if the notion of going to a top 20 dream school still beckons you, you can either apply to both (and many students do) or just pursue the traditional four-year pre-med/pre-dent path. Time, is required, though, to do a great job with this application process. This key factor may determine your decision.

Why apply if you are just going to throw your application together and hope for the best? You worked so hard thus far and doing a poor job on these applications will only earn you a rejection. So, this is the moment you need to decide and commit yourself to a direction.

# TOP 10 HIGHLY COMPETITIVE BS/MD & EAP PROGRAMS

*Selectivity, academic rigor, and transition from BS to medical school*

1. **Brown University** – Program in Liberal Medical Education (PLME)
   - o An 8-year program combining undergraduate and medical education.
   - o Acceptance rate: Approximately 2.19%.

2. **University of Rochester** – Rochester Early Medical Scholars (REMS)
   - o Offers early assurance to the University of Rochester School of Medicine.
   - o Focuses on research and clinical exposure.

3. **Case Western Reserve Univ.** – Pre-Professional Scholars Program (PPSP)
   - o Provides conditional admission to CWRU School of Medicine.
   - o Encourages exploration of diverse academic interests.

4. **University of Pittsburgh** – Guaranteed Admissions Program (GAP)
   - o Offers guaranteed admission to Pitt's School of Medicine for high-achieving undergraduates.
   - o Requires maintenance of specific academic standards.

5. **Stony Brook University** – Scholars for Medicine
   - o A combined 8-year program with the Renaissance School of Medicine.
   - o Emphasizes research and clinical experience.

6. **Hofstra University** – BA/MD Program with Zucker School of Medicine
   - o An 8-year program integrating a BA education with medical school.
   - o Focuses on early clinical exposure and community service.

7. **Wayne State University** – BS/MD Program
   - o Admits a select number of students annually.
   - o Emphasizes urban clinical experiences and community health.

8. **Florida Atlantic University** – Wilkes Medical Scholars Program
   - o A 7-8 year program combining undergraduate studies with the Charles E. Schmidt College of Medicine.
   - o Offers personalized education in a smaller cohort.

9. **Rutgers University** – BA/MD Program with Robert Wood Johnson Medical School
   - o Provides a pathway from undergraduate studies to medical school.
   - o Requires maintenance of academic standards and MCAT scores.

10. **University of Connecticut** – Special Program in Medicine
    - o Offers a combined undergraduate and medical school experience.

## TEN HIGHLY COMPETITIVE BS/DO PROGRAMS

1. **Nova Southeastern University BS/DO:** NSU offers both 3+4 and 4+4 tracks, integrating undergraduate education with osteopathic medicine.
2. **New York Institute of Technology BS/DO:** A 7-year program combining undergraduate studies with NYIT College of Osteopathic Medicine.
3. **Lake Erie College of Osteopathic Medicine (LECOM) Early Acceptance Program:** Offers flexibility with multiple campuses and pathways.
4. **Michigan State University Osteopathic Medical Scholars Program (OMSP):** Focuses on serving underserved communities.
5. **Philadelphia College of Osteopathic Medicine (PCOM):** Collaborates with various undergraduate institutions for combined programs.
6. **Rowan University School of Osteopathic Medicine:** Offers a 7-year BS/DO with early clinical exposure through Rowan-Virtua School of Medicine.
7. **A.T. Still University Kirksville College of Osteopathic Medicine:** Emphasizes whole-person healthcare and community service.
8. **University of New England College of Osteopathic Medicine:** UNE COM provides a comprehensive curriculum with a focus on primary care.
9. **Touro College of Osteopathic Medicine:** Touro COM accepts applications for its DO program across multiple campuses, including Great Falls, MT.
10. **Western University of Health Sciences College of Osteopathic Medicine of the Pacific (COMP):** Provides a holistic approach to medical education with diverse clinical rotations.

## SIX BS/DDS AND BS/DMD PROGRAMS

**University of Pennsylvania – *Bio-Dental Program:*** Highly selective 7-year program requires top academic performance and commitment to dentistry.

**University of Pittsburgh – *Guaranteed Admission Program (GAP):*** 8-year BS/DMD with only 6–8 students admitted annually; DAT not required.

**Case Western Reserve University – *Pre-Professional Scholars Program (PPSP):*** 7-year BS/DMD program, offering conditional admission to dental school.

**University of Connecticut – *Special Program in Dental Medicine:*** 8-year BS/DMD program emphasizing academic excellence.

**Stony Brook University – *Scholars for Dental Medicine:*** 8-year BS/DDS program with conditional acceptance to Stony Brook School of Dental Medicine.

**University of the Pacific – *Pre-Dental Advantage Program:*** Accelerated 5-, 6-, or 7-year BS/DDS tracks. One of the few 5-year programs; strong science background.

By systematically evaluating programs based on specified criteria, students and families can make informed decisions that align with their academic goals, personal preferences, and career aspirations. Remember, the best program is one that offers a pathway to medical/dental school and also supports you throughout the journey.

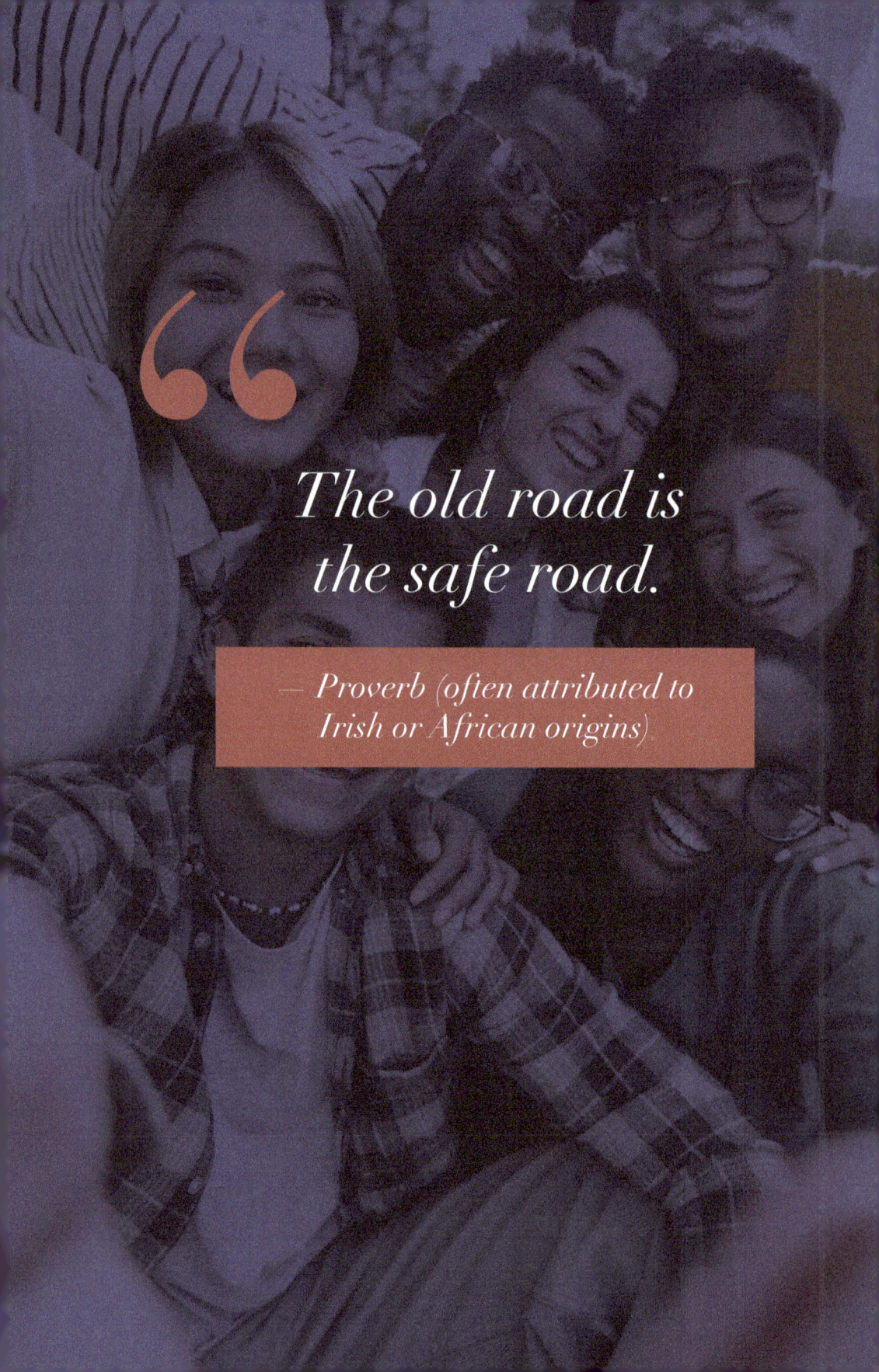

"

The old road is
the safe road.

— *Proverb (often attributed to Irish or African origins)*

CHAPTER THIRTY-TWO

# INTERNATIONAL STUDENT PATHWAY

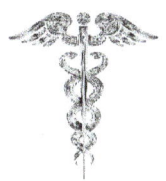

Pursuing a combined BS/MD, BS/DO, or BS/DDS as an international student presents unique challenges and opportunities. These programs offer a streamlined path to a medical degree, but for non-U.S. citizens or permanent residents, the journey is more complex.

## CHALLENGES FOR INTERNATIONAL APPLICANTS

**Limited Program Availability:** Most BS/MD, BS/DO, and BS/DDS programs are designed primarily for U.S. citizens, in-state students, or permanent residents. Only a select few programs consider international applicants, making the competition even more intense for these limited spots.

**Visa and Residency Issues:** Securing the correct visa status can be a hurdle. Some programs may require proof of the ability to obtain the necessary visas. Moreover, changes in immigration policies add uncertainty to the application, admission, and attendances processes.

**Financial Constraints:** International students often face higher tuition rates and limited access to financial aid or scholarships. Students must demonstrate the ability to finance their entire duration of the program by submitting financial documentation and bank statements.

**Standardized Testing and Curriculum:** Differences in grading and course systems mean that international students must meet standardized testing requirements like the SAT, ACT, and TOEFL while taking prerequisites that may not align with their previous education.

## PROGRAMS OPEN TO INTERNATIONAL STUDENTS

Despite the challenges, several programs do consider international applicants. Here are a few options you might consider.

**Brown University's Program in Liberal Medical Education (PLME):** An eight-year program that combines undergraduate education with medical school. It is the only Ivy League program and, it is open to international student applicants.

**Case Western Reserve University's Pre-Professional Scholars Program (PPSP):** Offers conditional admission to the university's medical school and is known to accept a limited number of international students.

**University of Rochester's Rochester Early Medical Scholars (REMS):** An eight-year BA/BS+MD program that has admitted international students in the past.

**New York Institute of Technology's BS/DO Program:** This seven-year program combines undergraduate studies with a Doctor of Osteopathic Medicine degree and is accessible to international students.

## ADMISSION STATISTICS

Admission rates for international students in these programs are notably low. For instance, Brown University's PLME program had an acceptance rate of 2.19% for the class of 2026, with international students comprising a small fraction of those admitted.

In general, international students face steeper competition due to the limited number of programs accepting them and the small number of seats allocated. Applicants often need exceptional academic records, high standardized test scores, and compelling personal statements to stand out.

## STRATEGIES FOR SUCCESS

**Early Preparation:** Begin preparing for standardized tests and gathering necessary documentation well in advance.

**Research Thoroughly:** Identify programs that accept international students and understand their specific requirements.

**Strengthen the Application:** Highlight unique experiences, especially those that demonstrate a commitment to the medical field, such as internships, research, or volunteer work.

**Secure Strong Recommendations:** Obtain letters of recommendation from individuals who can attest to your academic abilities and dedication to medicine.

**Demonstrate Financial Preparedness:** Be ready to show proof of financial resources to cover tuition and living expenses.

## FINAL CONSIDERATIONS

The path to BS/MD, BS/DO, and BS/DDS programs is highly competitive for students who live in the United States and with priority given to in-state residents for some schools, the road is even harder. Acceptance rates are 3 - 5 % for U.S. students and even lower for international students. Many programs have no international students at all, even if they accept applications from international students.

Thus, international students might consider applying in the United States as one option. However, there are similar direct-to-medical-school options in countries around the world. Most have a much higher acceptance rate for international students.

While the path to a BS/MD, BS/DO, or BS/DDS in the United States is more challenging for international students, it is not impossible. With diligent preparation, thorough research, and a strong application, international students can successfully gain admission to these competitive programs. It is essential to stay informed about each program's specific requirements and to seek guidance when needed to navigate the complex admissions landscape.

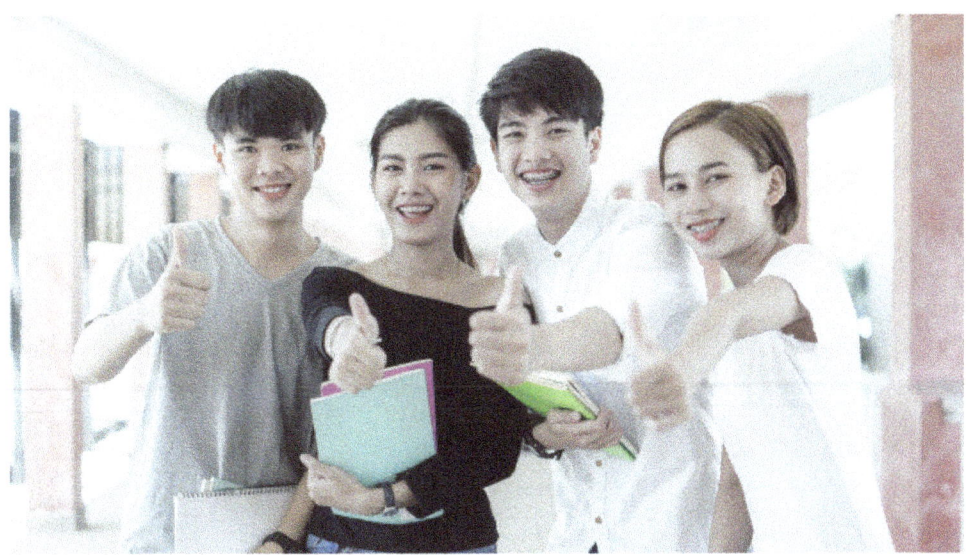

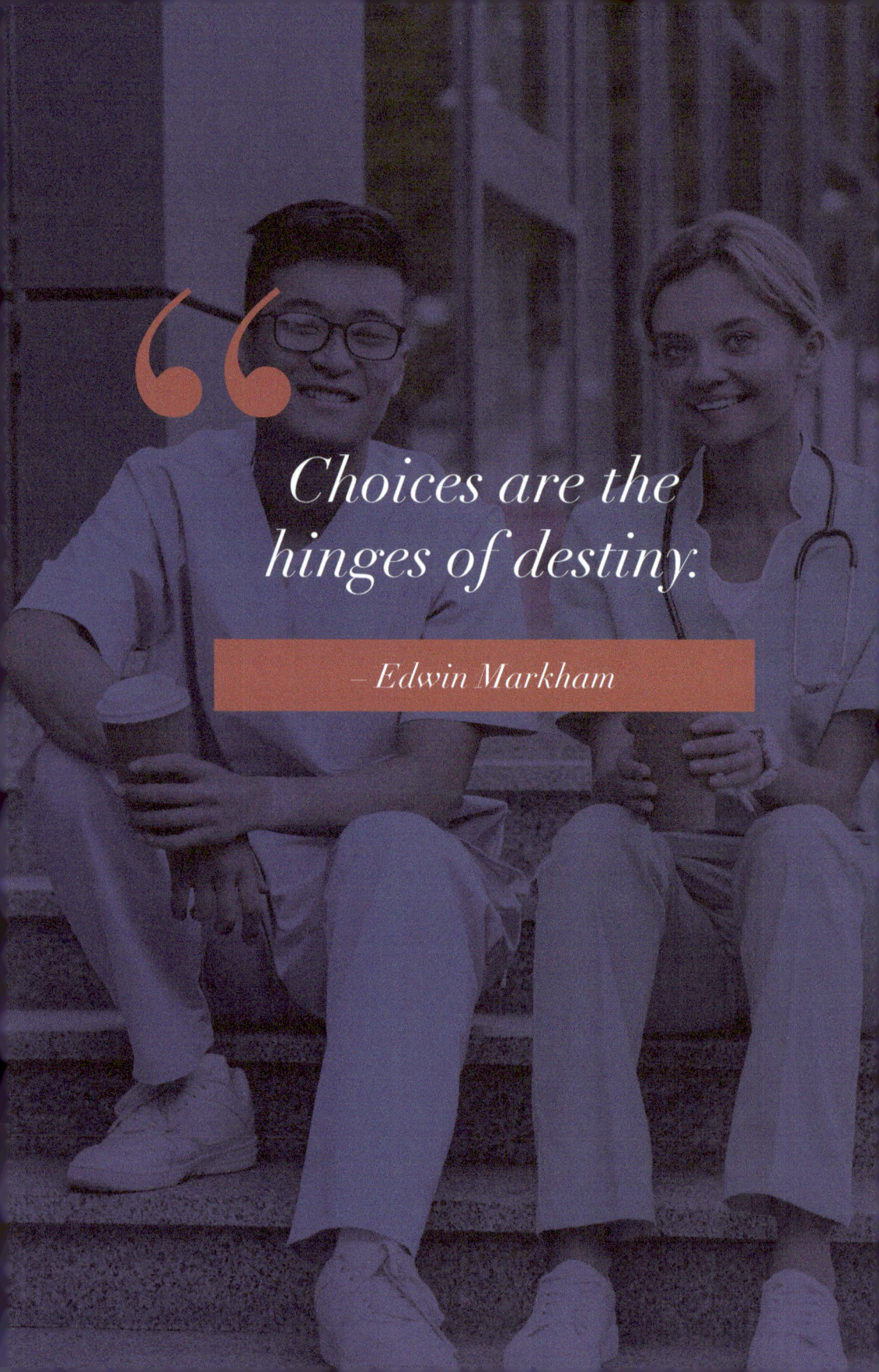

" Choices are the hinges of destiny.

*— Edwin Markham*

# CHAPTER THIRTY-THREE

# RECONSIDERING THE TRADITIONAL PATHWAY

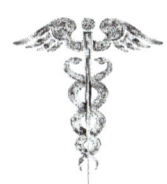

Now that you have learned how to research direct med options and have a sense of what these programs consider, let's take a look at the traditional pathway to medical school. After all, students who have the GPA, coursework, and test scores to gain admission to a direct med program are also prime candidates for the top four-year universities in the United States.

Think about what you seek in a university and whether that university is likely to be supportive in your quest to gain admission to medical school. You may want to attend a four-year program that is empowering, inspiring, and filled with academically motivated students who are friendly, collaborative, and interesting. After all, you will be there for four years taking challenging courses alongside students who are motivated, but also uncertain about their future.

While BS/MD, BS/DO, and BS/DDS programs offer appealing advantages such as a direct route to medical school and reduced admissions stress, the traditional four-year undergraduate pathway provides greater flexibility. Students cultivate maturity and perseverance as they explore their personal and academic interests. This time of learning and reflection can lead to a more well-rounded and resilient future physician.

Additionally, the traditional route offers academic flexibility. Students can take their time to explore a variety of majors and minors whether these sets of courses are in the sciences, humanities, or social sciences. Since the four-year undergraduate route also allows students to consider different career paths, students are not obligated to a singular route and may appreciate the flexibility to change their career objectives.

This freedom often results in a deeper intellectual curiosity and the chance to integrate other fields like public health, economics, ethics, or global studies into one's education. Many future physicians find their unique voice and career niche because of these broader academic explorations, whether this is in research, policy, or health equity.

The traditional path offers more time for growth. High school students admitted to BS/MD, BS/DO, and BS/DDS programs must commit to a medical/dental career as teenagers. In contrast, the traditional route allows students to mature emotionally, develop leadership skills, and gain more diverse clinical, research, and service experiences before applying to medical/dental school. This timeline can produce stronger applicants with richer personal narratives and more confident career goals.

Admission to BS/MD, BS/DO, and BS/DDS programs is highly competitive. There is limited flexibility to transfer or switch interests. The traditional route provides freedom to shift directions, reassess ambitions, and explore alternate careers if needed. Students may not have considered the myriad of alternative career paths while in high school.

Furthermore, traditional applicants often apply to more than one medical school, increasing the chance of receiving multiple acceptances and scholarship offers. In contrast, many BS/MD, BS/DO, and BS/DDS programs are "single school" commitments. Students may lack the ability to negotiate or compare medical school environments or financial aid packages.

Medical schools value applicants who take the traditional path and excel. The pressure to complete a specified medical/dental school oriented pathway associated with BS/MD, BS/DO, or BS/DDS programs is reduced. There is also less pressure to meet accelerated timelines or conditional GPA and MCAT requirements.

Navigating college while exploring interests and completing requirements often results in students who know where they are headed and why. The admissions process is designed to reward resilience, initiative, and demonstrated commitment. These traits are often cultivated over four years of undergraduate study.

On the other hand, the pressure to reach the high bars put up by direct med programs is not always bad since students are constantly aware of what they need to accomplish to reach their goals. Also, classmates often support each other. Since the direct med cohorts are small and the outcome is not a zero sum game with winners and losers, everyone can achieve their goal when they study together. This is not always true in a traditional four-year school.

Ultimately, the BS/MD, BS/DO, or BS/DDS path offers a fast track, while the traditional route provides broader exploration, personal growth, and long-term flexibility that may ultimately shape a more well-rounded and fulfilled physician.

## BEWARE OF COLLEGE STATISTICS

Be careful when you rely on the college's statistics regarding the percent of students accepted to medical school. While many colleges are transparent about their data, some are not. Students excitedly proclaim, "Wow, 95% of the students from College X were accepted to medical school! That's where I want to attend college."

Some colleges literally say, "95% of their medical school applicants are accepted each year." While it may be true that 19 out of 20 students who submitted their medical college application (AMCAS) gained admission, that may also be because the university only wrote committee letters of recommendation for 20 out of the 100 seniors who requested them.

Meanwhile, only 100 students even made it through the prerequisites with high enough grades to apply to medical school. The fact is, though, that 1,000 freshmen started out as pre-med students. Thus, 19 out of 1,000 freshmen who initially wanted to be doctors were ultimately accepted to medical school. Ultimately, the actual probability a freshman at College X is admitted to medical school is 1.9%.

## FIND THE RIGHT FIT

Some popular colleges are, ironically, not very friendly. The students fiercely compete against each other for a very few high grades. The rest receive Cs, Ds, and Fs. This environment is particularly hard on the student who has never received less than an A and has been told their whole life they are perfect. Without healthy doses of pragmatism and discipline, they flounder, watching their future vision fade into obscurity. Anxiety and frustration typically follow.

No matter where you attend college, determine if the school is a good fit for your personality. The environment, academics, and opportunities are equally important.

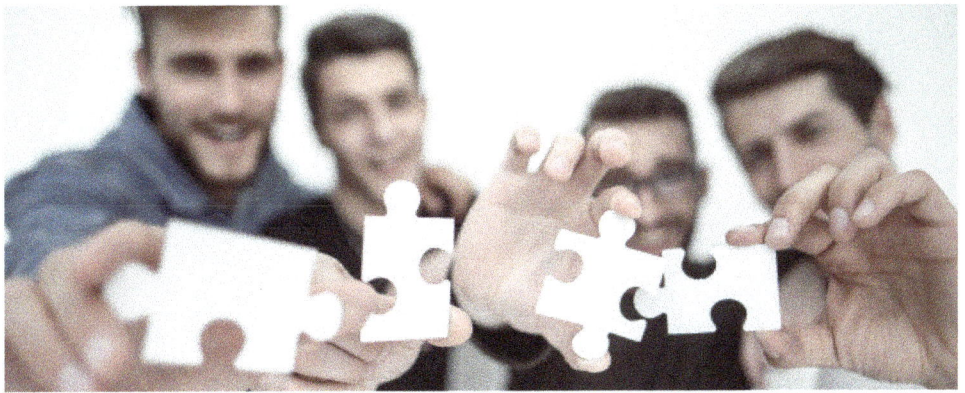

> " 
>
> *Wherever the art of medicine is loved, there is also a love for humanity.*
>
> — *Hippocrates*

# CHAPTER THIRTY-FOUR

# DENTAL SCHOOL, PA, PHARMD, VET SCHOOL

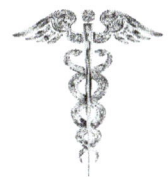

## EXPLORING ALTERNATIVE MEDICAL PURSUITS

For high school students aspiring to pursue medicine or dentistry, the traditional path to becoming a physician or dentist is well-known. However, it is essential to recognize that there are other rewarding and impactful careers within the healthcare industry Some choose college programs like Physician Assistant (PA), Pharmacy (PharmD), and Veterinary Medicine (DVM). These offer opportunities that may align more closely with individual interests, strengths, and lifestyle preferences.

## DENTISTRY

**Benefits:** Dentistry offers a blend of science, artistry, and patient interaction. Dentists often enjoy a balanced work-life schedule, the potential for private practice ownership, and the ability to specialize in areas like orthodontics or oral surgery. The profession allows for significant autonomy and the opportunity to build long-term patient relationships.

**High School Preparation:** Students should focus on science courses, particularly biology and chemistry, and seek opportunities for manual dexterity development, such as art or woodworking. Shadowing a dentist/orthodontist or participating in dental-focused programs can provide valuable insight.

**College Coursework and Admission:** Dental schools typically require prerequisite courses in biology, chemistry, physics, and math. Admissions committees look for strong academic performance, relevant experience, and a demonstrated commitment to the field.

**Testing:** The Dental Admission Test (DAT) offered by the American Dental Association is a standard requirement, though some school's testing requirements differ. A few may accept the MCAT in place of the DAT, particularly for students with a non-traditional background or those applying to dual-degree programs. Canadian, UK, and Australian dental schools have different but similar testing requirements.

**Challenges:** Dental school is rigorous, with a curriculum that demands both academic and clinical proficiency. The cost of education can be substantial, and establishing a practice requires business acumen and financial investment.

## PHYSICIAN ASSISTANT (PA)

**Benefits:** PAs are integral members of healthcare teams, providing diagnostic, therapeutic, and preventive services under physician supervision. The role offers flexibility in specialization and work settings, a shorter educational path compared to physicians, and a growing job market with competitive salaries.

**High School Preparation:** Emphasis should be on science and math courses. Volunteering in healthcare settings and obtaining certifications like CPR can be advantageous.

**College Coursework and Admission:** PA programs require a bachelor's degree with coursework in sciences such as anatomy, physiology, and microbiology. Clinical experience is often a prerequisite, and the Graduate Record Examination (GRE) may be required. Admission to PA schools is competitive, with programs seeking candidates with healthcare experience and strong interpersonal skills.

**Challenges:** The PA role requires adaptability, as responsibilities can vary by state and practice setting. Maintaining certification involves ongoing education, and the scope of practice is defined by supervising physicians and state laws.

## PHARMACY (PHARMD)

**Benefits:** Pharmacists play a critical role in patient care, focusing on medication management and counseling. The profession offers diverse career paths, including clinical, research, industry, academic, nuclear, managed care, and regulatory. Pharmacists often have stable hours and the opportunity to work in various settings.

**High School Preparation:** Students should concentrate on chemistry, biology, and math courses. Exposure to the healthcare environment through volunteering or part-time work in pharmacies can be beneficial.

College Coursework and Admission: PharmD programs require prerequisite courses in sciences and math. The Pharmacy College Admission Test (PCAT) may be required. Admissions committees look for academic excellence, communication skills, and a commitment to patient care.

Challenges: The pharmacy field is evolving, with increased competition and changes in the healthcare landscape affecting job prospects in certain areas. Staying current with advancements in pharmacology and healthcare regulations is essential.

## VETERINARY MEDICINE

Benefits: Veterinarians have the opportunity to work with a variety of animals, contributing to animal health and public safety. The field offers diverse specialties, including surgery, internal medicine, and public health. "Small animal" and "large animal" veterinarians can work in private practice, research, or government.

High School Preparation: A strong foundation in biology, chemistry, and math is crucial. Gaining experience with animals through volunteering at shelters, farms, or veterinary clinics is highly recommended.

College Coursework and Admission: Veterinary schools require extensive coursework in sciences. The Graduate Record Examination (GRE) is commonly required. Admission to DVM programs is highly competitive, with emphasis on academic performance, animal experience, and letters of recommendation.

Challenges: Veterinary education is demanding, and the cost of schooling can be significant. The emotional aspects of the profession, such as treating sick animals and empathizing their owners, can be challenging. Additionally, veterinarians often work long hours, including emergencies.

## FINAL THOUGHTS ON ALTERNATIVE MEDICAL PURSUITS

Exploring dentistry, physician assistant, pharmacy, or veterinary medicine offers high school and college students alternative pathways to fulfilling roles in healthcare. Each profession has benefits and challenges. Success requires dedication, academic excellence, and a genuine passion. By understanding the requirements and opportunities associated with each path, students can make informed decisions that align with their interests and goals in the healthcare industry.

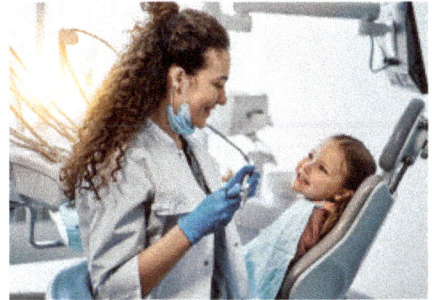

"

*There are no extra pieces in the universe. Everyone is here because he or she has a place to fill, and every piece must fit itself into the big jigsaw puzzle.*

*– Deepak Chopra*

# CHAPTER THIRTY-FIVE

# LOOKING AHEAD - MCAT, MED SCHOOL

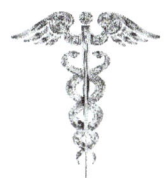

## INVESTIGATE MEDICAL SCHOOL REQUIREMENTS EARLY

Medical school may seem far away, but it is closer than you think. Without planning, you may need a couple of years after graduating from college to gain the academics and research/clinical experiences necessary to be a competitive candidate. Here are a few things to consider along the healthcare pathway.

When you apply, you will submit your application to:

AMCAS (American Medical College Application Service) - MD
AACOMAS (American Association of Colleges of Osteopathic Medicine Application Service) – DO
TMDSAS (Texas Medical and Dental Schools Application Service) - MD, DO, DDS, DMD
AADSAS (Associated American Dental Schools Application Service) - DMD, DDS
CASPA (Centralized Application Service for Physician Assistants) - PA
PharmCAS (Pharmacy College Application Service) - PharmD
VMCAS (Veterinary Medical College Application Service) - DM

Keep in mind your future college curriculum. Direct med programs may allow you to choose from a wide variety of majors, although you still need to take a set of standard requirements that could include anatomy, physiology, genetics, cell/molecular biology, microbiology, general chemistry, organic chemistry, biochemistry, physics, English, psychology, statistics, and calculus.

Check the BS/MD, BS/DO, or medical schools to which you plan to apply to see their specific requirements early enough in college to ensure that you are not missing a critical course. It does not hurt to research medical school academic requirements while you are in high school, well before you start college so you have a game plan. You may also want to seek counsel from your BS/MD, BS/DO, or premedical advisor, but the due diligence to know what is required is on your shoulders. Take responsibility to create an organized and manageable plan. You will have a course of action and appreciate the extra effort later.

You will want to be mentally and academically prepared for your future curriculum before you get into college. First, you do not want to be surprised, Second, you are likely to be required to take three years of college chemistry. The three toughest college classes are often, but not always, physics, organic chemistry, and biochemistry. This is why medical schools want to know how students fair in individual courses across a challenging curriculum.

Some students use AP credit to get out of taking college chemistry. Beware, jumping into a university OChem class is rarely successful. Also, physics is tough stacked alongside biology and chemistry, especially if you have not taken AP Physics in high school. AP Chemistry is extremely valuable. Especially at universities where classes are graded on a curve, you do not want to fall behind and have a difficult time reaching the higher end of the curve when most of your classmates already have a year or two of high school chemistry. Remember, BS/MD and BS/DO programs typically have a GPA requirement to remain eligible.

When you apply to medical school, the medical school application service, AMCAS, will verify and calculate a separate science GPA, called BCPM (Biology, Chemistry, Physics, and Math), which is very important for admissions. Thus, you want to be extra prepared by taking more challenging courses in high school and entering with the knowledge you need so that the classes you take or the competition you face does not overwhelm you. If you can manage this, you could even take two sciences in each of your last two years to lay a stronger foundation for what you will face ahead. The verified GPA chart will include:

## VERIFIED GRADE POINT AVERAGES

*GPA Calculations will appear only when your application status is Processed*

School Year   BCPM GPA   BCPM Hours   AO GPA   AO Hours   Total GPA   Total Hours

While you might be better served by completing requirements in college, a master's degree program in an affiliated area might be helpful. You might choose to earn an MPH (Master of Public Health) or an MS (Master of Science) in Biomedical Sciences, or other science/health fields. Other gap, bridge or interim options include Post-Bacc programs, research while gaining clinical exposure. These experiences may open the doors to alternative career options in case you are not admitted.

# WHAT DO MEDICAL SCHOOLS LOOK FOR IN AN APPLICANT?

Rigorous Curriculum - Challenging courses including required and recommended classes. Course Record on AMCAS - Standardized for each entry by school, year, grades, & credits. Verified GPA and Credit Hours - AMCAS list from high school to graduate school.

What Coursework is Considered When You Apply?
1. All courses in which you were ENROLLED whether or not you earned credit.
2. Courses from which you withdrew (W) or earned an incomplete (I).
3. Courses in which no grade was assigned.
4. Courses you repeated EVEN IF they were removed from your transcript for ANY reason.
5. Courses you failed, even if you repeated the class.
6. Courses in which you are currently enrolled OR EXPECT TO ENROLL before entering medical school.
7. Remedial/developmental courses.
8. College-level courses taken in high school, even if they were not counted toward a degree. This includes dual enrollment taught at your high school but offered by a college, and those AP courses in which you received college credit and appear on your transcript.
9. Courses taken at an American college overseas.

# ACADEMIC RECORD

You will input the following on AMCAS for each class in chronological order exactly as it appears on the original transcript(s). Note: *Semester Hours and AMCAS grades appear only when your application is processed.*

School Status Yr Term Course #  Type OT Hrs  Sem Hrs OT Grade AMCAS Gr & Use

# MCAT - MEDICAL COLLEGE ADMISSIONS TEST

Students must take the MCAT to apply to medical schools. This test includes multiple components and requires sufficient time to prepare. Scores are given from 118 to 132 on each of four sections with a total score range of 472 to 528. The mean for each section is 125 with a mean total score of 500 (Percentiles: 520 - 98th, 515 - 91st, 505 - 66th, 495 - 34th).

# CASPER AND PREVIEW TESTS

For MD and DO schools, you may need to take either the CASPer or PREview, which are situational judgment tests. You may need to take both tests. Note that the CASPer test is also required for some schools on TMDSAS as well as a few dental, PA, PharmD, and DVM applicants. Put this test on your very crowded schedule.

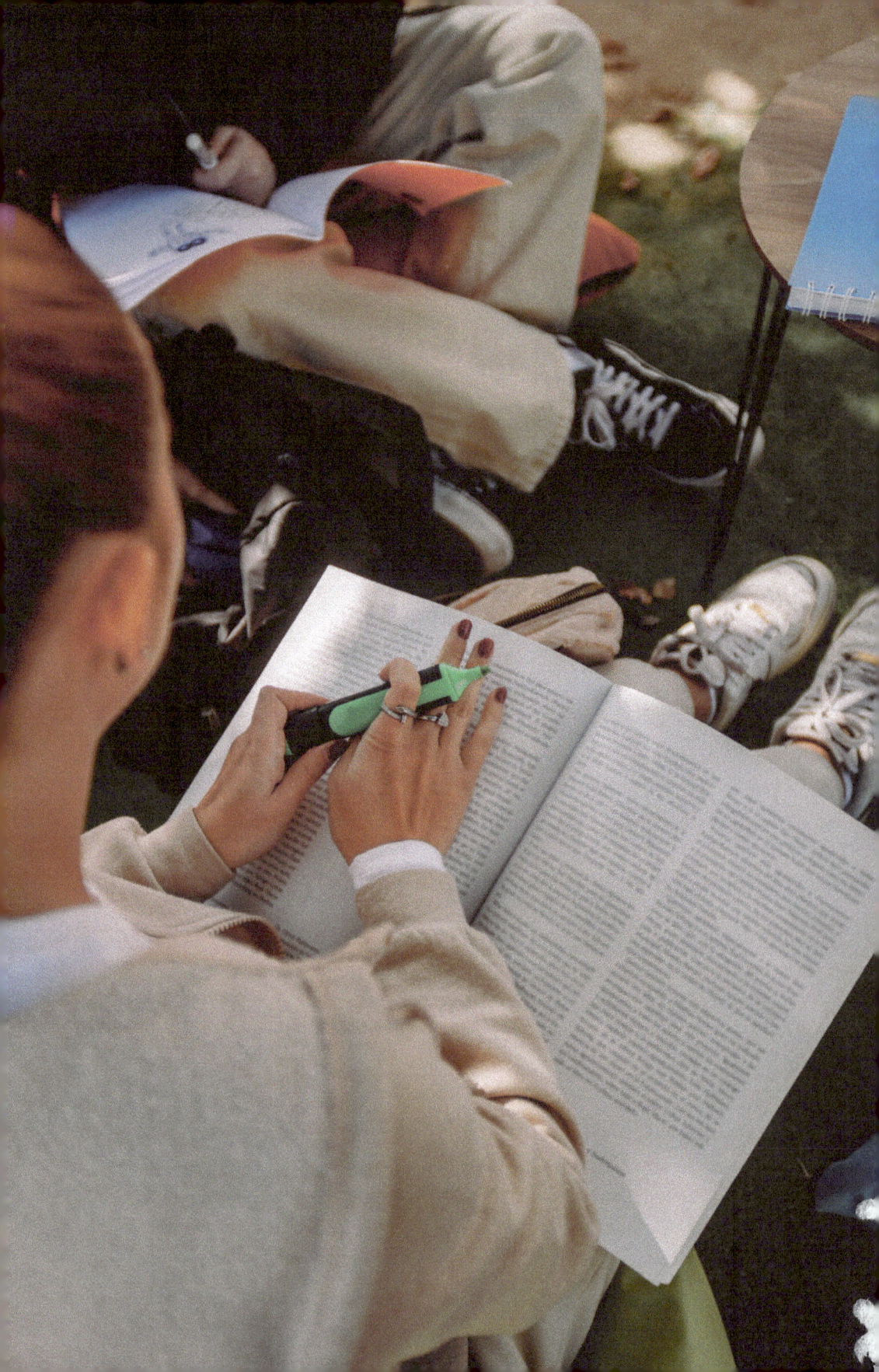

# PART FIVE

# APPLICATION & ADMISSIONS PROCESS

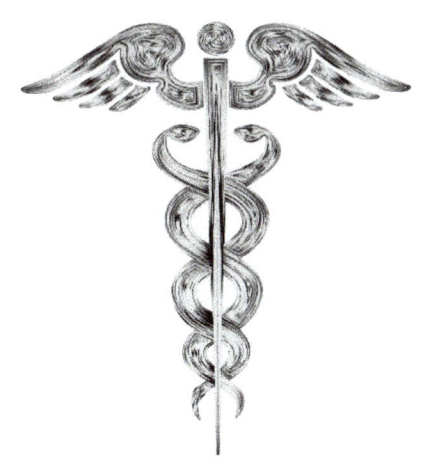

# COLLEGE APPLICATION

"Medicine is a science of uncertainty and the art of probability.

— William Osler

# CHAPTER THIRTY-SIX

# THE COLLEGE ADMISSIONS PROCESS

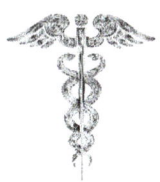

Applying for a BS/MD, BS/DO, or BS/DDS involves a multi-step, highly selective process that blends undergraduate and medical school admissions.

## STEP-BY-STEP PROCESS

### 1. Research and Build Your College List (Spring–Summer Before Senior Year)

Identify BS/MD and BS/DO programs that align with your interests, geographic preferences, and qualifications. Also, select four-year programs, considering:

* Program structure (6–8 years, conditional vs. guaranteed admission)
* MCAT requirements
* GPA/SAT/ACT thresholds
* Application platforms (Common App, Coalition App, institutional apps)
* Whether international or out-of-state students are accepted

### 2. Strengthen Your Academic/Extracurricular Profile (9th–11th Grades)

* Aim for a high GPA with advanced STEM coursework (AP/IB/honors, or college classes).
* Take the SAT or ACT. Most programs expect 1500+ SAT or 34+ ACT.
* Clinical experiences (volunteering, shadowing, internships, medical missions)
* Research (if possible, publish, present, journal clubs, literature reviews)
* Community service, homeless shelters, soup kitchens, disabled groups, the elderly, Red Cross, sports camps, refugee services, Habitat for Humanity
* Leadership, athletics, science competitions, robotics, rocketry, etc.

### 3. Prepare Materials (Summer Before Senior Year)

* Create a spreadsheet to track deadlines, essay prompts, and required materials. Draft a compelling Common App personal statement.
* Prepare supplemental essays for BS/MD or BS/DO components (e.g., "Why medicine?", "Why our program?", "What experiences do you have with diverse or rural populations?"
* Ask for letters of recommendation (usually 2–4), including one from a science teacher and one from a clinician or mentor.

### 4. Apply to Undergraduate Institutions (Aug–Nov of Senior Year)

* Use the Common App, Coalition App, or school-specific portals.
* Submit materials for undergraduate admission.
* Submit the supplemental applications to each BS/MD and BS/DO.
* Submit additional financial aid forms on the application or in the portals.
* Check to see if there are BS/MD applications and forms required after initial review.

### 5 Submit Medical School Essays and "Partner Medical School" Requirements

* Additional medical school" forms
* Additional essays
* A resume or CV
* A picture
* Short-answer questions about medical experiences or goals
* Tailor essays like "Why Medicine" and "Why This Program" to each school.

### 6. Interview Stage (Jan–March of Senior Year)

* Two sets of admissions interviews
  o Undergraduate programs
  o BS/MD, BS/DO, and BS/DDS program interviews by medical school faculty or committees
* Interviews can be MMI (Multiple Mini Interviews), traditional panel, or hybrid.
* Practice for your interviews, especially if your program uses MMIs or scenario-based interviews.

### 7. Notification and Decisions (Feb–April)

* Programs notify students in waves.
* Some offer undergraduate admission without BS/MD admission.
* Students to enroll in the college without the medical linkage.

* Stay motivated as you get responses. With acceptance rates between 2-10%, you are likely to get rejections. You can only attend one college anyway.

## 8. Choose and Commit (by May 1)

* Decide between:
  o BS/MD, BS/DO, and BS/DDS admission
  o Traditional undergraduate admission and later med school application

* Maintain Conditional Requirements (College Years)

* Once admitted, students must:
  o Maintain a required GPA (often 3.5+ science and cumulative)
  o Fulfill clinical, research, and volunteer requirements
  o In some cases, take the MCAT and score above a threshold

Every college's process is unique. However, there are a few commonalities. In 2025, approximately 1,100 colleges used the Common App; about 150 colleges used the Coalition Application. A few used both. The University of California system has its own application as do the California State Universities and the Texas schools. UT Austin and Texas A&M joined the Common App in 2023.

The Common App and Coalition App may be started early. In your junior year, consider getting a head start reviewing requirements. College-specific questions may change each year. However, the basic application is generally the same and can be created ahead of time. The application rolls over August 1. Toward the end of July, make a copy of the application you completed just in case.

Some schools admit on a rolling basis. 'Rolling' means that periodically, after all materials are received, the admissions committee determines who they will accept, and then sends the notification of the admissions decision. Some students are accepted as early as August. The thrill of acceptance cannot be overstated.

Throughout high school and college, stay organized. Keep track of your courses, experiences, supervisors, and hours. You may need this later if you apply via AMCAS, AACOMAS, or ADEA ADDSAS. Within a BS/MD, BS/DO, and BS/DDS program, there may be hurdles to jump over, courses that seem impossible, professors who are uncompromising, complex steps to handle, tons of information to manage, and separate deadlines. Find a way to keep track of information that works for you.

Finally, set up your organizational systems so you are not overwhelmed. Managing college is more complicated than high school. Ask for help if you feel stressed. you do not want to throw away this opportunity when a counselor, advisor, professor, or parent can help you find a solution.

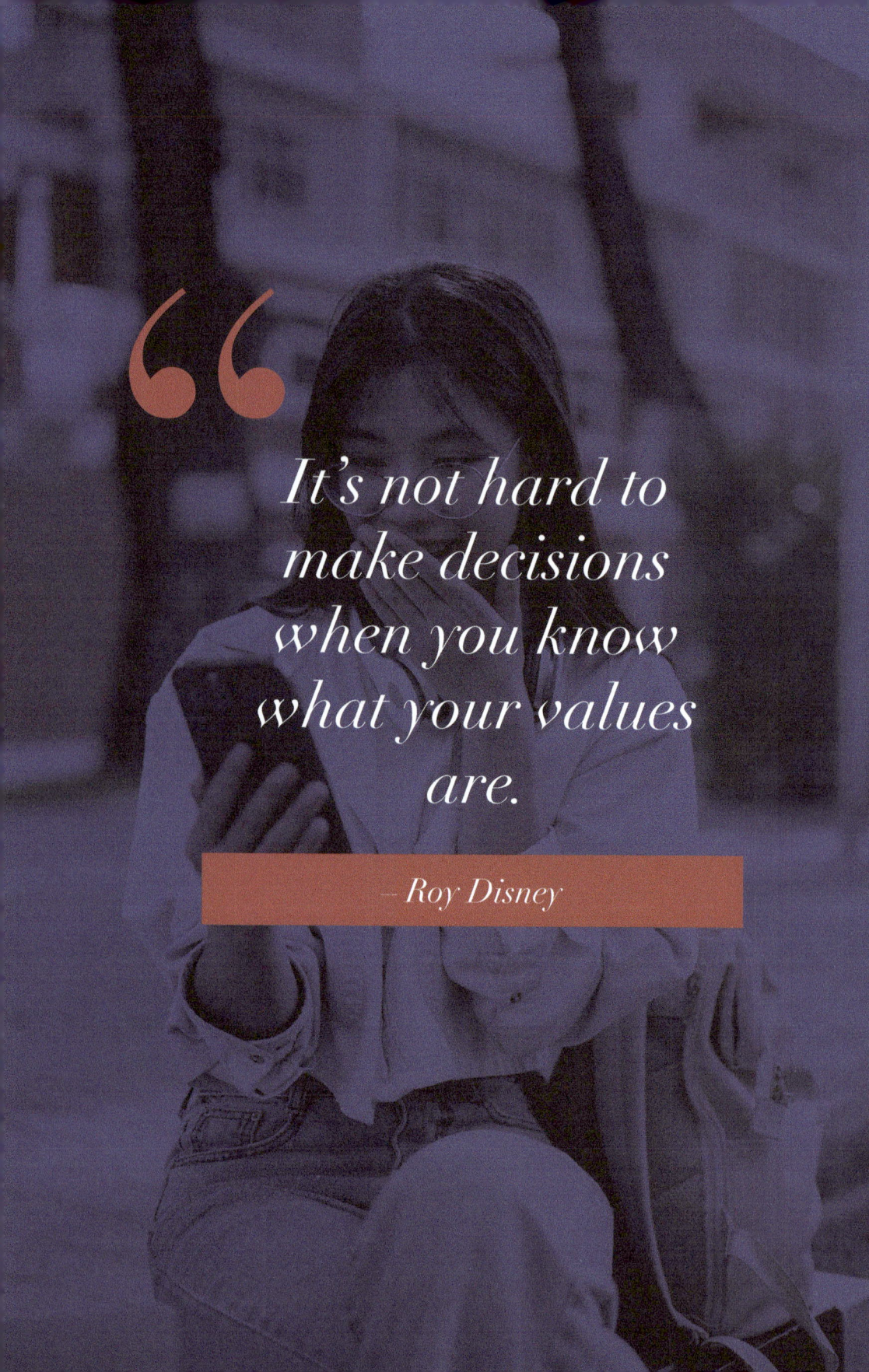

" It's not hard to make decisions when you know what your values are.

– Roy Disney

# CHAPTER THIRTY-SEVEN

# ED, EA, REA, RD, & ROLLING

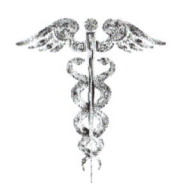

## EARLY DECISION (ED), EARLY ACTION (EA), RESTRICTED EARLY ACTION (REA)

With low acceptance rates, higher probably of admission for ED candidates, and changes in AP, IB, SAT, and ACT testing, students clamor to apply early to schools. Additionally, applications to the top schools have increased, resulting in colleges needing to make difficult admissions decisions in their quest to build a diverse, talented, and engaged student body. Furthermore, students applying early have access to many more scholarship options.

This confluence sent students in droves to apply early. This trend is likely to continue. In ED, EA, and REA, students apply to college in late summer or early fall and generally find out around winter break, though some decisions come out earlier and a few arrive later. This advantage not only gives students a chance for more scholarship money in some cases but the benefit of finding out early reduces the tension of the long waiting period until Regular Decision results arrive. Another benefit is that students might choose to apply ED II, which is a second early decision round.

EA and REA are different. In REA, a limitation is placed on the colleges you can apply to simultaneously. Many REA schools do not allow students to apply to other Early Action schools, though some will allow students to apply early to public colleges. Check the admissions sites to be sure. In addition, some schools like Georgetown will allow students to apply EA elsewhere but not to a binding ED program. However, most EA schools do not have these restrictions. Some students apply to a handful of EA schools during the admissions process.

# ADMISSIONS DATA TO CONSIDER

## The Ivy League Schools
## Comparison of Early vs Regular Decision Admit Rates and Waitlist Data

| Ivy League University | ED Admit Rate – Class of 2029 | Overall Admit Rate – Class of 2029 | ED Admit Rate – Class of 2026 | RD Admit Rate – Class of 2026 | Waitlist Admits Class of 2028 |
|---|---|---|---|---|---|
| Brown | 18% | 6% | 14.6% | 3.71% | 118 |
| Columbia | 11% | 4.3% | 10.3% | 3% | N/A |
| Cornell | 19% | 7% | 21.4% | 6.7% | 362 |
| Dartmouth | 17% | 6% | 20% | 4.8% | 29 |
| Harvard | 7.6% (previous yr) | 3% | 7.9% | 2.34% | 65 a previous year |
| UPenn | 14.5% | 4% | 15.6% | 4.2% | 40 |
| Princeton | No data available | | | | 40, 52 for class of '27 |
| Yale | 11% | 4.6% | 11% | 3.4% | 0 for class of 2027 |

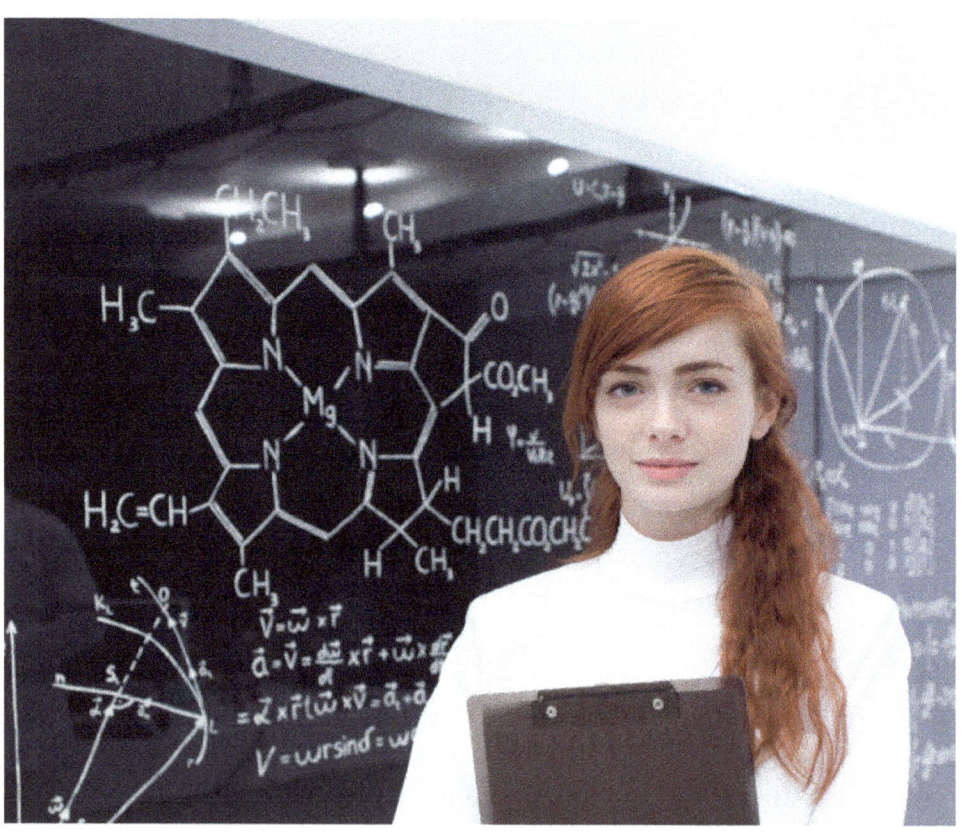

# ADMISSIONS DATA FOR TOP SCHOOLS - EARLY VS. REGULAR DECISION

| University | ED1/EDII/EA Admit Rate – Class of 2029 | RD/Total % Admit Rate – Class of 2029 | ED/EDII/EA Admit Rate – Class of 2026 | RD/Total % Admit Rate – Class of 2026 | Waitlist 2029 Spots, Accepted, Admitted |
|---|---|---|---|---|---|
| Amherst College | 27% (class of '27) | 7% | 32% | 6.1%/7% | 1,105, 623, 8 |
| Boston College | 31% | 13% | 28% | 16.7% | 13 accepted '27 |
| Boston Univ | 34% (class of '28) | 12% | 26%/25.3% | 13.4%/14.15% | 15,339, 8,996, 18 |
| Cal Poly SLO | N/A | 27.5% | N/A | 30% | 6,898, x, 2,905 |
| Claremont McK | 25% (class of '28) | 9.4% | 28.2%/29.5% | 7.5%/10.3% | 997, 621, 33 |
| College of W&M | 49.7% | 35% | 25.2% | 11.1%/17% | 4,232, 2,063, 207 |
| Colorado College | 32% (class of '28) | 19% | 49.3%/26%/15% | 11%/13.6% | 696, 140, 32 |
| Duke University | 12.8% | 3%, 4.8% overall | 21.3% | 4.3%/4.9% | N/A |
| Emory University | 30% | 10% | 36.5%/14% | 9.5%/10.7% | 6,98, 3,355, 109 |
| Georgetown | 11% | 12% | 10% | 12.11% | 2,690, 3,355, 109 |
| GWU | 64% | ~45% | 66.1%/65% | 48.2%/49% | N/A |
| Georgia Tech | 33% (in-state) 8.1% (out) | 30% (in-state) 9% (out) | 39% (in-state) 12% (out) | 17.14% | 6,491, 4,471, 201 |
| Harvey Mudd | 16% | 12% | 19.1% | 12.6%/13% | 663, 403, 53 |
| Johns Hopkins | 13.6% | 4% | 21%/14.8% | 5.9%/7.2% | 2,374, 1,614, 30 |
| MIT | 6% | 3.5% | 4.7% | 4% | N/A |
| Northeastern | 39% ED | ~5.1% | 32.6%/6% | 6%/6.8% | N/A |
| Northwestern | 20% | 5.3% | 22.1%/12.8% | 5.6%/7.2% | 83 accepted '27 |
| Notre Dame | 12.9% | 6.7% | 17.3% | 13% | 2,206, 1,385, 42 |
| NYU | ~38% | 7.7% | 38% | 12.2%/12.4% | N/A |
| Rice University | 13.2% (6% ED II) | 7.3% | 24%/18.8% | 7.7%/8.6% | N/A |
| SMU | -87% | ~35% | 70.9% | 50%/51.6% | 1,480, 607, 67 |
| Stanford | ~5% | 3.9% | N/A | 3.7% | 8 accepted '27 |
| Texas Christian | 29% | 43% | 70.4% | 55.3%/56% | 3,707, 909, 753 |
| Tufts University | N/A | 10.5% | N/A | 9.7% | 183 accepted '27 |
| Tulane University | 59.4% | 14% | 67.9%/17% | 7.9%/8.4% | 4,192, 2,290, 432 |
| UChicago | N/A | 4.5% | N/A | 5.4% | N/A |
| Univ of Miami | 59% | 19% | 56.7% | 17.6%/18.9% | 18,078, 7,364, 681 |
| Univ of So Cal | 8% | 12.5% | N/A | 11.9%/12% | N/A |
| Univ of Virginia | 29.5% (in-state) 21% (out) | 9.3% | 37.8% (in-state) 18.1% (out) | 18.7% | 10,470, 6,759, 242 |
| Vanderbilt | 15.2% | 3.7% | 24%/17.6% | 5.3%/6% | ~200 accepted '27 |
| Virginia Tech | N/A | 10.2% | 50% | 56% | xx |
| Wash U St. Louis | 25% | 8% | 25% | 8% | 168 accepted '27 |
| Wesleyan | 36% | 15.2% | 44% | 12.4% | 81 accepted '27 |
| Williams College | 26.6% | 7.3% | 31% | 8.5% | 2,303, 858, 113 |

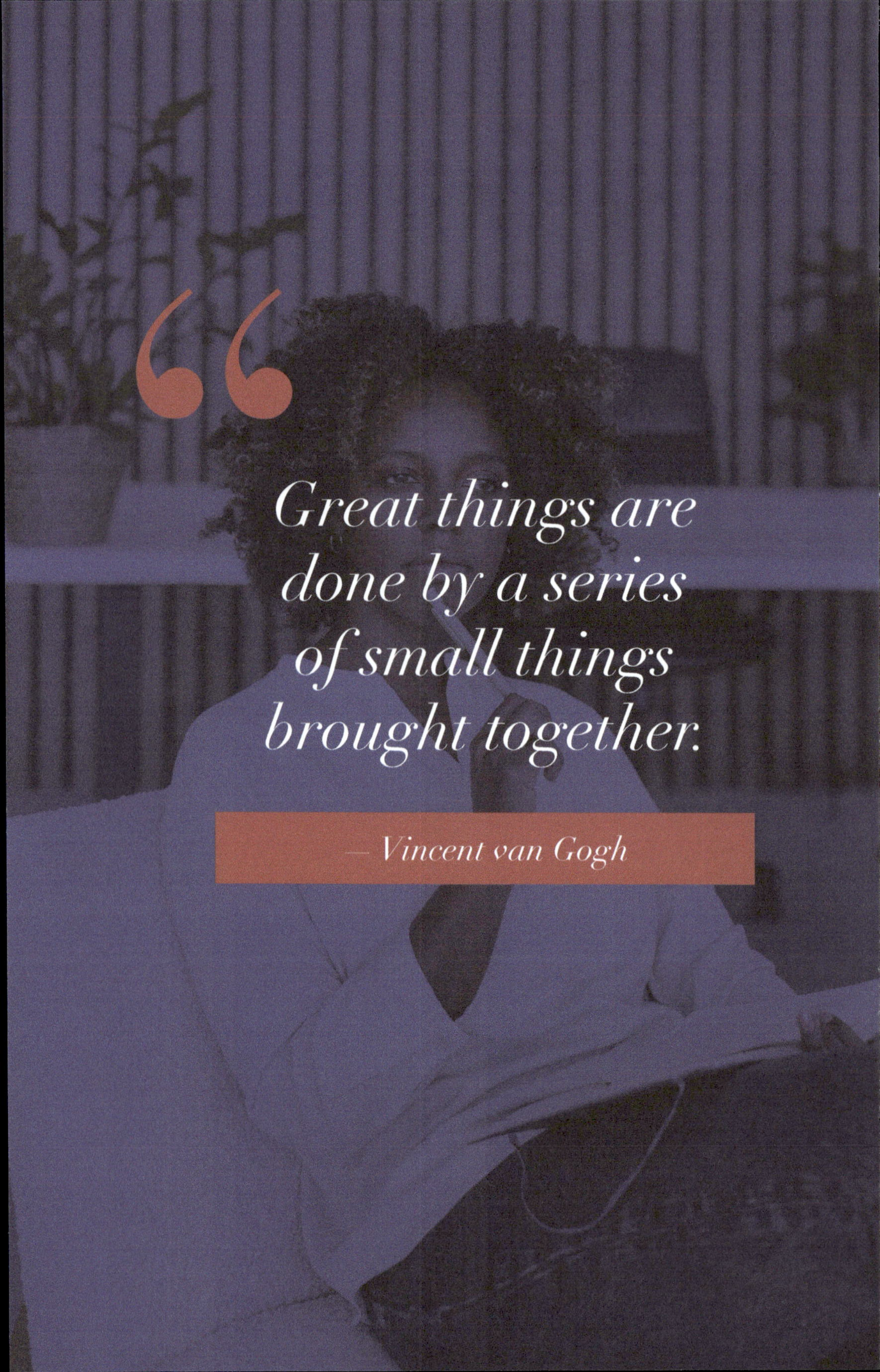

" "

*Great things are done by a series of small things brought together.*

— *Vincent van Gogh*

CHAPTER THIRTY-EIGHT
# YOUR COLLEGE COUNSELOR

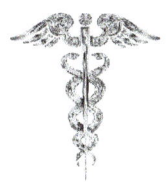

## PARTNERING WITH YOUR COUNSELOR

Throughout this journey, one of your most valuable allies will be your school counselor. This individual has helped countless students navigate the admissions process and can offer you structure and insight as well as critical support when you need it the most. In fact, this person will write one of your most crucial recommendation letters, including explanations about your coursework, GPA, leadership, character, consistency, and commitment.

Your counselor is an advocate and may speak to colleges if asked to clarify information on your application or share an explanation about your coursework or circumstances. If you stumbled academically, make sure they know why. Get them on your side. So, share your story with them so they can see your progress turnaround or how you learned from a failure.

Meet with your counselor early. Ask questions about the various pathways you can take to reach your goal. Share your interests regarding urban settings, academics, independent learning, quarter vs. semester system, student body, social life, sports, school spirit, support services, special programs, financial aid, and scholarships. Be open with your counselor about what you want in a school and whether you want to live at home or move away. It is perfectly okay to ask questions about your future.

It would be beneficial for you to analyze your academic profile: grades, test scores, rank, activities, and leadership with your counselor. While you should not let them discourage you, you should consider their wisdom. At this point, whatever grade level you are at while reading this book, you should create a resume. Share your resume with your counselor to get feedback.

While your counselor may be either enthusiastic or critical, they often have a few good ideas. Take their advice and use the parts that make sense for you and your family. However, you need them on your side for college. Your counselor can recommend you to Girls State, Boys State, HOBY, and leadership programs. Demonstrate the qualities of compassion, thoughtfulness, and leadership. Demonstrate these in your extracurricular activities and add them to your resume.

You can use your resume for a job, send to interviewers, or sometimes upload to college applications. Most schools want to know what activities you have pursued, supported, and led. Right now is a good time to make an organized list. Your counselor can share what you might be missing. Since they have typically worked with thousands of students, they often have some great tips and new ideas about what you can do to broaden your horizon.

What can you do now to gain a greater awareness of your community? What hospitals or clinics are accepting volunteers? Are there domestic violence shelters, rape crisis centers, or soup kitchens looking for volunteers? What biomedical research centers are in your local community? Your counselor might know of professors or faculty at a local college who are seeking interns or lab assistants for the summer.

Set up a clear timeline. Share your goals and reflections. A well-structured plan, guided by those who believe in your potential, will allow you to stay focused, confident, and prepared to step fully into the next stage of your medical journey. Let your passion be the spark while allowing strategy and reflection to serve as your compass.

## A STRATEGIC CHECKLIST FOR BS/MD PREPARATION
### Key Topics to Discuss with Your Counselor

On your BS/MD, BS/DO, BS/DDS journey, counselors can provide tailored advice, coordinate essential documentation, and connect you to the opportunities that strengthen your application.

However, direct med pathways are rare, and not all counselors are familiar with their specific demands. This it is crucial to take the initiative and schedule regular meetings with your counselor, using a clear checklist to guide those conversations.

1. **Academic Rigor and Course Selection**
   Ensure your four-year plan includes advanced science and math courses (AP, IB, or dual enrollment) to demonstrate preparedness for college-level STEM coursework. Push yourself, but only as much as you can handle.

2. **GPA Monitoring**
   Ask your counselor to help you confirm you are meeting the GPA, testing, and activity requirements for BS/MD, BS/DO, BS/DDS competitiveness.

3. **Standardized Testing Strategy**
   Discuss SAT, ACT, TOEFL plans. Determine a study plan, test prep, and timelines. Ask whether or when AP scores should be sent to colleges.

4. **Health Career Interest Documentation**
   Have your counselor note your long-term interest in medicine in your school report or counselor letter.

5. **Extracurricular and Leadership Tracking**
   Review your activities to ensure you are consistently involved in service, leadership, STEM research, and clinical exposure.

6. **Shadowing and Clinical Experience Support**
   Ask for help identifying local clinics, hospitals, or alumni connections where you can shadow physicians or volunteer.

7. **Research Opportunities**
   Inquire whether your high school partners with universities or labs where you might gain exposure to biomedical or public health research.

8. **Letters of Recommendation**
   Confirm which teachers are best positioned to write strong letters for you. Coordinate timing so your counselor can help avoid overlap or delays.

9. **Essay Planning**
   Discuss how the BS/MD, BS/DO, BS/DDS personal statement differs from general college essays and brainstorm ideas that demonstrate maturity and commitment to medicine.

10. **Special BS/MD, BS/DO, BS/DDS Forms and Application Supplements**
    Some programs require institutional forms or secondary essays. Ask your counselor to help you determine a submission timeline.

11. **Financial Aid and Scholarships**
    Ask if your school offers scholarship nominations, fee waivers, or workshops on financial planning for pre-med/pre-dent students.

12. **Application Timeline**
    Build a customized calendar with your counselor that includes BS/MD, BS/DO, BS/DDS deadlines (many of which are earlier than regular college apps) and interview preparation checkpoints.

Partnering with your high school counselor is an important part of your college planning, especially with the complexities of gaining admission to BS/MD, BS/DO, and BS/DDS programs.

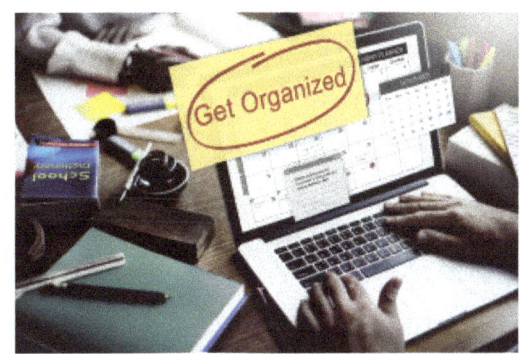

"

*Even when you think you have your life all mapped out, things happen that shape your destiny in ways you might never have imagined.*

— Deepak Chopra

# CHAPTER THIRTY-NINE

# CHOOSING A MAJOR

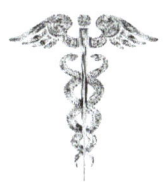

Except when BS/MD, BS/DO, or BS/DDS programs require candidates to pursue prescribed areas of study, students can literally major any field and gain admission to medical school, provided all prerequisites are met. While the prevailing notion is that majoring in Biology is the direct path to medical school, that is not the case. Ironically, Biology majors do not have the statistically highest probability of admission. So, choose a field in which you are passionate and one that will inspire you toward your aspirations.

Ultimately, medical schools seek a class of empathetic, talented, and diverse students who are well prepared, have experience with medicine, and are likely to be collaborative and brilliant physicians no matter what major they choose. To make well-informed choices, aspiring students should assess the university's prerequisites along with tangible skills and proficiencies.

According to the American Association of Medical Colleges (AAMC), medical school admission is not tied to a specific undergraduate major. Instead, admissions committees appreciate applicants with diverse academic backgrounds, mirroring medical schools' acknowledgment of healthcare's complexity. The crucial factor is fulfilling the prerequisite coursework.

Consequently, while prospective medical school students have the freedom to choose from a range of majors, they must ensure their coursework includes medical school prerequisites and probably also recommended courses. This approach aligns with the evolving healthcare landscape, where interdisciplinary cooperation is increasingly prized for its potential to drive innovation, use cutting edge technologies, and tackle complex health issues.

Furthermore, the inclusion of majors beyond traditional sciences underscores the significance of holistic viewpoints in medicine. Areas like social sciences and humanities offer insights into human behavior, cultural contexts, and ethical considerations, all crucial for effective patient care.

Similarly, the American Association of Colleges of Osteopathic Medicine emphasizes a holistic, patient-centered philosophy that considers not only the physical body, but also the mental, emotional, and spiritual dimensions of health. As a result, DO programs welcome applicants from a wide range of academic backgrounds, recognizing that excellence in osteopathic medicine is grounded in a comprehensive understanding of the whole person. With a focus on the body's innate ability to self-regulate and heal, the interconnectedness of structure and function, and the application of evidence-informed, rational treatment, osteopathic medicine invites future physicians who are committed to treating patients, not just symptoms, with empathy, curiosity, and a deep respect for human complexity.

According to a recent edition of the Medical School Admission Requirements, (MSAR), published by the Association of American Medical Colleges, students "should select a major area of study that is of interest and will provide a foundation of knowledge necessary for the pursuit of several career choices." As such, medical schools do not prioritize a specific pre-med major, despite popular opinion. However, if you choose a major that genuinely interests you, you are more likely to earn better grades, which is extremely important.

The AAMC goes on to state, "It should be strongly emphasized that a science major is not a prerequisite for medical school, and students should not major in science simply because they believe this will increase their chances for acceptance...." Thus, the AAMC recommends is a broad academic background that includes courses in the natural sciences, the social sciences, and the humanities. Chemistry, physics, and mathematics are highly valued, problem solving majors. However, the AAMC also notes, "For most physicians...the undergraduate years are the last available opportunity to pursue in depth a non-science subject of interest, and all who hope to practice medicine should bear this in mind when selecting an undergraduate major." Still, you also want to ensure you are fully prepared for the academic rigor and knowledge base required.

It is interesting to note that in a recent year, 50.2% of Philosophy majors were accepted to medical school, which is much higher than, say, Biology majors which was 39.9%. In the previous year, the acceptance rate for Philosophy majors was 53%! Philosophy majors make interesting applicants. Consider how many Biology Majors with a 4.0 apply to Med School. In contrast, a successful Philosophy major is thoroughly trained in a broad range of useful skills including critical thinking, ethical reasoning, intellectual history and both oral and written communication. In short, provided all required courses are completed, Philosophy majors tend to be well-rounded and well-educated.

You might want to read, "Major Anxiety: If You Think Biochemistry is your Ticket Into Medical School, Think Again" by Paul Jung, M.D. Open your scope and look through the lens of options that intrigue and inspire you to read, investigate, and learn.

Referring back to page 15 of this book, here is the data for percent admitted to the class of 2028 that entered in the fall of 2024.

| ACADEMIC FIELD | MATRICULANTS | APPLICANTS | PERCENTAGE |
|---|---|---|---|
| Biological Sciences | 12,050 | 30,054 | 40.09% |
| Humanities (Phil., Rel., Lit., etc.) | 861 | 1,661 | 51.83% |
| Math & Statistics | 180 | 344 | 52.33% |
| Other | 3,767 | 9,064 | 41.56% |
| Physical Sciences | 2,094 | 4,228 | 49.53% |
| Social Sciences (Psych., Soc., Anthro.) | 2,065 | 4,844 | 42.63% |
| Specialized Health Sciences | 964 | 2,382 | 40.47% |

In conclusion, take advantage of the chance to learn as much as you can while you are in college. Explore your interests. Unless your program restricts you to a specific major, you are in the driver's seat of your education. You control the steering wheel. You might discover that you have a passion for investigating healthcare policy, access to medical services, public health initiatives, or innovations in biotechnology. You might have a curiosity for kinesiology, prosthetics, or neural implants.

Your road to medical school may take you to an MD/MPH, MD/JD, MD/Ph.D. where you expand your education into areas where you can serve communities holistically, navigate the legal aspects of medicine, or focus on laboratory research. Medicine is on a course toward significant and exciting changes. Artificial intelligence and quantum computing are likely to transform the way physicians diagnose and treat patients.

You have the chance to be on the cutting edge of these changes, leading the way toward a tomorrow of unlimited potential.

"

*A dream becomes a goal when action is taken toward its achievement.*

—Bo Bennett

# CHAPTER FORTY

# RECOMMENDATIONS

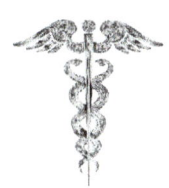

**M**ost colleges on the Common App and Coalition App, though not all, request letters of recommendation from a counselor and one or more teachers. Admissions officers in STEM programs, particularly BS/MD, BS/DO, BS/DDS, and direct med, typically want recommendation letters from academic teachers in mathematics, science, or humanities. Plan for this.

Occasionally, there is a section for optional recommendations too. In this location, you might request a recommendation from a summer program leader clinical research coordinator, or someone with whom you held a job or completed a hospital internship. If you participate in a sport, you might choose a coach or, if you are an artist or musician, you might chose your teacher. For those who are active in a church, synagogue, mosque, or temple, you might select a religious leader who can speak to your responsibility, commitment, and integrity. Live your values. Interact and communicate thoughtfully.

Each college has a different set of requirements regarding letters of recommendation, though there are standardized forms in the Common App, Coalition App, MIT application, Georgetown application, and ApplyTexas. Look at the requirements or the desired recommendation criteria for each school's application.

Some BS/MD, BS/DO, and BS/DDS programs and talent-based programs require additional recommendations that are separate from the main university application. Be sure to check if the schools you are considering have special recommendation or requirements specifically for that school, e.g. a college may want a recommendation from a life science, physical science, and mathematics teacher.

# COMMON APP TEACHER RECOMMENDATION FORM

Your teachers will write a letter of recommendation. They will relay to the college the grade you were in, courses they taught you, and the level of difficulty. They are prompted with this: "Please attach additional comments that address what you think is important about this student, including a description of academic and personal characteristics, as demonstrated in your classroom. We welcome information that will help us to differentiate this student from others."

The form they complete also includes a section where teachers assess students across various attributes using a standardized rating scale. This area provides checkboxes to help admissions committees use a comparative perspective to evaluate a student's performance and character traits. See this chart below:

| | Below Average | Average | Good (Above Average) | Very Good (Well Above Average) | Excellent (top 10%) | Outstanding (top 5%) | One of the top few in my career |
|---|---|---|---|---|---|---|---|
| Academic Achievement | | | | | | | |
| Intellectual Promise | | | | | | | |
| Quality of Writing | | | | | | | |
| Creative Orig. Thought | | | | | | | |
| Productive Class Discussion | | | | | | | |
| Respect by Faculty | | | | | | | |
| Respect by Students | | | | | | | |
| Disciplined Work Habits | | | | | | | |
| Maturity | | | | | | | |
| Motivation | | | | | | | |
| Leadership | | | | | | | |
| Integrity | | | | | | | |
| Reaction to Setbacks | | | | | | | |
| Concern for Others | | | | | | | |
| Self-Confidence | | | | | | | |
| Initiative | | | | | | | |
| Overall | | | | | | | |

To expand these words a bit so that you can read this better, here is the list of criteria in which students are evaluated.

Academic Achievement Intellectual Promise Quality of Writing
Creative Original Thought
Productive Class Discussion Respect Accorded by Faculty Respect Accorded by Students Disciplined Work Habits Maturity
Motivation

Leadership
Integrity
Reaction to Setbacks
Concern for Others
Self-Confidence
Initiative
Overall Evaluation

As you choose the teachers who will write your recommendations, ask yourself which teachers will more likely checks the boxes "Outstanding" or "One of the Top Few in My Career"?

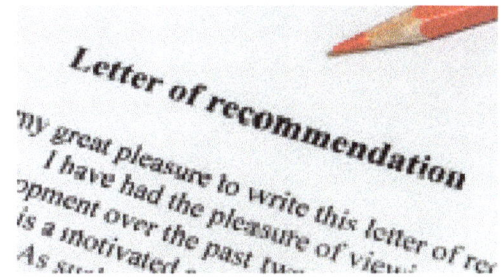

If you are a freshman, sophomore, or junior, look at the list. How do you demonstrate those qualities, attributes, or skills? The time is now to contribute to discussions, demonstrate characteristics like leadership, maturity, integrity, concern for others. Do not be disingenuous, but congruous with your genuine self. This is the time to step up to the plate and help others in your class, show initiative, and demonstrate self-confidence. Be authentic, grateful, and responsible in all you do.

In the Common Application, "Other Recommenders" are individuals who can provide additional insights into your experiences and character outside the traditional academic context. When inviting an Other Recommender, you must select their role from a predefined list. The available categories for Other Recommenders include:

**Arts Teacher:** An instructor who has taught you in disciplines like music, theater, visual arts, film, or dance.

**Clergy:** A religious leader who can speak to your moral character and community involvement.

**Coach:** An athletic coach familiar with your teamwork, leadership, and dedication.

**College Access Counselor:** A mentor or advisor who has guided you through the college preparation process.

**Employer:** A supervisor from a job or internship who can attest to your work ethic and responsibilities.

**Family Member:** A relative who can provide personal insights into your character and background. (Note: I do not generally advise using this one.)

**Peer:** A fellow student or friend who can offer a perspective on your interpersonal skills and contributions. (Note: While I do not advise this either, some colleges have specifically asked for a peer recommendation.)

**Other:** Any individual not fitting the above categories but who can provide a unique perspective on your qualifications. (This could be a family friend who has known you since childhood and can offer insights that academic teachers do not have.)

**Note:** Not all colleges accept letters from Other Recommenders. To determine if a specific college allows additional recommendations, check the "Recommenders and FERPA" section for that institution within your Common App account.

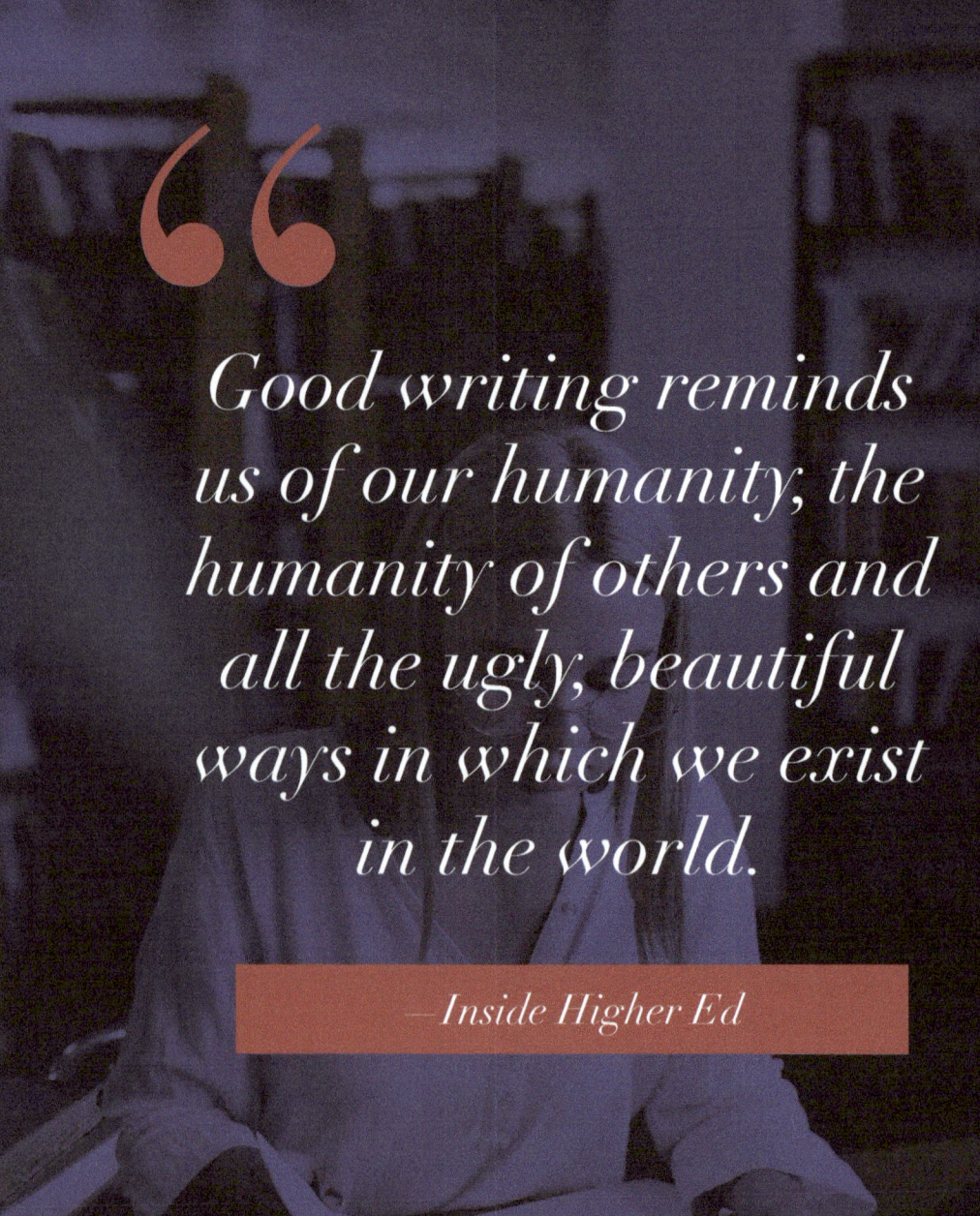

"

*Good writing reminds us of our humanity, the humanity of others and all the ugly, beautiful ways in which we exist in the world.*

*—Inside Higher Ed*

CHAPTER FORTY-ONE

# ESSAYS, SUPPLEMENT ESSAYS, AND AI

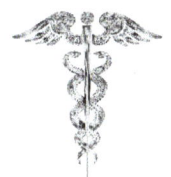

## ESSAYS

The Common Application and Coalition essays are often posted months ahead of time. Since this main essay is required or recommended for nearly all Common Application and Coalition Application schools, the personal statement is an excellent place to start thinking about what you might want to say to colleges.

In addition to the main essay on the Common Application and Coalition Application, more than half of the colleges have their own specific questions or essays. In August, most admissions applications are open and ready for you to dive into the supplemental college-specific questions, though many of the essay topics are available earlier, and some schools hold out until later for their big essay reveal.

Essays can be prepared ahead of time too. One popular question is, "What activity is most important to you and why?" Another is "Why did you choose your major?" A third common question is, "Why do you want to attend our school?" For others, you should prepare or at least consider the topics of diversity, adversity, and personal challenges since these topics have become increasingly important in the admissions process. Everyone has a challenge they needed to overcome, especially during the pandemic. What did you learn from your experiences?

Complete the application fully. Think carefully about optional sections. Typically, universities offer you the chance to provide the school with just the right cherry on top of the sundae, allowing you to share something unique about you. If you have absolutely nothing to say, leave it blank. There is an additional information section on the main Common App, Coalition Application, and University of California application. This location is not a place to write another essay, but you can include information that cannot be adequately explained in the rest of the application.

There are also schools that include scholarship essays within the supplement part of the application. Start early. Paint a clear picture. Let colleges get to know you!

## TIPS FOR THE COLLEGE ESSAY

Let's look at some step-by-step advice on college entrance essays.

### Step 1: Read the Prompt Carefully

Answer the question fully and completely.
Check the word or character count.
Re-read the prompt to understand themes.
Teamwork, diversity, challenges, community, or goals are important.
Where do you fit into that college?
What is the intersection of your interests and what they offer?

### Step 2: Brainstorm Ideas

List hobbies, passions, and influences.
Reflect on your life stories and events.
What areas fit with the college's culture?
What were pivotal moments, challenges, or achievements?

### Step 3: Find a Unique Angle

Be creative and interesting but also authentic.
Do not copy, augment, or adapt someone else's story.
Going outside of the box is fine, but remember, simple is fine too.
They just want to get to know you.
Some students focus on uniqueness at the cost of being relatable.

### Step 4: Focus on Key Moments

Focus on key moments rather than generalities.
Remember: Show, don't tell.
Make the story compelling and meaningful.
What experience changed your perspective?

### Step 5: Create an Outline

This is an essay after all.
What is your catchy introduction?
What body paragraphs provide examples for your thesis?
Conclude with a reflection that ties the story together.

**Step 6: Start with a Hook**

    A quote, shock, epiphany, or idea can help introduce your story.

    Connect your story to the prompt.

**Step 7: Write a Draft and Wrap it with a Bow**

    Tie the hook with a story.

    Tie the story to your life experiences.

    Tie the body paragraphs to the prompt.

    Tie the loose ends in a bow and memorable idea.

    Avoid cliches and generalities.

**Step 8: Edit for Clarity**

    Check spelling, grammar, and ideas.

    Make sure your essay aligns with the college.

    Remember, readers must digest and evaluate thousands of essays.

    Create smooth paragraph transitions.

    Maintain focus.

**Sept 9: Seek Feedback**

    The reader is not a teenager.

    What you think is funny or amusing may not appeal to an adult.

    However, parents may not be in-tune with colleges.

    Think through the feedback. Trust your instincts.

**Step 10: Revise, Proofread, and Submit**

    Remember to use your unique voice.

    Format as directed – font, spacing, word count.

    Read it over one more time and submit.

**Final Notes:**

- Optional rarely means optional. In most cases, do it.
- If there is a COVID and Natural Disasters essay, tell your story.
- Write in complete sentences.
- Research the school. Every school is different.
- Do not just write the same essay for each school.
- Don't complain about a teacher, even if it is true.
- Don't lie or tell untruths in your essay or application.

**Additional Information Section**

    Do not put essays in the additional information section, but you can use this section to clarify elements in your application that need explanation, like low grades, a bad semester, family emergencies, additional activities, honors/awards, or why you earned a W or did not take a class that you really should have completed.

> *A résumé should be more than a list of jobs. It should tell the story of who you are and what you can become.*

— Paul Sloane

# CHAPTER FORTY-TWO

# RESUME

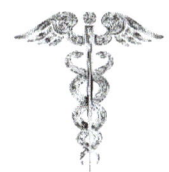

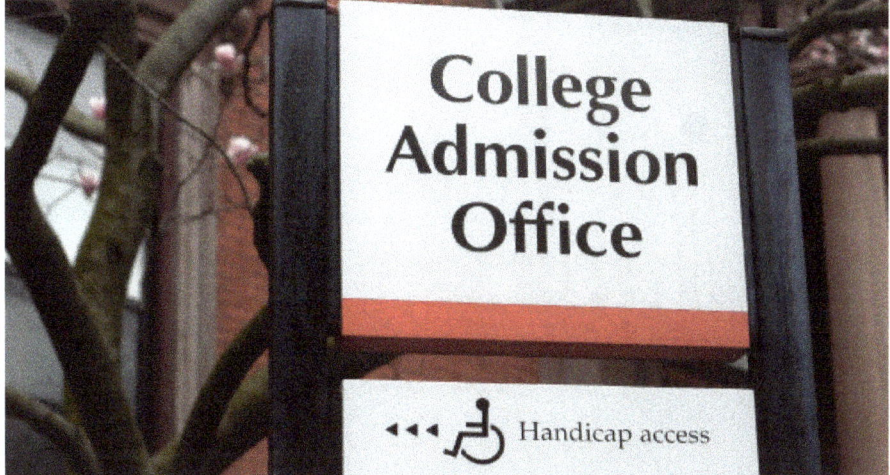

## STUDENT RESUMES FOR COLLEGE ADMISSION

1. **Decide on a clean, easy-to-read format**
   - One page is best.
   - Most people will only read the first page.
   - Being long-winded and wordy is not helpful.
   - Arial, Calibri, or Times New Roman are easy to read. "Cute" fonts may reflect your personality, but may not be legible.
   - Font sizes should not be too small.

2. **Pictures are okay for a freshman admissions resume**

3. **Name, E-Mail, and Phone Number**
   - Do not include your home address.

4. **Educational Experiences or Academic Background**
   - High School(s), dates, location(s)
   - Colleges Attended, dates, location(s)
   - Academic Programs/Training
   - Languages

5. **Honors, Awards, Certifications**
   - Academic Honors
   - Awards
   - Certificates
   - Acknowledgments
   - Extraordinary Accomplishments

6. **Extracurricular Activities**
   - Clubs/Activities
     - Bulletpoint each accomplishment with past tense verbs.
     - Focus on achievements, consistency, and leadership.
   - Sports/Athletics – Separate if extensive

7. **Community Service**

8. **Work Experience**

9. **Hobbies**

**Final Notes**
- You might add a goal/vision statement at the top or a quote that defines your destiny or vision.
- Avoid writing paragraphs since people will not read these.
- Proofread by double-checking for spelling and errors.
- Ask for feedback.
- If you have time, tailor the resumes to each school.
- Add a LinkedIn URL, Portfolio Link, or Personal Website.

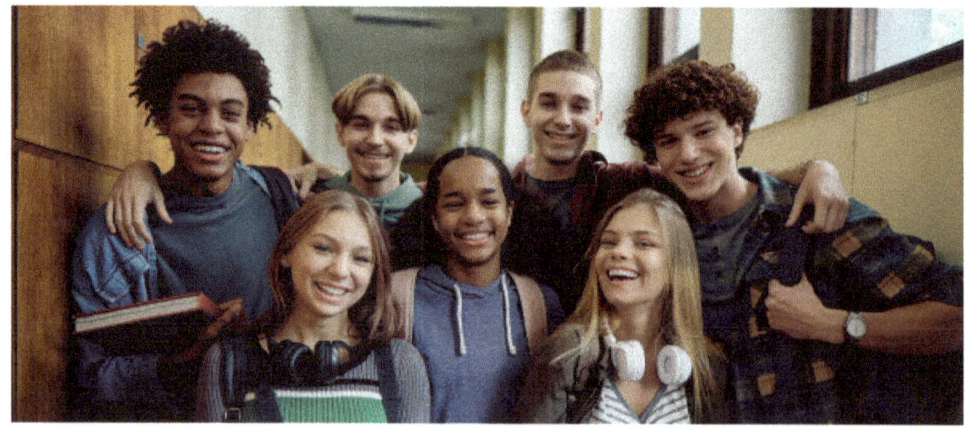

# CRAFTING IMPACTFUL RESUMES INCORPORATING CLINICAL AND RESEARCH EXPERIENCES

Since applying to a BS/MD, BS/DO, or BS/DDS program as a high school student requires more than high grades and test scores, your resume should highlight evidence of a sincere, sustained interest in healthcare. To stand out, applicants must not only seek meaningful clinical exposure and research experience, but also present their experiences with maturity and depth.

Clinical exposure can range from hospital volunteer work and shadowing physicians to assisting in dental offices or community health fairs. Even escorting patients or preparing rooms offer valuable insight into how healthcare teams communicate, the pace of clinical environments, and the compassion required to treat patients. Seek mentors who will allow you to observe procedures and debrief you afterward. Take notes and reflect on patient interactions, physician's tone of voice, and professional responsibilities.

Next, find summer programs, university labs, or virtual research internships that align with your curiosity. If you lack access to formal labs, consider independent projects such as data analysis, literature reviews, or presenting at local science fairs. Show initiative by asking questions, troubleshooting, and learning from failure.

When listing these on your resume, describe what you did, what you learned, and why it matters. Use concise bullet points beginning with active verbs (e.g., "Observed laparoscopic procedures and documented post-operative protocols."). Include outcomes (e.g., "Created a patient brochure on diabetes prevention used by the clinic's patients."). Reflect on takeaways like empathy, precision, attention to detail, resilience, and ethical reasoning.

Finally, in interviews or essays, be ready to tell a story behind your resume entries. Describe a patient who shaped your perspective, a mistake that taught you a lesson, or a mentor who inspired your path. Show that you are not just fulfilling required service hours but informing your future in medicine with depth, humility, and insight. Show your readiness for an accelerated path to medicine.

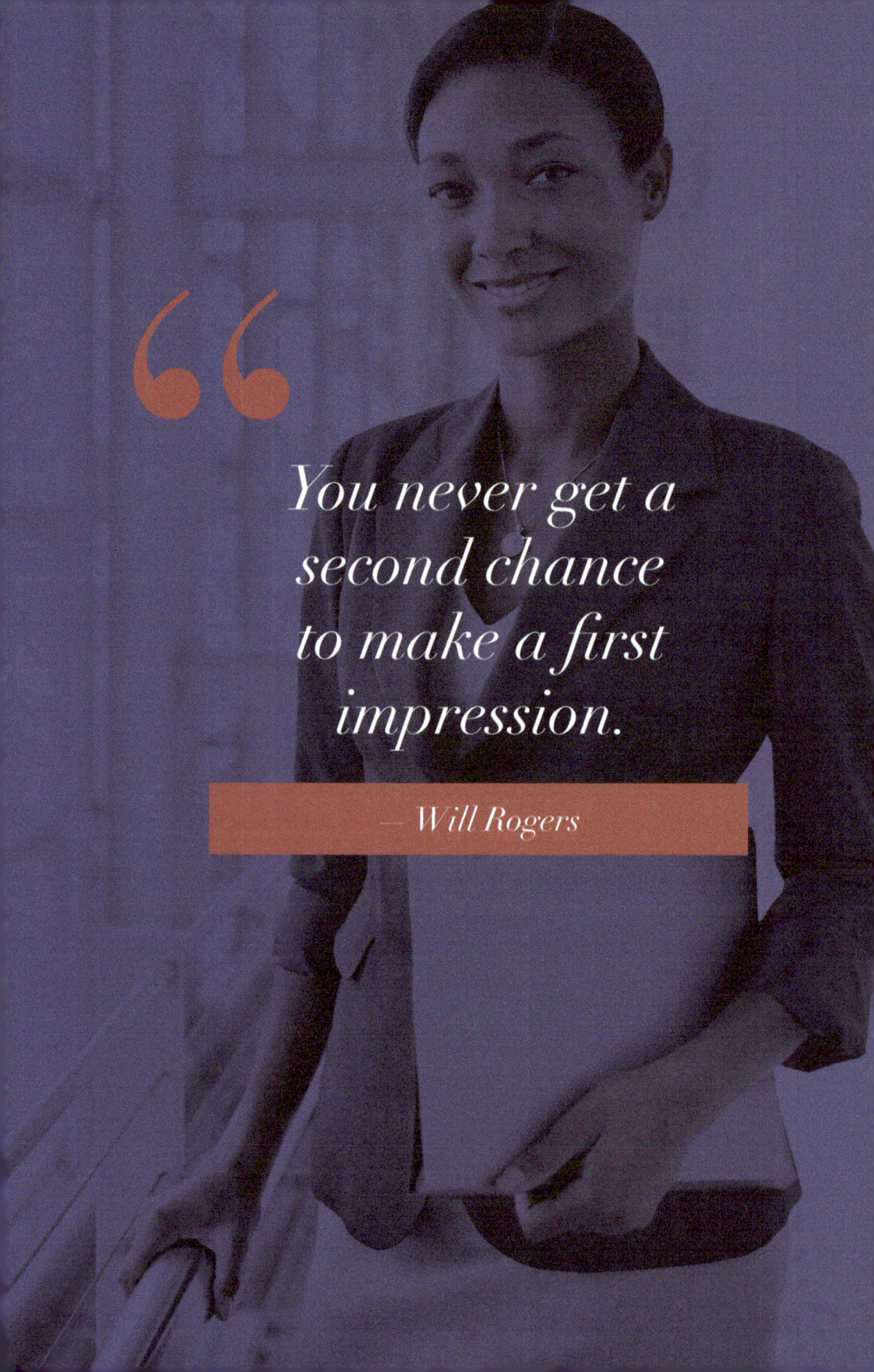

"

You never get a
second chance
to make a first
impression.

— Will Rogers

# CHAPTER FORTY-THREE

# PORTFOLIOS, ABSTRACTS, TALENT

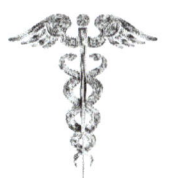

## SHOWCASING EXCELLENCE, EXPERIENCE, AND TALENT

In an increasingly competitive college admissions landscape, students seek ways to distinguish themselves beyond GPA, test scores, and volunteer hours. One often overlooked yet powerful tool is a portfolio. This opportunity can by submitted through platforms like SlideRoom, college-specific portals, and the additional information section. A well-curated portfolio can showcase talents in art, music, dance, creative writing, film, or academic research, illustrating intellectual vitality, discipline, creativity, passion, and depth of character.

## THE VALUE OF PORTFOLIOS IN PRE-MED ADMISSIONS

While portfolios are traditionally associated with arts-based admissions, they are increasingly being recognized as meaningful supplements to applications in STEM fields, including pre-med tracks. Many colleges and combined medical programs now provide optional spaces for students to submit portfolios to demonstrate excellence in areas not captured by transcripts or test scores.

According to the AAMC, medical schools seek applicants who possess strong communication skills, cultural competency, resilience, and a capacity for growth. A student who presents a portfolio of published literature reviews, award-winning compositions, or independently conducted laboratory research not only exhibits intellectual curiosity but also a proactive, integrative mindset, qualities closely aligned with the AAMC's Core Competencies for Entering Medical Students.

## WHAT TO INCLUDE IN A PRE-MED PORTFOLIO

A pre-med applicant's portfolio may vary based on strengths, but it may include:

- **Research Abstracts and Posters:** Highlight lab-based or social science research. Include purpose, methodology, and results.

- **Creative Writing or Literature Reviews:** Demonstrate analytical thinking, medical humanities perspective, or ability to synthesize scientific information.

- **Published Papers or Conference Presentations:** These scientific articles, papers, or publications signal initiative and professionalism.

- **Art, Film, or Music:** Showcase creativity, talent, discipline, and innovation.

- **Dance or Theater Performances:** Reflect discipline, body awareness, communication, and dedication.

- **Awards or Recognitions:** Competitions, certificates, trophies, ribbons, grants, acknowledgments, or arts residencies.

- **Service Projects or Public Health Campaigns:** Creative health outreach efforts, especially those that involve visual or multimedia components.

## PLATFORMS AND SUBMISSION TOOLS

- SlideRoom is the most commonly used platform for portfolio submissions and is integrated into the Common App and Coalition App. SlideRoom allows students to upload images, documents, and multimedia files along with descriptions and captions.

- ZeeMee for profile sharing with a social media component.

- College-specific portals that allow PDF uploads or direct embedding of links to digital projects or publications.

- LinkedIn or Personal Websites for long-term hosting and professional development.

## WHY THIS MATTERS FOR BS/MD, BS/DO, & BS/DDS APPLICANTS

BS/MD, BS/DO, and BS/DDS programs are highly selective, often admitting fewer than 5% of applicants. Successful candidates must demonstrate maturity, a clear commitment to medicine, and exceptional abilities that predict future success. Portfolios provide additional evidence of:

- **Depth and Breadth:** Applicants who balance academic rigor with creative or research excellence stand out.

- **Commitment:** Time-intensive projects show follow-through and dedication, which are key qualities for a career in medicine.

- **Narrative Coherence:** A student who presents a portfolio that supports their personal statement (e.g., a future physician who creates a short film about end-of-life care) demonstrates clarity of purpose.

## STUDENT SUCCESS STORIES

- A BS/MD admit to Brown University included a SlideRoom portfolio with a short documentary on immigrant health care access, which complemented her public health advocacy.
- A Johns Hopkins pre-med student submitted abstracts from two summer research internships and a published article in the *Journal of Emerging Investigators,* reinforcing his scientific acumen.
- A violinist accepted at Northwestern submitted video performances, demonstrating discipline and stress management.
- A creative writer submitted personal essays on medical ethics, which helped her stand out in the BS/DO pool.

## DOES AAMC ENDORSE PORTFOLIOS?

While the AAMC does not ask for a portfolio, they do encourage the inclusion of diverse experiences in applications and essays, especially those demonstrating core competencies like service orientation, cultural awareness, and communication. For applicants to undergraduate universities, these portfolios can strengthen a student's narrative and prepare them for future AMCAS applications.

## SCHOLARSHIPS AND ENRICHMENT

Portfolios can also be submitted to qualify for merit scholarships. For example, institutions like Emory, USC, and NYU consider artistic and research excellence in awarding full or partial scholarships. Additionally, portfolios can help students gain entry to summer research institutes, honors programs, or national competitions like Regeneron ISEF or the Scholastic Art & Writing Awards.

Finally, portfolios are not just for art majors. For students bound for medical school, a portfolio provides a canvas to illustrate the qualities you bring to school that will make you an exceptional caregiver and scholar. Whether capturing the precision of a scientific abstract or the empathy behind a painting, portfolios offer admission committees a fuller picture of your potential. Start early, curate thoughtfully, and let your multidimensional self shine.

## A FEW UNIVERSITIES & PROGRAMS WITH SLIDEROOM OR RESEARCH SUBMISSION PORTALS

**Brown University – Program in Liberal Medical Education (PLME)**

- o Uses SlideRoom for academic or artistic supplements.
- o Students can upload science research abstracts, videos, or published papers.

**Case Western Reserve University – Pre-Professional Scholars Program in Medicine (PPSP)**

- o Accepts research supplements through the Common App or SlideRoom.
- o Strong emphasis on undergraduate research makes this highly valuable.

**Columbia University**

- o Allows the submission of visual arts, music, film, dance, and theater supplements via SlideRoom.
- o Academic research may be submitted as a supplement under STEM achievements, especially if published.

**Harvard University**

- o Allows the submission of artistic portfolios, academic research, and creative writing.
- o Upload documents (PDFs, images, links) directly to the Common App or via a Harvard-specific upload portal, not SlideRoom.
- o Research abstracts, publications, or scholarly work can be added under the Additional Information section or emailed.

**Northwestern University**

- o Northwestern accepts academic and research supplements through SlideRoom.
- o Research posters, abstracts, and scientific writing are encouraged.

**Princeton University**

- o Accepts arts supplements (e.g., visual arts, dance, music, theater) via SlideRoom.
- o While Princeton does not have a formal academic research supplement, students may include publications or abstracts in the Additional Information section.
- o Discuss research experience in essays or recommendation letters.

**Rice University**

- o Rice University accepts research supplements via SlideRoom.
- o Students can showcase independent or mentored research.

**Stanford University**

- o Accepts arts portfolios via SlideRoom in music, dance, theater, and visual arts.
- o Academic supplements or research papers are not accepted separately, but can be submitted elsewhere.

- o Research can be described in the Activities section or Additional Information area.
- o Link to a personal website is sometimes permitted.

**Stony Brook University – Scholars for Medicine (BS/MD)**

- o Allows applicants to upload research documentation and abstracts in their supplemental application section.
- o Also accepts e-mailed supplements if properly labeled.

**SUNY Upstate Medical University – Early Assurance & BS/MD Pathways**

- o In partnership with institutions like Syracuse University and SUNY Albany, portfolios and research projects may be submitted via college portals or as part of supplemental applications.

**Tufts University – Early Assurance Program**

- o Tufts uses SlideRoom for arts, research, and creative work.
- o Particularly valuable for students submitting lab research or scholarly writing.

**University of Pittsburgh – Guaranteed Admissions Program (GAP) for Medicine**

- o Offers a space in the application portal to describe and attach scientific research experiences.
- o Students can list published work and conference presentations.

**University of Rochester – Rochester Early Medical Scholars (REMS)**

- o Accepts research papers and abstracts through SlideRoom or via Common App upload.
- o Rochester encourages showcasing STEM-related creative work.

**University of Southern California – Keck School of Medicine Pathways**

- o USC has a SlideRoom portal for talent and research submissions.
- o Students can submit research PDFs, media, and detailed descriptions.

**Yale University**

- o Arts supplements may be submitted through SlideRoom in visual arts, music, film, theater, dance, and architecture.
- o While Yale does not formally accept academic research as a supplement, students can describe projects in the application activities, essays, or the additional information section.
- o Exceptional research achievements (e.g., publication or competition) may be noted in letters of recommendation.

"

*Always remember the privilege it is to be a physician.*

*—Daniel P. Logan*

# CHAPTER FORTY-FOUR

# INTERVIEWS

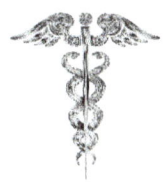

## COLLEGE INTERVIEW TIPS AND PREPARATION

Not all colleges offer interviews. Check with each admissions office. If so, determine the location, process, and timing. While many colleges interview on campus, some interview online, while others meet locally by alumni or regional representatives. BS/MD, BS/DO, and BS/DDS interviews are by invitation only. Traditional college interviews are offered on a first-come, first-served basis.

For example, to obtain an interview at one of the Claremont Colleges, go to their website and choose a date and time early. The most desired times are taken by the end of August. Harvard, Yale, Columbia, Georgetown, and MIT interview candidates after the application is submitted. If there are no representatives available, the student is not disadvantaged in the process.

Interviews may be either informational or evaluative. If informational, the goal is for students to have their questions answered. So, be prepared with questions. If evaluative, the representative will write up and submit and evaluation of the candidate. Either way, set an appointment, prepare, and interview.

Here is an interesting tidbit. Colleges may say that they do not interview, but on a campus visit you can often meet the regional representative who will read your application. Make a good impression. It may make a difference.

If a university interviews, the meetings are typically held in November for early action and January for regular decision. Read about the college's programs ahead of time and consider questions you might want to ask. Dress appropriately - clean, neat, and polished. Shorts, t-shirt, or revealing clothing are discouraged.

# HOW TO HAVE A SUCCESSFUL INTERVIEW

**Preparation**

*   Read materials about the college ahead of time.
*   Get a sense of the student body and type of school environment.
*   When interviewing on campus, you may be able to schedule appointments with coaches, faculty in your major, religious leaders, program representatives, students, or other people of interest. If you can't, don't sweat it.
*   Know whether the interview is evaluative (they will determine whether or not you would be a good fit) or informational (they are only 'interviewing' you to provide you with more information about the school).
*   Tour before you interview if the meeting is held on campus.
*   Dress to impress. Remember, this is an interview. You want to make a positive impression with the adult interviewer. Avoid baggy pants, jeans, showing skin, sneakers, sandals, or flashy accouterments. You do not need to wear a suit, but a sweater, slacks, and conservative clothes are appropriate.
*   Parents are sometimes invited, but they must NOT dominate the conversation. Many times it is better if they are not in the interview room. Remember, most colleges want you to demonstrate independence.
*   Be sure that you are not hungry or tired when you arrive.
*   Smile. You want them to get a sense of your charming personality.
*   Be sure to leave the interviewer with a great impression.

**Greeting**

*   When the interviewer calls your name, greet him or her with a handshake and a smile. Be relaxed and friendly.
*   Make eye contact and create a connection.
*   Introduce your parents or siblings if they are with you.

**The Interview**

*   Be prepared to tell the interviewer more about yourself.
*   Research the school first so you can ask questions about the college.
*   Bring a pad or folio with a pad. Jot notes before you go to remind yourself of key questions. You might also want to take notes during your interview.
*   Body language tells much about a person. Use good posture; leaning, slouching, or looking away makes you appear disinterested.
*   Use correct grammar and appropriate vocabulary.
*   Avoid inappropriate language like swearing, politically incorrect terminology or usage such as "you know" or too many "ums."
*   Think before you answer questions, but try to remain relaxed.

* Exude confidence. Do not act overconfident.
* If you are truly interested in the school, be authentic and demonstrate that interest and enthusiasm.
* This is your chance to impress. Arrive early. Surprisingly, many students arrive late. Some do not even come. Others do not appear to take the interview seriously and are unprepared. It is better if the interviewer is late, not you.
* Be friendly, but not flirtatious or overly casual. Shaking hands is appropriate.
* Do not badmouth counselors, teachers, fellow students, religions, cultures, races, genders, or political groups.
* Do not memorize answers; try to sound natural and conversational.
* Do not chew gum.
* Do not eat food during the meeting unless you are at a restaurant and requested or offered to do so.
* Do not wear lots of cologne or perfume.
* Do not respond with only "yes" or "no" answers.
* Ask for a business card at the end of the interview. Write the name of college representative and the meeting date on the back.
* Thank the interviewer after the meeting and shake their hand.
* Always follow up later with an e-mail or a thank you note.

## Be Prepared to Answer These Questions
* What led you to pursue medicine? Describe your clinical experiences.
* What three adjectives describe your commitment to heathcare? Humanity?
* Describe your favorite class? Your least favorite? What subjects inspire you?
* What activity is most important to you and why?
* After touring our campus, what factors are most appealing about our school?
* What is the greatest contribution you could make to our student body?
* What is your greatest strength? What is your greatest weakness?
* Why do you want to go to college? What are you looking forward to most?
* Where do you envision yourself in ten years? twenty years?

## After the Interview
* Write a short thank you note to your interviewer and send it within 24 hours.
* In the note, include a reference to something specific from the interview. You want some specific point to stand out so that they remember you.
* If you have a question that was not answered, include that in the note.
* Also, send the interviewer an e-mail with a question about special services/ opportunities in order to learn more and create a dialogue.

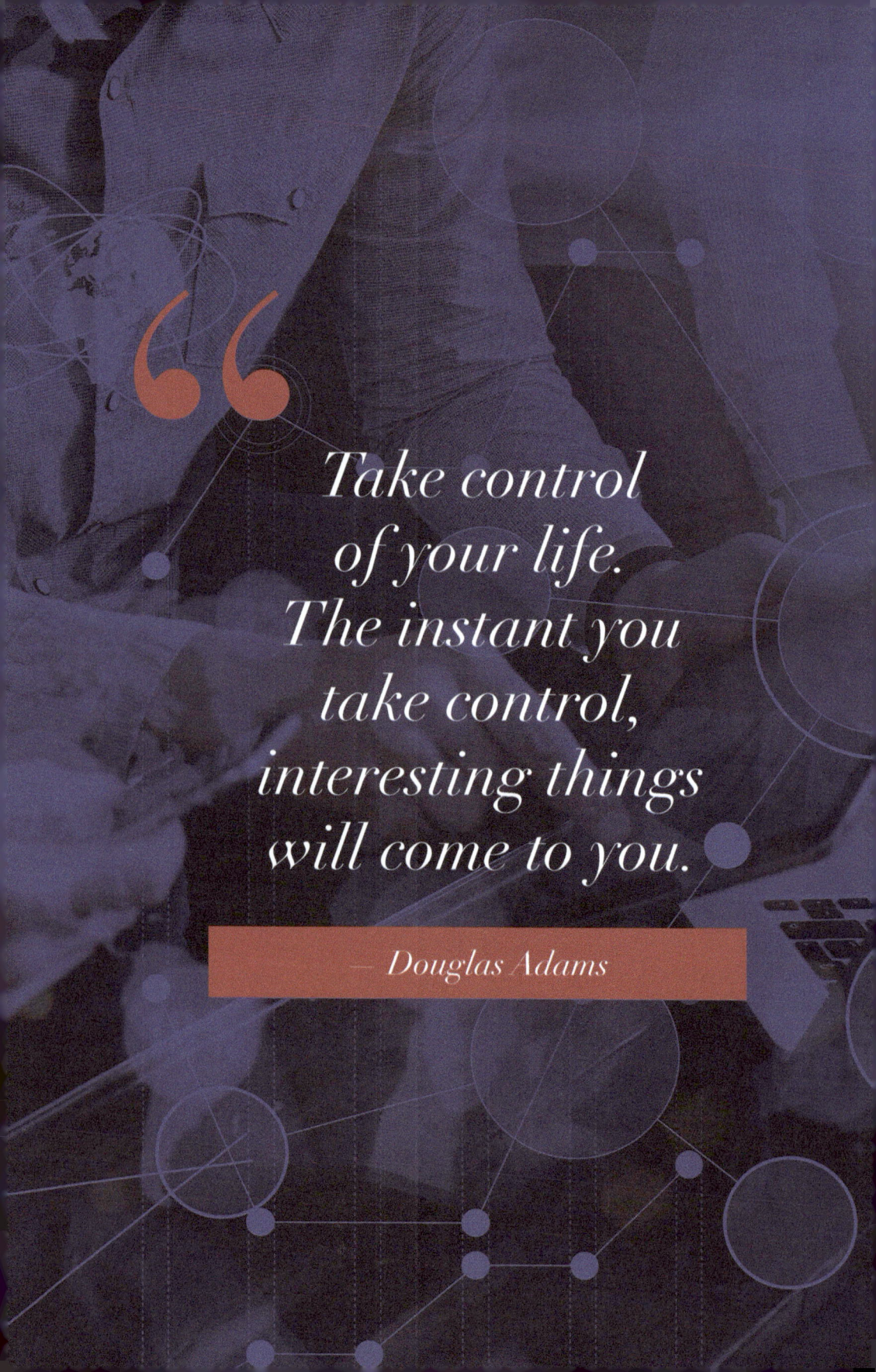

"

*Take control of your life. The instant you take control, interesting things will come to you.*

— *Douglas Adams*

## CHAPTER FORTY-FIVE

# PORTALS, VERIFICATION, VALIDITY

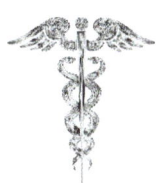

When applying to colleges, especially highly selective BS/MD, BS/DO, and BS/DDS pathways, students must navigate several digital systems to complete and monitor their applications. One of the most important tools in this process is the college application portal. A few days after the submission of the Common App or Coalition App, students are sent an e-mail requesting that they set up a link to the college, typically with a user name and temporary passcode. This direct connection is called the portal.

This is a crucial step, so be sure to check your e-mail and connect. The college will send you a "Bear ID" or a special login that is typically unique to that college. In your Google Doc or Google Sheet you will keep the individual logins for each of the colleges to which you applied. Check your portals regularly. If you do not follow through with college requests by a certain date, the school may delete your entire application. Seriously!

For students who do not check their e-mail often or delete college e-mails as spam or ignore college communication because they are too busy, their inaction spells disaster. Though frequently overlooked, these portals serve as a central hub for communication between the applicant and the institution.

### WHAT ARE COLLEGE APPLICATION PORTALS?

An application portal is a secure, personalized webpage created for each applicant after they submit their initial college application via Common App, Coalition App, or a school-specific form. Once created, the portal provides access to:

* Confirmation that your application was received
* Updates on required or missing documents (e.g., transcripts, test scores, recommendations)
* Financial aid submission statuses (FAFSA, CSS Profile, tax forms)
* Opportunities to upload a resume, website link, research, papers, or supplemental materials
* Scholarship opportunities
* Honors program invites
* Interview invitations
* Admission decisions and financial aid offers

Portals often serve as the final authority for application completeness and admissions decisions. However, for BS/MD, BS/DO, and BS/DDS programs, where timelines can be accelerated and interview invitations are limited, missing a portal update can mean a lost scholarship or program opportunity.

## WHY CHECKING PORTALS IS CRITICAL

Colleges may send e-mails to reach you. However, critical updates often appear first (or exclusively) on your portal. If you forget to check, you might miss a:

* Deadline to submit supplemental essays or materials
* Request to verify an activity or prove you did not use AI
* Interview scheduling window
* Financial aid verification request
* Change in application status or required information

For BS/MD, BS/DO, and BS/DDS programs, the process often involves multiple rounds, including the university admission, supplemental application, interview requests, and medical school reviews. These portals may also separate updates for each program component. A student admitted to the university but rejected from the BS/MD, BS/DO, or BS/DDS track may not learn this unless they review their portal.

## BEWARE OF MISINFORMATION & ARTIFICIAL INTELLIGENCE

The University of California announced in their November 13, 2024 *Counselors & Advisors Bulletin* that they would randomly check applications for verification of information in mid-December and then notify students via their portal and other methods that they will need to verify what they submitted by January 31 or else their application would be canceled. Additionally, the essays (UC Personal Insight Questions) would also be reviewed for plagiarism or artificial intelligence. Students had two weeks to respond with proof of authenticity. Failure to respond resulted in their application being canceled. Check your portals!

## HOW OFTEN SHOULD STUDENTS CHECK?

During peak application season (October to April), students should:

* Check each application portal once per week after submission.
* Increase this to 2–3 times per week as decision dates or interviews approach.

Set calendar reminders and use a spreadsheet to track usernames, passwords, and last login dates.

## WHAT SHOULD STUDENTS CHECK FOR?

When reviewing your application portal, look for:

1. **Checklist Completion:** Ensure transcripts, test scores, recommendations, and portfolios are marked as received.
2. **Supplemental Requests/Requirements:** Some schools release program-specific forms or short essays through the portal after submission.
3. **Interview Notifications:** For BS/MD, BS/DO, or BS/DDS programs, interviews may be posted to the portal and not sent via e-mail.
4. **Financial Aid Requests:** Institutions might ask for tax documents, W-2s, or other verification forms.
5. **Decision Releases:** Admissions decisions are often posted first to the portal before e-mails are sent.

## HOW COLLEGES VERIFY APPLICATION INFORMATION

Colleges use multiple methods to confirm the authenticity of student submissions:

1. **School Reports & Transcripts:** Verified and sent by guidance counselors.
2. **Recommendation Letters:** Sent directly from teachers and uploaded through secure systems.
3. **Standardized Test Scores:** Must be sent from official testing organizations (e.g., College Board, ACT).
4. **Interviews:** Help verify character and consistency in application materials.
5. **Social Media Audits:** In rare but increasing cases, colleges review publicly available content tied to a student's name.
6. **Plagiarism Detection Tools:** Some institutions run essays through software to detect AI use or copied content.

Discrepancies or red flags (e.g., essays written in a noticeably different voice from other materials) may prompt further review or disqualification.

## THE RISKS OF USING AI OR MISREPRESENTATION

With the rise of tools like ChatGPT, some students are tempted to use artificial intelligence to write college essays. While AI can be helpful for brainstorming or grammar checking, submitting an AI-generated essay as your own work violates academic integrity policies.

Admissions officers are trained to recognize inauthentic or overly polished writing that lacks personal insight. For BS/MD, BS/DO, and BS/DDS applicants, whose essays must convey emotional maturity, long-term commitment to medicine, and personal motivation, AI-generated content often falls flat and appears generic.

Additionally, falsifying activities, awards, or research experiences can lead to revocation of offers. Some programs contact research mentors or use honor code verification forms to confirm the extent of participation.

## THE IMPORTANCE OF HONESTY IN APPLICATIONS

Truthfulness is especially important in medicine-related programs. BS/MD, BS/DO, and BS/DDS applicants are being considered for a career that demands ethical integrity, trust, and compassion. Admissions committees are evaluating not only your academic and extracurricular success but your character and authenticity.

Colleges often state that dishonesty in an application, once discovered, is grounds for:

* Immediate rejection
* Revocation of admission (even after enrollment)
* Notification to other schools via shared platforms
* Ineligibility for future application cycles

## REAL CASES OF REVOKED ADMISSIONS OR ACADEMIC MISCONDUCT

1. **Harvard University (2017):** Ten admitted students had their offers rescinded after sharing offensive memes and comments in a private Facebook group. The university deemed the content inconsistent with its standards.
2. **Stanford University (multiple years):** Several students had offers rescinded after it was discovered they exaggerated or fabricated their research experiences.

3. **BS/MD Program (undisclosed):** A student had their offer withdrawn after claiming to have interned at a hospital that reported they had never heard of the applicant. The program notified other schools about the misconduct.

4. **University of Rochester:** An applicant submitted a personal essay largely written by ChatGPT. The admissions committee flagged it due to unnatural phrasing and lack of detail, then verified it using plagiarism software. The student was denied.

5. **Columbia University Ph.D. Revocation:** In 2011, Columbia revoked the Ph.D. of a biochemistry graduate after discovering the individual fabricated data in their dissertation. This case underscores the seriousness with which academic institutions treat research misconduct, even after graduation.

6. **University of Minnesota Expulsion:** A former student filed a lawsuit after being expelled for allegedly using ChatGPT on an exam, a claim the student denies. This incident highlights the complexities and challenges institutions face in addressing AI-related academic misconduct.

7. **Texas A&M University Cheating Incident:** A professor at Texas A&M failed an entire class after suspecting students of using ChatGPT to complete assignments. This drastic measure, based on AI detection tools, sparked controversy and discussions about the reliability of such tools.

8. **Medical School Applicant's Institutional Action:** A medical school applicant shared on a forum that they faced an institutional action for participating in an e-mail thread discussing test questions. This action illustrates how academic misconduct can jeopardize medical school admissions.

These examples underscore the seriousness with which admissions officers view integrity, trust, honor code violations, and abiding by agreements, such as not using artificial intelligence to represent your work. Your patients, fellow students, professors, and colleagues rely on you for their life and the lives of others. They need to trust you.

For students pursuing BS/MD, BS/DO, and BS/DDS admission, this diligence is especially important. You are applying not just for admission, but for early entry into one of the most trusted professions. Let your application, recommendations, and essays, reflect the professionalism and responsibility of the doctor or dentist you aspire to become.

In the end, colleges and your future colleagues need you to follow through. Whether this is by taking responsibility to complete your applications, following the rules, or checking your college application portal. These serve as digital handshakes between you and your future college and medical institutions. Take ownership of your application and ensure every aspect is an authentic representation of your journey.

> "A formal education will make you a living; self-education will make you a fortune.

— *Jim Rohn*

CHAPTER FORTY-SIX

# FINANCIAL AID & SCHOLARSHIPS

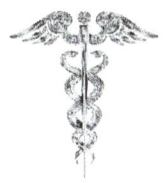

Financial aid is one of the most important questions for students and their parents. Navigating financial aid is a critical part of the college application process, especially for families managing educational expenses. From determining eligibility to submitting forms and receiving aid offers, understanding the timeline and requirements can make the process smoother and less stressful.

Unless your family's tax returns show significant income and assets, you may qualify for financial aid. Complete the Free Application for Federal Student Aid (FAFSA) at https://studentaid.gov/h/apply-for-aid/fafsa, You may also need to complete the CSS Profile, available through the College Board URL where you sign up for the SAT. Apply as soon as the sites open if possible, even if you must estimate your income and revise the amount later. Note that some colleges have their own forms or additional required documents.

## FINANCIAL AID TIMELINE

The financial aid process typically begins in the fall of a student's senior year. The FAFSA typically becomes available October 1. Families should submit the FAFSA before the school's deadline, which may be in November for Early Action.  Some states also have specific dates for state aid.

Many colleges also require the CSS Profile, especially for institutional aid, with similar deadlines. Check each college's financial aid webpage for exact dates, as some schools have early deadlines aligned with admission plans like Early Action or Early Decision.

# COLLEGES WITH FREE TUITION

Several elite universities offer free tuition or full financial aid to students from families below certain income thresholds. For example:

Harvard, Princeton, Yale, Cornell, Dartmouth, and Stanford offer free tuition as well as room and board to families earning under $75,000. For a few universities, the threshold is $200,000 for free tuition. Columbia, Brown, and Duke offer generous aid to families earning under $100,000. The University of North Carolina and University of Texas provide aid for families under certain state-defined income caps.

Amherst, Pomona, MIT, and many other schools meet 100% of demonstrated need, often with no loans. There are numerous examples, but you should know that if your income is less than $200,000, frequently funding opportunities are available.

# REQUIRED APPLICATION MATERIALS

To apply for financial aid, most colleges require:

* The FAFSA for federal/state aid and some scholarships
* The CSS Profile for institutional aid (some public and many private colleges)
* Tax returns, W-2s, and bank statements for verification

Some schools may require institutional forms or IDOC submission (College Board's document collection service).

# DEADLINES AND NOTIFICATION

Deadlines vary by school but often align with admission timelines.

Typically, FAFSA and CSS Profile should be submitted by:

* Nov 1–15 for Early Action/Early Decision.

* Jan 1–Mar 1 for Regular Decision.

Colleges usually notify students of their financial aid eligibility around the time they receive their admission decision.

# WHAT IS WORK-STUDY?

Federal work-study is a type of financial aid that allows students to earn money through part-time campus or community jobs. These extra funds help students cover personal or academic expenses without adding to loan debt. These jobs pay competitive wages and are often positions students would have done as a volunteer like working in a research lab or gaining career experiences.

## DOES AID IMPACT ADMISSION CHANCES?

At need-blind schools, requesting financial aid does not impact your chance of admission. However, need-aware schools consider financial need in the decision process, particularly for borderline applicants.

## WILL MY AID LAST ALL FOUR YEARS?

If your financial situation remains the same and you remain in good standing academically, most schools will continue to meet your demonstrated need annually. You must reapply each year with updated FAFSA and CSS Profile forms. Some merit scholarships may have GPA or enrollment requirements to remain eligible.

## STATE FINANCIAL AID AND PAYMENT PLANS

Many states offer their own aid programs (e.g., Cal Grant, NY TAP, Florida Bright Futures), often requiring FAFSA or a separate state form. Additionally, most colleges offer monthly tuition payment plans that allow you to divide semester-by-semester billing requirements into installments.

## MEDICAL SCHOOL FINANCIAL BURDEN

Medical school tuition and living expenses for four years can range from $300,000 to $500,000. The American Association of Medical Colleges website in May 2025 states that the median debt for medical students is $204,000.

Some medical schools like NYU and Kaiser have relieved the debt burden to some or all medical students, which is a major step. Furthermore, since some specialties like surgery and orthopedics require years of additional training, research has shown that this easing of debt encourages students to pursue areas where salaries are often double 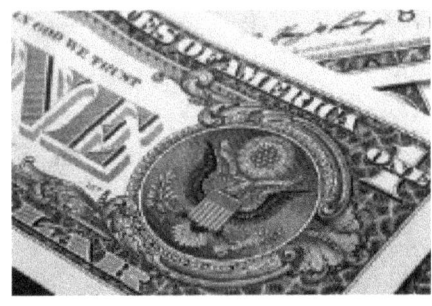 the average income of a general practitioner, despite the extended time.

One option to pay for medical school is the National Health Service Corps Scholarship Program. This scholarship covers full tuition, fees, and a monthly stipend and requires a return service commitment of years in an underserved Health Professional Shortage Area.

Additional options include the Public Service Loan Forgiveness (PSLF) program, which provides debt relief for doctors who choose to pursue public service. This incentivizes physicians to serve in areas where there is the greatest need. Other choices for debt relief include service with the Department of Veterans Affairs, the National Institutes of Health, the Indian Health Service, and the U.S. military.

With the motto, "Learning to Care for Those in Harm's Way," the Uniformed Services University is affiliated with the U.S. military. Located in Bethesda, Maryland, at Walter Reed National Military Medical Center, the Uniformed Services University is not only free, but students are paid for their medical training in exchange for paid service upon graduation. Since the program is year-round, students gain more than 700 hours of additional training beyond what is offered at traditional medical schools.

Therefore, quite a few options are available; some that are reasonably priced.

## FINDING ADDITIONAL AID SOURCES

Scholarships are offered by service organizations, international corporations, community foundations, non-profit organizations, veteran's groups, employers, and colleges. In addition to going to your high school counseling office which should have a list of current scholarship sources, there are scholarship search engines like Fastweb, Cappex, or BigFuture that provide lists. College financial aid offices typically also have information regarding outside scholarship opportunities.

## SCHOLARSHIPS

Merit scholarships are frequently available through colleges, private donors, or corporations. These are based upon academic success, background, talent, or life experiences. Scholarships may require additional forms, recommendations, essays, and proof of academic success. Note: A few universities, particularly the highest-ranked schools, do not offer merit scholarships, though most colleges do.

Check each college website for their financial aid process. For example, some colleges require students to submit the CSS Profile to be awarded merit money while others consider students automatically. However, many college scholarships require the submission of an SAT or ACT, even when the college admissions process is test optional. To help you get a sense of available scholarships, I selected three schools from the options listed in the profile section.

# PRIVATE SCHOLARSHIPS FOR STEM STUDENTS

## Prestigious Scholarships

**Barry Goldwater Scholarship** - This $7,500 scholarship is for college students, but high schoolers can plan early - 400 scholarships awarded.
**Davidson Fellows Scholarship** - Awards of $100,000, $50,000, and $25,000 for high school research in science, technology, literature, and philosophy.
**Regeneron Science Talent Search (STS)** - Top award is $250,000.
**Siemens STEM Day Innovation Challenge**
**U.S. Presidential Scholars** – Nomination required; medallion awarded.

## STEM & Research-Based Scholarships

**AISES Intel Growing the Legacy Scholarship** - Although AISES has Native American roots, Intel partners provide STEM scholarships that are open to general applicants in college or graduate school ($5-10,000).
**American Society of Human Genetics Essay Contest** - Science writing-based competition for high school students with thirteen scholarships.
**Cognizant Making the Future Scholarship** - Science and technology
**Lockheed Martin STEM Scholarship** - $10,000 renewable for high school seniors pursuing STEM.
**S.C.R.U.B.S. Healthcare Scholarship** – For students pursuing healthcare.

## Health/Medicine/Pre-Med-Focused Scholarships

**ACF Visionary Scholarship** – Open to all high school students; judged on essays, vision, and leadership.
**Anthem Essay Contest by The Ayn Rand Institute** - Not science-specific but highly respected and critical thinking focused.
**Healthcare Leaders Scholarship** – This $1,500 essay-based award is for high school or college students pursuing healthcare.
**National CPR Foundation Healthcare Scholarship** - This essay-based scholarship is for high school or college students pursuing medicine.
**Tylenol Future Care Scholarship** - Ten $10,000 and twenty-five $5,000 scholarships for college seniors pursuing health-related graduate school.

## General STEM & Tech Scholarships

**EngineerGirl Writing Contest** – Essay contest combining communication and STEM skills with elementary, middle, and high school categories.
**Microsoft Disability Scholarship** - For STEM students with disabilities.

**NCWIT Aspirations in Computing** - AI/cognitive science technology.
**NSHSS STEM Scholarship** - STEM-focused HS seniors can submit an application and personal statement for this $1,000 scholarship.
**Society of Women Engineers Scholarships** - HS seniors and college women in STEM majors - 320 scholarships ($1.5+ million annually).

## Research & Innovation-Based Scholarships

**ExploraVision Science Competition** - Collaborative research contest for futuristic science solutions.
**Genes in Space** - Challenge with real-life science application. Winners get their experiments run on the International Space Station.
**Junior Science and Humanities Symposium** - State/regional competition; focus on student research.
**Science Without Borders Challenge** - Combines science and hand-drawn or hand-painted to promote conservation - two HS age category scholarships.
**Toshiba/NSTA ExploraVision Award** - Prestigious K-12 STEM innovation competition with awards of $5,000 - $10,000 and a computer.

## General Academic Scholarships

**Burger King Scholars Program** - Burger King employees or their children can obtain one of these 21 scholarships of $60,000, $10,000, & $5,000.
**Coca-Cola Scholars Foundation** - $20,000 for leadership and academics.
**Elks National Foundation Most Valuable Student Scholarship** - Merit-based; considers leadership, need, and academics.
**GE-Reagan Foundation Scholarship** - High-achieving HS seniors who exemplify leadership, drive, integrity, and citizenship - $10,000/year for each.
**Jack Kent Cooke Foundation College Scholarship** - Up to $55,000/year for HS seniors whose family income is less than $95,000 - competitive.

## Lesser-Known

**American Fire Sprinkler Association Scholarship** - Five $1,000 awards for HS students who answer 8-question MC quiz - random drawing.
**College JumpStart Scholarship** - Open to 10th–12th graders, strong academic/research potential valued.
**Create-A-Greeting-Card Scholarship** - Art messaging and creativity.
**E-Waste Scholarship** - Environmental awareness for science students.
**Flavorful Futures Scholarship** - No major requirement, $5,000 award.
**Hutchinson Medical School Scholarship** - This $2,000 scholarship for

pre-med students; must have regional ties to Silicon Valley.

**Niche "No Essay" Scholarship** - Monthly random drawing; takes one minute to apply.

**Tall Clubs International Scholarship** - This $1,000 - $2,000 scholarship is for women who are at least 5'10" or who are at least 6'2".

**Technology Addiction Awareness Scholarship** – Psychology, neuroscience, and biotech - $1,000 & $500 award - HS or College

**Unigo $10K Scholarship** - Easy essay prompt; accessible to all students, no field restrictions - one HS student chosen.

## PRIVATE SCHOLARSHIPS

Private individuals, corporations, and endowments offer outside scholarships. Some offer full tuition. Here are a few of the thousands to consider.

### AQHA and AQHF – $25,000 - $35,000 (Dec 1) Quarter Horse Members

A few scholarships for journalism, communications, agricultural studies, and equine research.

### Alzheimer's Foundation of America

HS seniors impacted by Alzheimer's disease submit a 1,500-word essay or 4-min video describing the impact of Alzheimer's/dementia. Amount: $5,000 Due: April 1.

### American Legion National Oratorical Contest

HS juniors/seniors prepare an oration on the U.S. Constitution and citizenship. State Winners: $2,000, National Winner: $20,000 - $25,000.

### Ayn Rand Essay Contest - 455,000 student winners; $2,200,000 given out

Read and analyze one of three books (Anthem, Fountainhead, Atlas Shrugged) by Ayn Rand to win this contest. Multiple awards given out. Amount: $2,000  Due: April

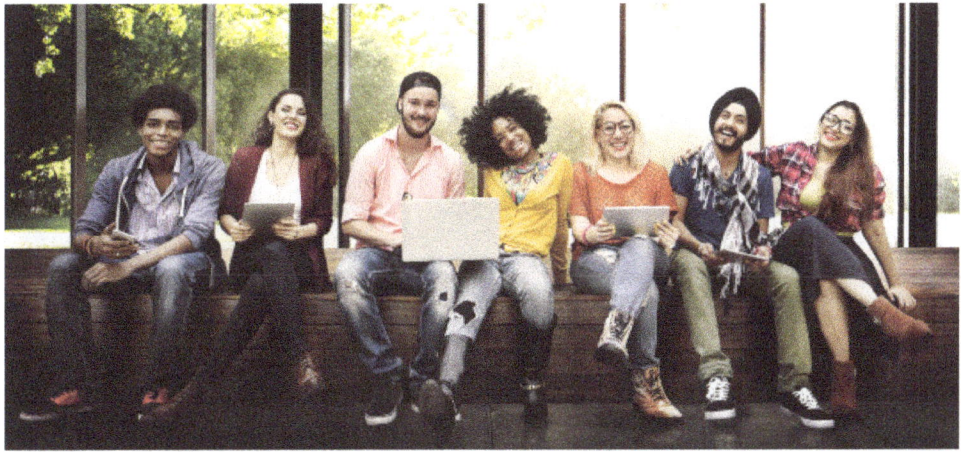

### Blaze Your Own Trail Scholarship

HS seniors and college students submit a 600-800-word essay describing a challenge you faced, how you overcame it, and your experience. Amount: $1,000 Deadline May

### Boren Scholarships ($8,000 - $25,000) and Boren Fellowships ($12,000 -30,000) – Foreign Language Study

The National Security Education Program (NSEP) awards funding for students to study one of about 65 languages the U.S. deems necessary for national security through a study abroad program. Applications open from mid-August to early February. Approximately 300 students are selected.

### Brower Youth Awards

Environmental activism awards are granted to 6 winners; each receives $3,000.

### Coca Cola Scholarship

1,400 students are selected to receive scholarships. The total amount awarded annually is approximately $3,550,000. 150 students receive $20,000 scholarship.

### Comcast NBC Universal Leaders and Achievers Scholarship

More than 800 high school student winners each year win a $2,500 scholarship.

### Dell Scholars Program – 500 students selected – $20,000 - First-Generation

This scholarship is awarded to students who exhibit grit, potential, and ambition.

### Doodle for Google Contest

This art/imagination contest is for K-12 students. Use any medium to describe your wish for the next 25 years. Amount: $5,000  Due: March 14.

### Gates Millennium Scholarship

These scholarships cover the full cost of attendance and are granted to 300 African American, American Indian/Alaska Native, Asian Pacific Islander, or Hispanic American student leaders.

### GE-Reagan Foundation Scholarship Program $40,000 (10 students)

Each year, 25 students ages 8 – 18 receive $10,000 for community service projects.

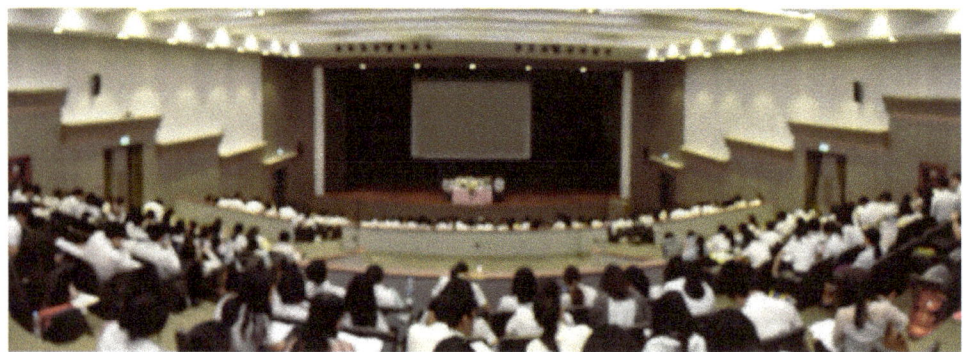

### Gloria Barron Prize for Young Heroes

25 students each year ages 8 – 18 receive $10,000 for community service projects

### Grit Award Scholarship

HS seniors with a GPA of 3.0+ must show GPA improvement and describe why they now have academic promise. Amount: $500 Due: May.

### Hispanic Scholarship Fund

Approximately 10,000 winners - $30,000,000 awarded annually.

### K-12 Educator Scholarship

This scholarship is for children with parents who teach in the K-12 system.

### Karcher Founders Scholarship

College-bound HS seniors that live near a Carl's Jr. Award: $10,000 Due: April 4.

### LULAC (League of United Latin American Citizens)
### Ford Driving Dreams Scholarship, ExxonMobil Scholarship
### NBC Universal Scholarship

The LULAC National Scholarship Fund along with corporations (Walmart, CocaCola, Nissan, Danaher, etc.) provide hundreds of scholarships for high school and college students.

### Minecraft Scholarship

HS/college students submit an essay of 500+ words, detailing how Minecraft can be a positive influence on education and careers. Amount: $2,000 Due July 31.

### NAACP – National Association for the Advancement of Colored People

African Americans - about 170 students receive awards of $3,000 to $15,000.

### NASSP – National Association of Secondary School Principals

600 Scholarships awarded per year, 1 national winner ($25,000), 24 national finalists ($5,625 each), 575 national semifnalists ($3,200 each). Apply Oct-Dec 1.

### Optimist International Essay Contest

HS students submit a 700-800-word essay on how optimism connects people. Amount: $2,500 Due: February 28.

### Parent Employment

Many companies offer scholarships for their employees and their children.

### Project Yellow Light Video Contest Scholarship

High school juniors and seniors, plus FT undergrads create a 10 or 25 second video that discourages texting while driving. Award: $8,000 Due: April 1.

### Prudential Spirit of Community Award ( Prudential Emerging Visionaries)

25 students in grades 5 to 12. Amount: $1,000 - $5,000 award for community service.

### Questbridge Scholarship

$200,000 is granted to each of 1,464 students to be used over 4 years.

### Race to Inspire Essay Contest

Student runners (5k, 10k, half marathons, or marathons) submit a 1,000-2,000 word essay detailing why they run and challenges/lessons. Amount: $500  Due in August.

### Rover College Scholarship

HS seniors/college students submit a 400-500-word essay on how growing up with a pet impacted the person they are today. Award: $2,500  Due May 1.

### ROTC

These military scholarships are not given to everyone in  ROTC. A select group of outstanding candidates is given tuition, fees, textbooks, plus a monthly stipend.

### Scholastic Art and Writing Competition

**Herblock Award** - $1,000 scholarships for editorial cartoons

**New York Life Award** - $1,000 writing award about personal grief and loss

**One Earth Award** - $1,000 scholarship for writing about human-caused climate change

**PortfolioScholarships** – Up to $10,000 granted for top portfolios

**Civic Expression Award** - $1,000 scholarships for writing on political and social issues

**Best-In-Grade** – Juror favorite awards receive $500 scholarships

**Art & Writing  Scholarships** - https://www.artandwriting.org/scholarships/

### #ScienceSaves High School Video Scholarship

HS seniors create a 20-30 second video about science and what it does for people. Amount: $10,000 Due May 6.

### Service/Leadership/Focused Organization Scholarship

Lions Club, Moose Club, Elks Club, Rotary Club, Soroptimists Club, Mensa

### Student Veterans of America

These scholarships are awarded to veterans. The funds granted to not interfere with GI Bill grants or other financial aid.  Scholarships total over $100,000 yearly.

### Susan Thompson Buffet Foundation Scholarships

This scholarship for high school and undergraduate students in Nebraska provides $3,200 plus a book allowance.

### Target Scholarship

HBCU Design Challenge for African Americans – Students submit designs for Black History Month. Target Scholars Program – 1,000 students get $5,000 each.

### Thurgood Marshall College Fund

Approximately 500 scholarships are awarded per year to engaged and motivated African American students. The average is $6,200 per year.

### Unboxing Your Life Video Scholarship

High school seniors and college students create a 5-minute video describing who they are as they unbox their life. Award: $4,000 Due: March 31.

### Vegetarian Resource Group Scholarship

HS students who actively promote vegetarianism and peace while demonstrating compassion, courage, and commitment. Amount: $5,000-$10,000 Due Feb 20.

### Walgreens Expressions Challenge

High school students between 13 and 18 are challenged to describe their world through words, visual arts, media arts or creative writing. Award: $1,500 - $2,000 This application is due in March.

### Walmart Scholarship Program

Employees and dependents can obtain up to $13,000 in scholarships to be used over four years. Complete the online application. Qualified candidates will be considered depending on their financial needs and academic performance.

### We The Future Contest

HS/college students submit an essay, song, project, film, social media, or PSA on a topic related to the Constitution. Amount: $1,000-$5,000 Due May 31.

### Final Note:

Like Walmart, many corporations offer scholarships for employees and dependents. For example, with Starbucks College Achievement Plan, students can receive 100% upfront tuition coverage for a first-time bachelor's degree through Arizona State University's online program. Starbucks partners can choose from over 100 diverse undergraduate degree programs.

Other prominent examples include AT&T whose deadline is in March. The AT&T Ability ERG Scholarship provides $1,500 to support students enrolling in accredited undergraduate programs. Pepsi provides 400 new scholarships each year for postsecondary education for children of PepsiCo associates. If your parent works for a corporation, check with their human resources department.

Also, many organizations like the American Legion, Elks Club, Exchange Club, Kiwanis International, Knights of Columbus, Lions Club, Moose International, National Grange, Jaycees, National League of Masonic Clubs, Optimist International, and Rotary Club, offer scholarships. These are typically offered through the branch clubs in your local area.

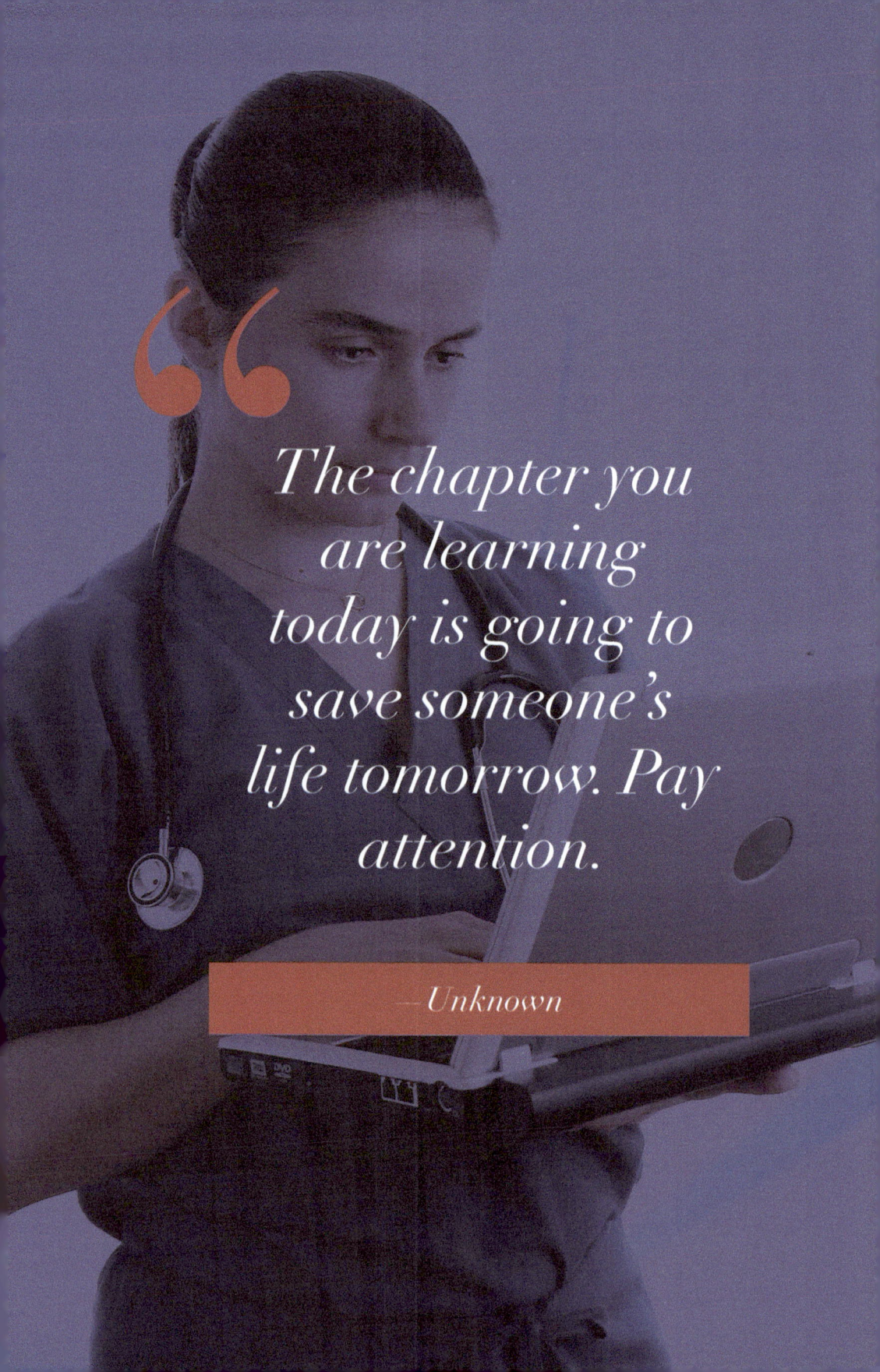

The chapter you are learning today is going to save someone's life tomorrow. Pay attention.

—*Unknown*

# CHAPTER FORTY-SEVEN

# DEFERRALS, WAITLISTS, & DECISIONS & WAITLISTS

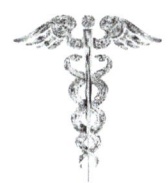

You may be deferred in the early decision or early action round. Do not give up hope. Consider applying ED II to a school, unless the programs you have applied to prevent this option. You can also apply regular decision. Most ED II and regular decision deadlines are between January 1 - 15.

Even if you reach the end of the application process and are waitlisted, know that many students do get off waitlists. At some schools, more than a hundred students are given an acceptance after being waitlisted.

## DECISIONS, DECISIONS: WAITING FOR A RESPONSE

The period between submitting your application and getting your admissions results requires patience and diligence. Most schools will send you a link to a portal where you will see what the college is missing, follow through with honors programs or scholarships, and check the results. Go into the site every couple of weeks in case the college requires a recommendation or has offered you the chance to apply for an extra scholarship.

Check your portal regularly. Additionally, note the college portal updates and correspondence sent through your e-mail. Waiting from November to April is agonizing. Your life is on the line and you just want to know where you are headed. However, colleges typically list the date they will send admissions results on the portal and on the college website. Other popular web locations post admissions decision notification dates too. You will find out soon.

## THICK OR THIN ENVELOPE

Students eagerly check each day as winter turns to spring, waiting to hear via e-mail, the college portal, or the mail for a welcome packet or denial letter. You know spring has come as regular decision admissions results steadily roll in, one at a time. In March, every day seems to last 26 hours - two extra hours for the period that lingers until that day's announcement. With each school announcing, one-by-one, the slow drip torture as you wait is exacerbated by the uncanny way each college picks a different day in March or April to announce their decision.

At some point you will know. That statement may seem like little solace in the middle of the fray. You have until May 1 to make a decision, though with limited housing available and a first-come, first-served basis of selection, the pressure is on to choose. Even so, visiting the college is vital, despite the fact that AP tests and finals are just around the corner and there seems to be no time. However, this decision influences where you will live, eat, study, make friends, take classes, and get involved for four years. Do you want to base your next four years on a few college-selected pictures and the tweets or newsfeeds of other people?

There are many variables to consider. This is why forward thinking at the beginning of the application process is valuable and even necessary to seek scholarships, merit money, or opportunities for financial aid. This proactive planning is especially needed with the spike in college applications at selective schools and the ever-changing landscape of test-optional admissions. MIT, Stanford, and Ivy League schools, for example, resumed their test requirement.

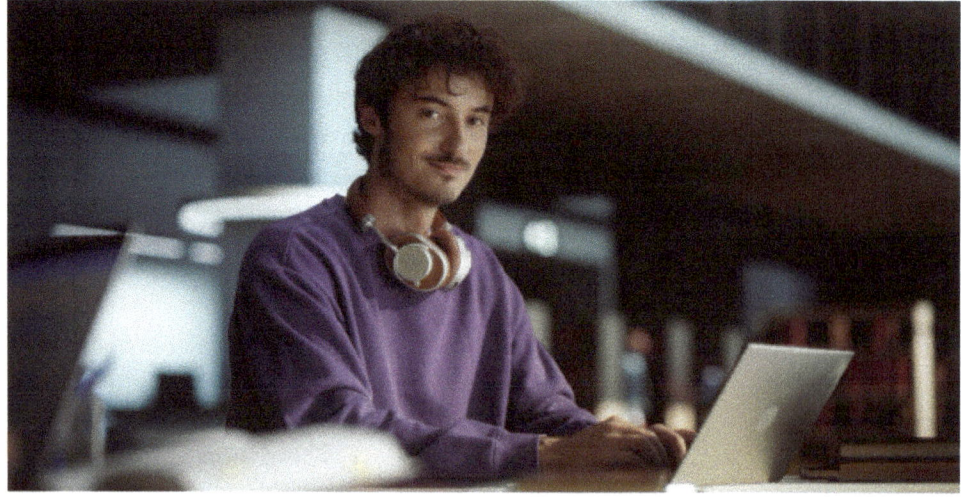

Plan ahead. The college application period is not a good time to procrastinate. The fall of your senior year is tough, especially with a demanding course load. It is even tougher for athletes who compete in a fall sport. However, throughout your life you will work on time management, organization, and goal setting. This is a good time to start so you do not miss thousands of dollars in financial aid and scholarships. Time management proved challenging for students who adjusted their lifestyles with self-paced classes, Zoom meetings, and online assignments.

## CELEBRATING ACCEPTANCES AND DEALING WITH REJECTION

Acceptance is not guaranteed. The sad fact is that many highly qualified candidates are rejected. Colleges seek students who are wholly committed to their education, talents, and learning experiences. Unfortunately, even for dedicated students, the probability of acceptance is low at the most highly selective schools where students have won national awards, competed on the international stage, and have produced novel technologies and published research. Your commitment, work ethic, and planning make the outcome sweeter when you are accepted. Celebrate each step along the way. You can do this. Get help. Think critically and logically. Be willing to work for it.

Congratulations! When you are accepted, you have colleges on your list of options. Check your financial aid and scholarship packages. Money is often an important factor in making your final decision. Even if you cannot visit the campus, ask the college for student contact names in your major. Many students apply to college merely by someone's recommendation, *U.S. News and World Report* ranking, Google photos, or posts on a website.

Nothing replaces the actual campus visit. After all, you will spend a few years there. Be selective as to where you apply, You may decide after visiting you do not want to apply. Understandably, the pandemic's uncertainty added more question marks to an already complicated set of admissions processes.

The buzzword for 2025-2035 is resilience. It is never easy to be rejected. However, rejection happens. You will survive this. Note: Many colleges still accept applications in April, May, and June long after most school's applications are closed. If you did not get accepted, look up colleges that still have openings. Some schools on the list may surprise you and may be good options. In April and May, Google "College Openings Update" to see schools that still have open spots.

## WAITLISTS: THE ART OF WAITING

Immediately confirm if you are given a waitlist spot and still want to attend. There is often a deadline. You do not want to miss this. If you are no longer interested or you have placed a deposit at another school, go into the portal and turn down the offer. Someone else is bound to be thrilled by your "anonymous gift".

If you are still interested, find the designated location on the portal and update them on what you have done since applying – accomplishments, awards, extra classes, honors, art shows, or films. Only add what they have not yet seen, but if you have taken the initiative to do something more than what you originally stated on the application, by all means, tell them. Some let you write a "love letter."

## UNIVERSITY OF CALIFORNIA WAITLIST DATA

| UC Campus | Waitlist Offers | Waitlist Opt-Ins | Admitted from Waitlist | Admit Rate |
|---|---|---|---|---|
| UC Berkeley | Not specified | Not specified | 26 | ~0.3% |
| UCLA | Not specified | 11,725 | 1,404 | 12% |
| UC San Diego | Not specified | 19,372 | 2,634 | 13.6% |
| UC Santa Barbara | 15,677 | 9,670 | 5,506 | 57% |
| UC Irvine | 16,743 | Not specified | 3,031 | ~18% |
| UC Davis | Not specified | 10,988 | 4,453 | ~41% |
| UC Riverside | Not specified | 3,891 | 1,151 | 29.5% |
| UC Santa Cruz | Not specified | Not specified | 8,206 | Not specified |
| UC Merced | N/A | N/A | N/A | N/A |

You could just wait for their decision, but you are better off showing that you really want to be at their school. Students do get off the waitlists at most schools. Be proactive! How much do you want to attend? Meanwhile, you will have to deposit somewhere else before the May 1st "National Candidate Reply" deadline. Stay hopeful. This next year is a significant step along your journey. Relax!

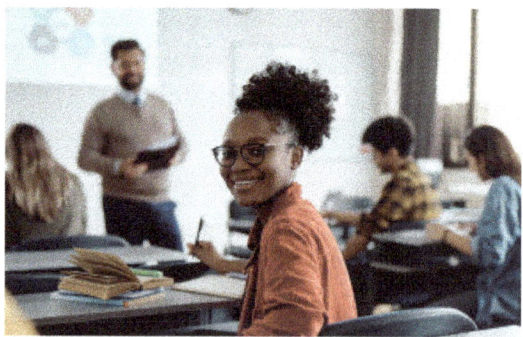

# WAITLIST DATA FOR SELECT U.S. UNIVERSITIES

| University | Waitlist Offers | Waitlist Opt-Ins | Admitted from Waitlist | Admit Rate |
|---|---|---|---|---|
| Boston University | 15,033 | 8,907 | 34 | 0.40% |
| Cornell University | ~6,000 | Not specified | 192 | ~3.2% |
| Dartmouth College | ~2,500 | Not specified | 51 | ~2.0% |
| Georgia Institute of Technology | 5,809 | 4,016 | 60 | 1.5% |
| Harvard University | ~2,000 | Not specified | 27 | ~1.4% |
| Princeton University | ~1,300 | Not specified | 23 | ~1.8% |
| Stanford University | ~1,400 | Not specified | 37 | ~2.6% |
| Tufts University | 2,565 | 1,324 | 200 | 15% |
| University of Miami | 21,869 | 7,758 | 215 | 2.8% |
| University of Michigan | 24,804 | Not specified | 973 | ~3.9% |
| University of North Carolina at Chapel Hill | ~2,800 | Not specified | 82 | ~2.9% |
| University of Pennsylvania | ~3,000 | Not specified | 57 | ~1.9% |
| Yale University | ~1,000 | Not specified | 46 | ~4.6% |

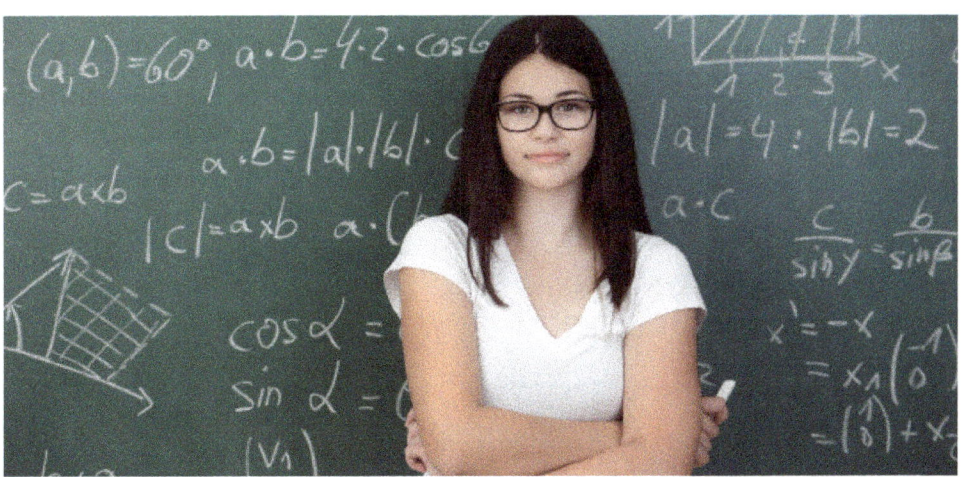

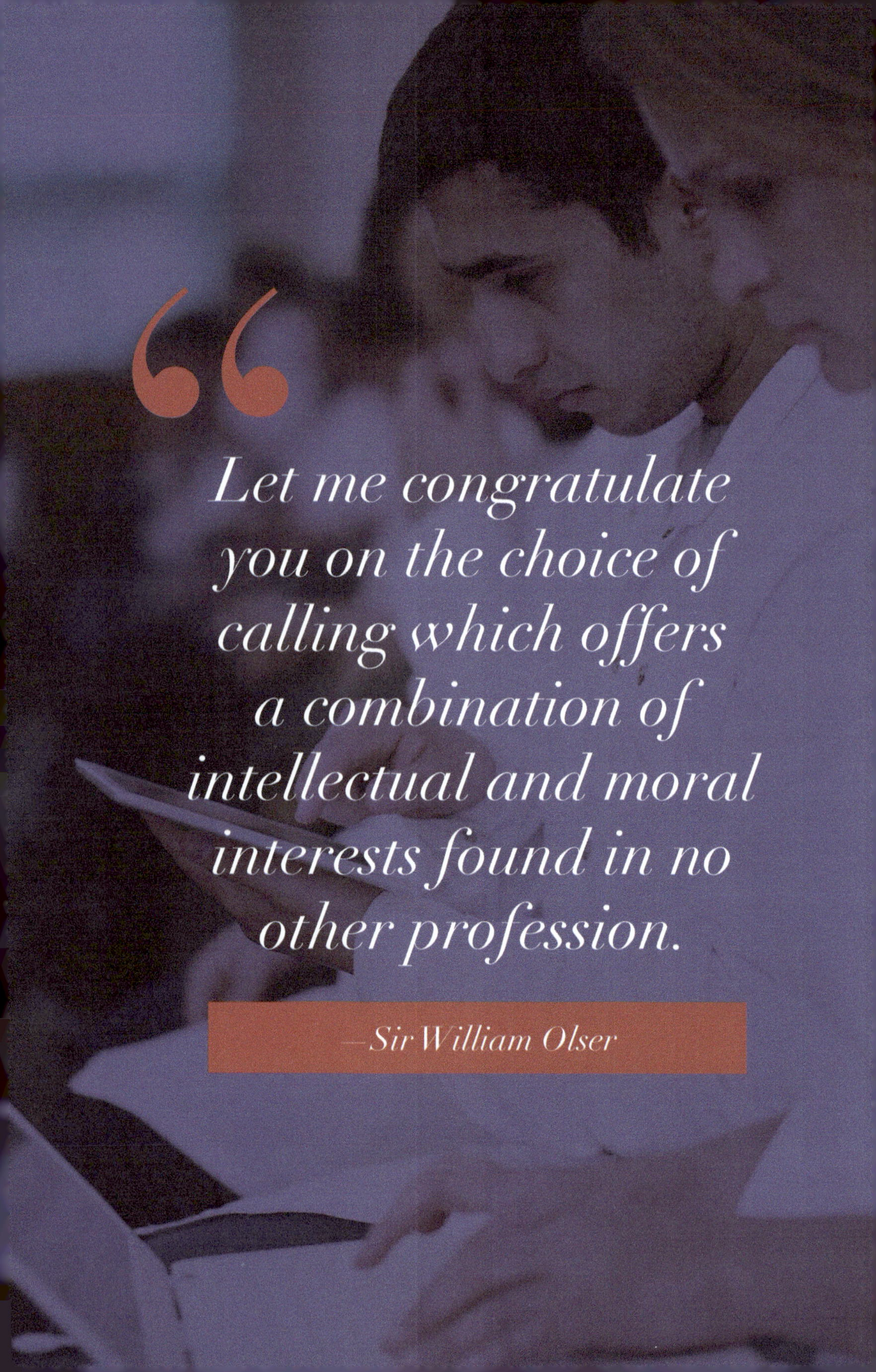

> " Let me congratulate
> you on the choice of
> calling which offers
> a combination of
> intellectual and moral
> interests found in no
> other profession.

—Sir William Olser

# CHAPTER FORTY-EIGHT

# NEXT STEPS: TRANSITIONING TO COLLEGE

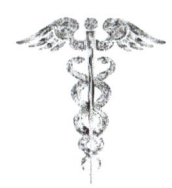

C hoosing a college is a major milestone. For students entering as part of a BS/MD, BS/DO, BS/DDS, or beginning the traditional pre-med track, the transition from high school to college marks the start of an exciting but more demanding journey. Most students are essentially on their own to navigate their way, advocate for themselves, and ensure they are taking the right steps. There is help, but you may need initiative to locate resources.

You are never alone, though, since there are advisors, faculty, counselors, tutors, classmates, and your parents who can help you make smart decisions. There is nothing wrong with asking for help. And, frankly, help will likely save you when you encounter tough junctures. You are likely to get stuck somewhere no matter how smart you are. Starting with college, you choose your direction.

Now that the excitement of acceptance has settled and you have chosen the school you will attend, it is time to plan for success. This chapter outlines key considerations to help you navigate your early college years with purpose, balance, and insight.

## ROOMMATES AND RESIDENTIAL LIFE

Where you live and who you live with can shape your first-year experience. Most colleges allow you to submit preferences or profiles to match with compatible roommates. While BS/MD, BS/DO, and BS/DDS programs often have highly focused cohorts, traditional pre-meds may be placed with students in different majors. Discuss expectations with your roommate early regarding study habits, sleep schedules, shared responsibilities, and communication styles. A stable living environment reduces stress and allows more focus on academics.

Avoid competitive comparisons with roommates or peers in your major. Pre-med clubs are often competitive. Remember, everyone starts out with their own unique talents and skillsets. Everyone's path is different, even within the same major. Internalizing or focusing on others' progress can be distracting and demoralizing. Avoid following the path of others. Instead, go forth and leave a trail.

## CURRICULUM PLANNING: BUILDING A STRONG FOUNDATION

Whether you are in a BS/MD, BS/DO, BS/DDS or on the traditional route, medical schools expect mastery in core science and humanities courses. Work with your academic advisor to:

* Create a course plan of required pre-med courses (biology, chemistry, organic chemistry, biochemistry, physics, calculus, and statistics).
* Balance science-heavy semesters with manageable workloads to avoid burnout.
* Take advantage of research, seminar, and thesis-based courses for deeper learning.

BS/MD, BS/DO, and BS/DDS students often have prescribed majors, especially in accelerated programs. Many choose biology, chemistry, biochemistry, or neuroscience. Traditional pre-meds should select a major they enjoy, while ensuring their coursework covers the necessary prerequisites for medical school.

## AP CREDIT: USE WITH CAUTION

Some colleges allow AP credit to replace introductory social science and humanities courses. Others require students to retake courses, even when the student earned a 5 on the AP test. However, if your school accepts AP Biology or Chemistry, you still want to retake the course in college. Consider these:

* You need to feel comfortable in all science disciplines before moving on.
* These topics are on the MCAT if you need to take that test.
* Medical schools often prefer applicants who take core pre-med classes in college.

* AP courses vary in rigor across high schools.

* Repeating the class may strengthen your GPA and deepen your understanding. This will be imperative for the MCAT and medical admissions.

Speak with a pre-health advisor to decide whether to apply AP credit or repeat foundational coursework.

## WHAT MEDICAL SCHOOLS LOOK FOR

Know medical school admissions criteria. This will help you plan effectively. Key qualities include:

* **Strong GPA and MCAT:** A competitive GPA (3.8+) and MCAT score are essential for traditional applicants.

* **Clinical Exposure:** Shadowing physicians, hospital volunteering, scribing, EMT/phlebotomy/medical assistant certifications show commitment.

* **Research Experience:** Laboratory work, abstracts, literature review, and publications reflect curiosity and discipline.

* **Service and Leadership:** Tutoring, mentoring, or community health outreach demonstrate compassion.

* **Personal Growth:** Authentic essays and letters of recommendation are grounded in reflection and lived experience.

BS/MD, BS/DO, or BS/DDS students may not need the MCAT/DAT for their formal application process, but maintaining GPA and professionalism is crucial for progression into the medical/dental school phase.

## STAYING ON TRACK: MILESTONES AND MINDSETS

**First Year**

* Adjust to the academic pace and develop time management skills.
* Join student organizations and get involved in scientific research.
* Attend workshops, explore research labs, and look for shadowing opportunities.

**Sophomore Year**

* Deepen your involvement in clinical and volunteer activities.
* Begin/continue research or long-term service projects.

* Apply for summer programs, medical mission trips, or research opportunities.
* Build relationships with professors for future recommendations.

## Junior Year

* For traditional pre-meds, prepare and take the MCAT.
* Talk to those who may write your letters of recommendation.
* Consider gap year planning. If you submit your AMCAS when you graduate, you have a year to gain experience.
* Take leadership roles and apply for national scholarships and summer programs.

## Senior Year

* Finalize application materials if you apply to med school in May or June.
* Reflect on academic and personal growth.
* Sign up for the CASPer and PREview if required.
* For BS/MD students, prepare for transition to the medical curriculum.

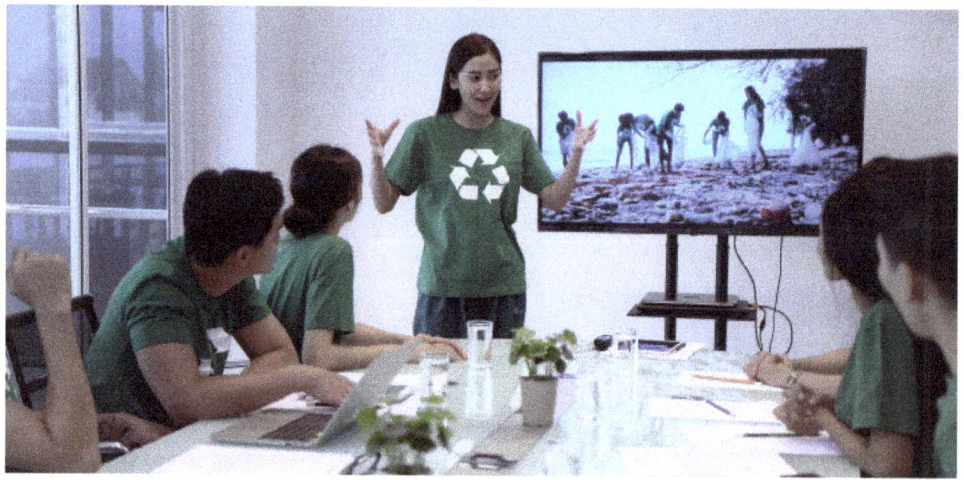

## CAUTIONARY ADVICE

* **Avoid Overcommitting:** Depth matters more than quantity. Do not stretch yourself too thin with an overload of classes, research projects, clinical opportunities, clubs, leadership, and jobs.
* **Watch for Burnout:** Sleep, nutrition, and exercise can improve your performance and well-being.
* **Manage Setbacks with Perspective:** A tough semester is not the end. Learn, recover, and adapt.

* **Uphold Academic Integrity:** One incident of dishonesty can derail your medical career before it begins.

## MAKE USE OF CAMPUS RESOURCES

* Pre-health advising offices offer program planning, MCAT prep timelines, and mock interviews.
* Writing centers can support personal statements and lab reports.
* Career services help with summer internships, research positions, and job shadowing.
* Mental health and wellness centers offer counseling, support groups, and stress-reduction tools.

## CULTIVATING PROFESSIONALISM EARLY

Medical schools expect maturity, reliability, and humility. Start building your professional identity by:

* Responding to emails promptly and respectfully.
* Showing up prepared and on time to commitments.
* Reflecting on mistakes and learning from them.
* Practicing empathy in team and classroom settings.

Whether you are guaranteed a medical school seat or working your way toward one, the transition to college is an opportunity to reset, recalibrate, and grow. The goal is to consistently make progress toward your goal. Engage deeply, ask questions, and build a network of mentors and peers. The habits, relationships, and choices you make now will echo throughout your journey toward becoming a physician.

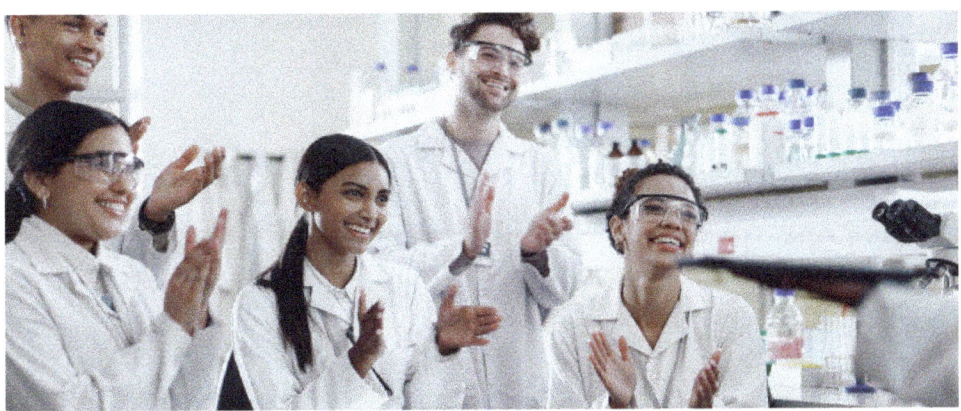

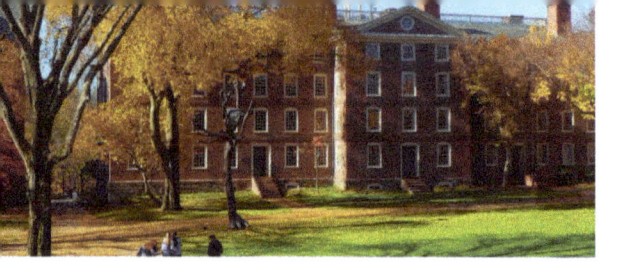

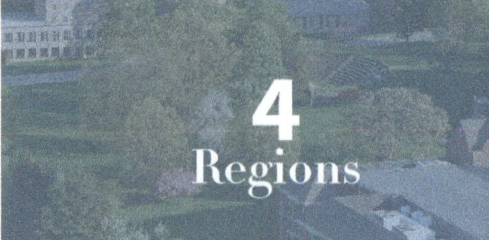

**4**
Regions

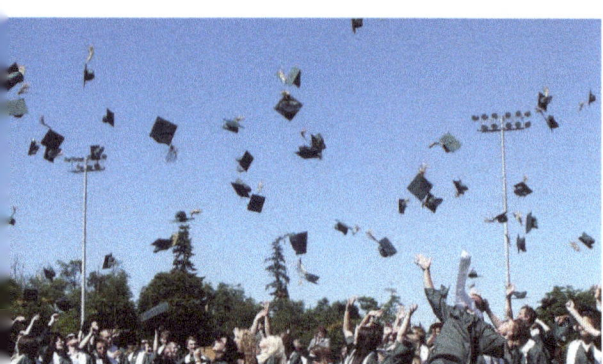

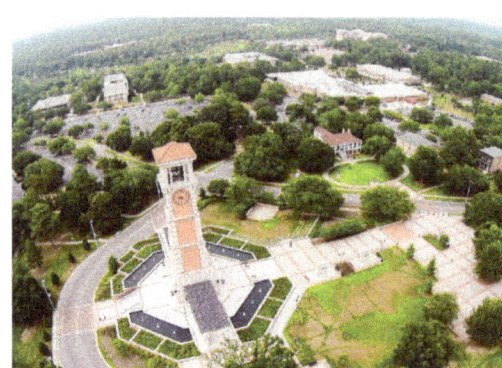

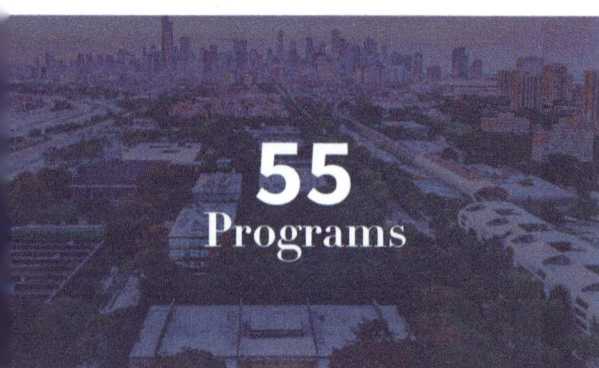

**55**
Programs

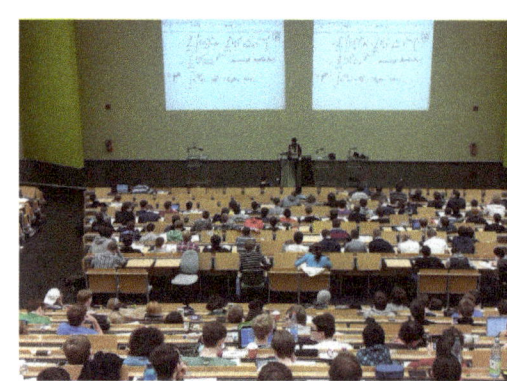

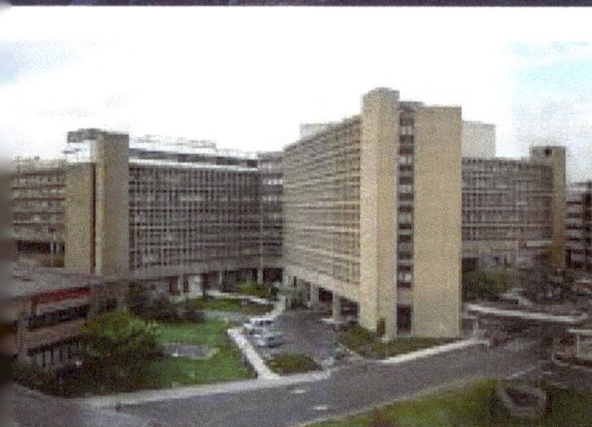

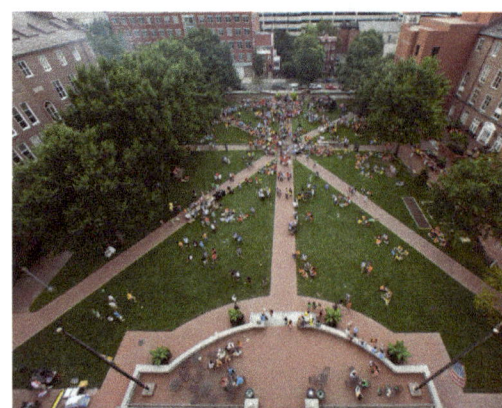

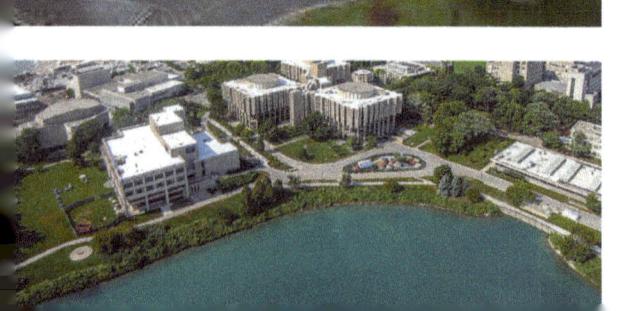

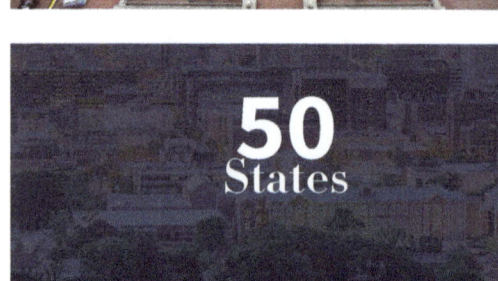

**50**
States

# PART SIX

# PROFILES OF BS/MD, BA/MD, BS/DO PROGRAMS

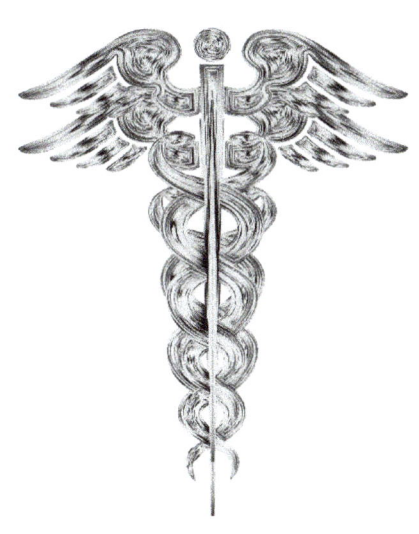

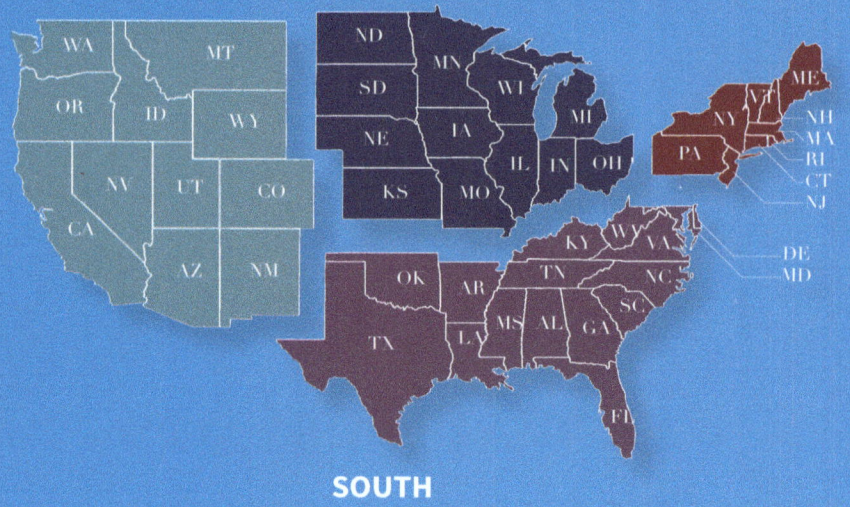

# BS/MD PROGRAMS BY REGION
## U.S. CENSUS BUREAU CLASSIFICATIONS

### REGION 1 – NORTHEAST

Connecticut, Maine, Massachusetts, New Hampshire, New Jersey, New York, Pennsylvania, Rhode Island, and Vermont

### REGION 2 – MIDWEST

Illinois, Indiana, Iowa, Kansas, Michigan, Minnesota, Missouri, Nebraska, North Dakota, Ohio, South Dakota, and Wisconsin

### REGION 3 – SOUTH

Alabama, Arkansas, Delaware, District of Columbia, Florida, Georgia, Kentucky, Louisiana, Maryland, Mississippi, North Carolina, Oklahoma, South Carolina, Tennessee, Texas, Virginia, and West Virginia

### REGION 4 – WEST

Alaska, Arizona, California, Colorado, Hawaii, Idaho, Montana, Nevada, New Mexico, Oregon, Utah, Washington, and Wyoming

## CHAPTER FORTY-NINE

# LIST OF BS/MD AND BS/DO PROGRAMS

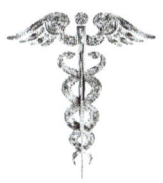

The BS/MD and BS/DO programs listed on the following pages are ONLY those where students apply as a high school student and not after currently enrolled in college. Those where students apply while they are already in a university like CWRU, Howard, FIU, FL Tech, Loma Linda, Marshall. Michigan State, Temple, Tufts, U. of AZ, UMiami, UTSA Health, and UCR are not listed.

This list is current as of June 2025. Note that popular programs like Baylor/Rice, BU, Northwestern, USC, University of Florida, and University of Central Florida have been discontinued. A few are left out because their program information was unavailable. However, more than fifty U.S. programs are listed to give you some excellent options to consider.

Pursuing a BS/MD or BS/DO is not for everyone. Although immensely rewarding, success in these programs, even if you are accepted is difficult. Some have MCAT requirements with thresholds in above the 75th percentile, meaning that the road requires you to not only keep up your grades but also spend significant time during your four year journey mastering the MCAT.

Thus, I have also included lists in the back of other program options you might consider. Keep this book handy since few lists of related opportunities may be valuable in the future. Creating lists is often tedious and cumbersome. These colleges and universities were gathered for you to help you with this task.

Some requirements may have changed by the time you read this book. Nevertheless, this information is a great place to start.

I wish you the best as you pursue this journey. You are in an exciting place where you have lots of choices. Go forth and conquer!

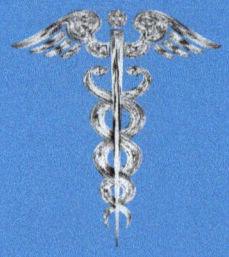

# REGION ONE

# NORTHEAST

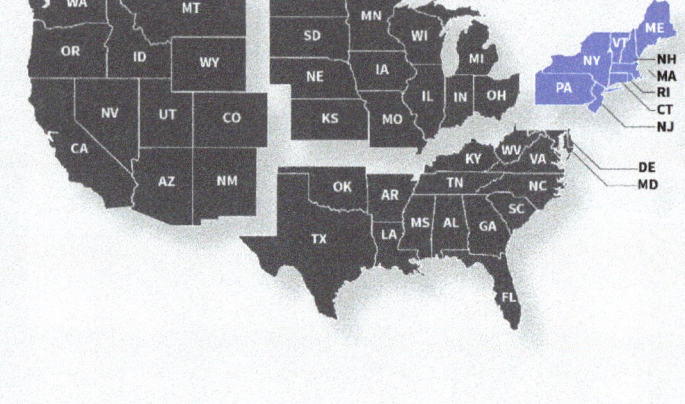

**CONNECTICUT**

**MAINE**

**MASSACHUSETTS**

**NEW HAMPSHIRE**

**NEW JERSEY**

**NEW YORK**

**PENNSYLVANIA**

**RHODE ISLAND**

**VERMONT**

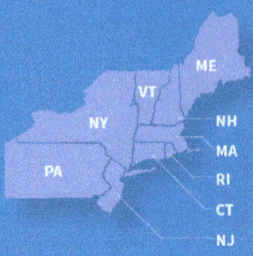

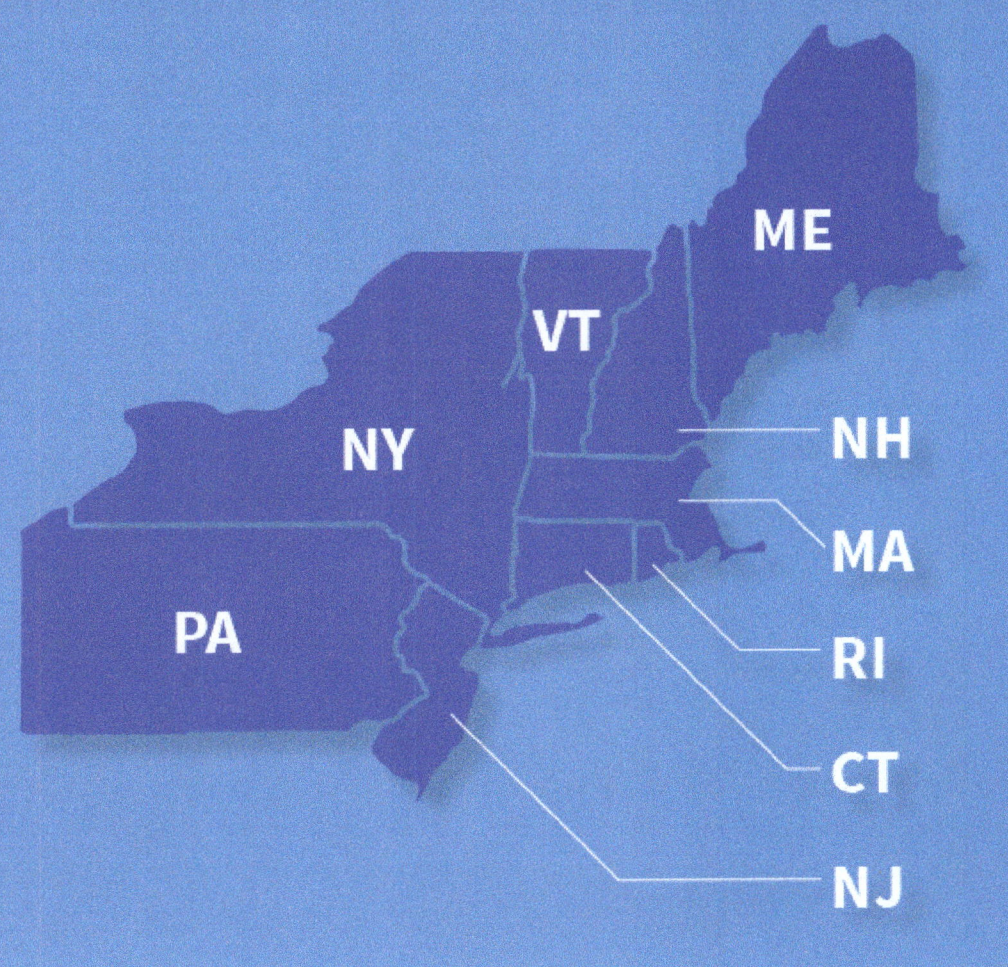

# 25 Programs | 9 States

1. CT – University of Connecticut - BS/MD (SPiM)
2. MA – Massachusetts College of Pharmacy and Health Sciences (MCPHS) – BS/DO
3. NJ – New Jersey Institute of Technology - BS/MD
4. NJ – Rowan University - BS/MD and BS/DO
5. NJ – Rutgers University, Camden - BS/MD and BS/DO
6. NJ – Stevens Institute of Technology - BS/MD and BS/DO
7. NJ – Stockton University - BS/DO
8. NY – Adelphi University - BS/MD and BS/DO
9. NY - Brooklyn College - BA/MD
10. NY - City College of New York - BS.MD
11. NY – Hofstra University - BS/MD
12. NY – New York Institute of Technology - BS/DO
13. NY – Rensselaer Polytechnic Institute - BS/MD
14. NY – Siena College - BS/MD
15. NY – St. Bonaventure University - BS/MD and BS/DO
16. NY – Stony Brook University - BA/MD SPM
17. NY – SUNY Old Westbury - BS/DO
18. NY – Union College Leadership in Medicine - BS/MD
19. NY – University of Rochester REMS - BS/MD
20. PA - Drexel University - BS/MD
21. PA – Duquesne University - BS/MD and BS/DO
22. PA - Gannon University - BS/DO
23. PA - Penn State University Accelerated Med PPM - BS/MD
24. PA - University of Pittsburgh - BS/MD
25. RI – Brown University PLME - BS/MD

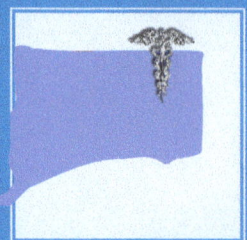

**CONNECTICUT**

**MAINE**

**MASSACHUSETTS**

**NEW HAMPSHIRE**

**NEW JERSEY**

**NEW YORK**

**PENNSYLVANIA**

**RHODE ISLAND**

**VERMONT**

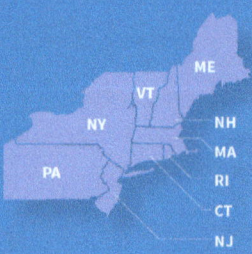

# UNIVERSITY OF CONNECTICUT
## BS/MD (SPiM) (8-YEARS)

**University of Connecticut Special Program in Medicine**
2131 Hillside Road Storrs, CT  06269
**Affiliated Medical School:** UConn School of Medicine
**Request Information:** *https://connect.uconn.edu/register/join*
**Phone:** (860) 679-2000 | **E-Mail:** *admissions@uchc.edu*
**International Students:** Considered
**Preference to In-State Residents:** Yes
**Application Deadline:** November 15
**Ave SAT/ACT:** 1500/34 | **GPA:** 3.9+ (unwt) | **MCAT:** Yes

## COST OF ATTENDANCE

**Tuition & Fees:** ~$20,000 (in-state), ~$46,000 (out of state)
**Addl Exp:** $25,000 | **Total:** $45,000 (in-state), $71,000 (out-of-state)
**Scholarships:** Merit-based, need-based, and special program scholarships are available.

## ADDITIONAL INFORMATION

Interviews are offered to select candidates. Students can apply to the Special Program in Medicine directly through the Common App. The admissions committee evaluates applicants based on academic achievements, extracurricular activities, leadership roles, community service, and a demonstrated commitment to the field of medicine. Students may choose from over 110 majors. Although there are no state residency requirements, Connecticut residents will receive special preference.

# MASSACHUSETTS COLLEGE OF PHARMACY AND HEALTH SCIENCES (MCPHS) BS/DO (8-YEARS)

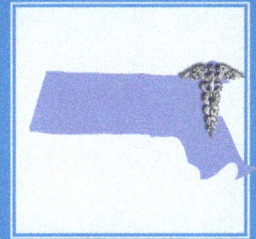

**Massachusetts College of Pharmacy and Health Sciences**
179 Longwood Avenue, Boston, MA 02115
**Affiliated Medical School:** A.T. Still University or Lake Erie College of Osteopathic Medicine
**Request Information:**
*https://www.mcphs.edu/request-for-information?inquiry*
**Phone:** (617) 879-5964 | **E-Mail:** *admissions@mcphs.edu*
**International Students:** Considered
**Preference to In-State Residents:** No
**Application Deadline:** Admission is on a rolling basis.
**Min SAT/ACT:** 1200/26 | **GPA:** 3.5+ | **MCAT:** Yes (No for LECOM)

## COST OF ATTENDANCE

**Tuition & Fees:** ~$44,000 | **Addl Expenses:** $44,000 | **Total:** ~$88,000
**Scholarships:** All first-year applicants are automatically considered for merit scholarships based on academic performance.

## ADDITIONAL INFORMATION

Prospective students should apply through the MCPHS undergraduate admissions process, indicating their interest in the BS/DO pathway. MCPHS has 12 distinct healthcare schools with over 100 programs across more than a dozen distinct health fields, including pharmacy, nursing, PA, optometry, acupuncture, physical therapy, occupational therapy, and more.

CONNECTICUT

MAINE

MASSACHUSETTS

NEW HAMPSHIRE

NEW JERSEY

NEW YORK

PENNSYLVANIA

RHODE ISLAND

VERMONT

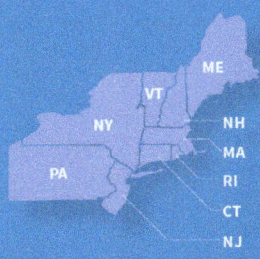

NORTHEAST

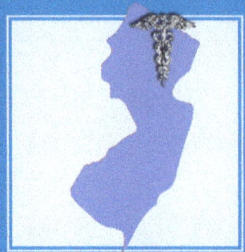

# NEW JERSEY INSTITUTE OF TECHNOLOGY BS/MD (7-YEARS)

**New Jersey Institute of Technology**
Fenster Hall, Room 100, University Heights, Newark, NJ 07102
**Affiliated Medical School:** Rutgers New Jersey Medical School
**Request Information:** *https://connect.njit.edu/register/rfi*
**Phone:** (973) 596-3300 | **E-mail:** *admissions@njit.edu*
**International Students:** Considered
**Preference to In-State Residents:** No
**Application Deadline:** November 1
**Min SAT/ACT:** 1490, 33 | **GPA:** 3.92+ | **MCAT:** Yes

## COST OF ATTENDANCE

**Tuition & Fees:** ~$21,000 (in-state), $36,000 (out-of-state)
**Addl Exp:** $25,000 | **Total:** $46,000 (in-state), $61,000 (out-of-state)
**Scholarships:** Approximately 95% of NJIT students receive scholarships, and financial aid.  All applicants are automatically considered for merit scholarships

## ADDITIONAL INFORMATION

Through NJIT's Albert Dorman Honors College, high school seniors apply by Nov 1 via the Common App, selecting both the Honors College and the 7-year BS/MD accelerated pathway. This program typically receives about 350 applications and offers ~28 seats annually.

Admitted students enter NJIT, complete a rigorous three-year bachelor's plan (any major, provided they maintain semester GPA ≥3.5 with B or better in all pre-med courses), and then matriculate directly into NJMS's medical school without a formal secondary application, though taking the MCAT is required by spring of the third year, with no minimum score but under probation if coursework weakens.

Admissions standards are extremely competitive. All applicants must submit SAT (min 1490) or ACT (min 33) from a single test date (not a superscore), and average admitted students is SAT ~1504 and GPA 4.0 (unweighted).

The interview process includes two rounds: NJIT and NJMS.  Students are considered holistically, including passion for medicine and leadership with an emphasis on academic excellence, commitment to service, and thoughtful essays. Advice to students:f clearly articulate why the accelerated track suits you, demonstrate community engagement and leadership, and lean into NJIT's abundant research and advising support in both STEM and humanities contexts.

**CONNECTICUT**

**MAINE**

**MASSACHUSETTS**

**NEW HAMPSHIRE**

**NEW JERSEY**

**NEW YORK**

**PENNSYLVANIA**

**RHODE ISLAND**

**VERMONT**

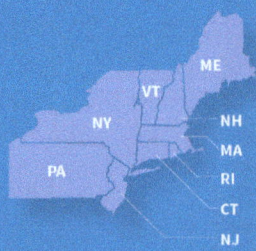

# ROWAN UNIVERSITY
## BS/MD AND BS/DO (7-YEARS)

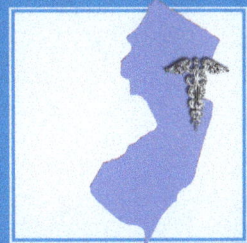

**Rowan University:** 225 Rowan Boulevard, Glassboro, NJ 08028
**Affiliated Medical School:** BS/MD w/Cooper Medical School of Rowan University (CMSRU) BS/DO with Rowan-Virtua School of Osteopathic Medicine
**Request Information:** *https://admissions.rowan.edu/request-information.html*
**Phone:** (856) 256-4200 | **E- mail:** *admissions@rowan.edu*
**International Students:** BS/DO - Yes, BS/MD - No
**Preference to In-State Residents:** Yes, but all are considered.
**Application Deadline:** November 1
**Min SAT/ACT:** 1350 | **GPA:** 3.5 + | **MCAT:** Yes

## COST OF ATTENDANCE

**Tuition & Fees:** ~$18,000 (in-state), ~$30,000 (out-of-state)
**Addl Exp:** $25,000 | **Total:** $43,000 (in-state), $55,000 (out-of-state)
**Scholarships:** Merit-based scholarships awarded to eligible first-time students enrolled full-time during the fall semester. Applications submitted before January 31 are reviewed for scholarship eligibility.

## ADDITIONAL INFORMATION

Students can apply via the Common App, Coalition App, or Rowan App. Select interest in the 3+4 medical program. Complete the supplemental application.

# RUTGERS UNIVERSITY
## CAMDEN - BS/DO, NEWARK - BA/MD

**Rutgers University, Camden** - 406 Penn Street, Camden, NJ 08102
BS/DO w/Rowan-Virtua School of Osteopathic Medicine
**Rutgers** - 195 University Ave, Newark, NJ 07102
**BA/MD** w/Rutgers New Jersey Medical School
**Request Information:** *https://www.ugadmissions.rutgers.edu/forms/InfoRequest.aspx*
**Phone:** (856) 225-6104 | **E-mail:** *admissions@camden.rutgers.edu*
**International Students:** Not eligible
**Preference to In-State Residents:** Yes, but all are considered.
**Application Deadline:** November 1
**Min. SAT/ACT:** 1400/31| **GPA:** top 10% | **MCAT:** Yes

## COST OF ATTENDANCE

**Tuition & Fees:** ~$19,000 (in-state), $39,000 (out-of-state)
**Addl Exp:** $25,000 | **Total:** $44,000 (in-state), $64,000 (out-of-state)
**Scholarships:** BA/MD Presidential Scholarship: Available to students accepted into the 7-year BA/MD Program. Covers in-state tuition, room, and board annually during the three years of undergraduate coursework. Students are expected to live on campus.

## ADDITIONAL INFORMATION

Apply and select "Newark College of Arts & Sciences." and "Med Joint BA/MD" Supplemental application also due by November 1

CONNECTICUT

MAINE

MASSACHUSETTS

NEW HAMPSHIRE

NEW JERSEY

NEW YORK

PENNSYLVANIA

RHODE ISLAND

VERMONT

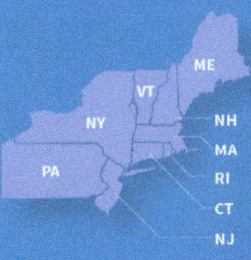

NORTHEAST

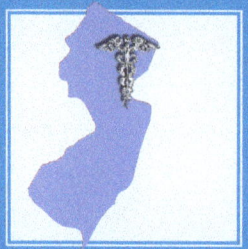

**CONNECTICUT**

**MAINE**

**MASSACHUSETTS**

**NEW HAMPSHIRE**

**NEW JERSEY**

**NEW YORK**

**PENNSYLVANIA**

**RHODE ISLAND**

**VERMONT**

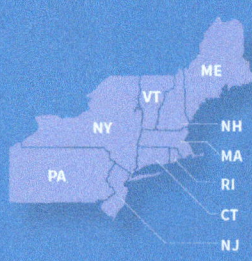

# STEVENS INSTITUTE OF TECHNOLOGY
## BS/MD AND BS/DO (7-YEARS)

**Stevens Institute of Technology BS/MD and BS/DO**
1 Castle Point Terrace. Hoboken, NJ 07030
**Affiliated Medical Schools:** MD - Rutgers NJ Medical School and NY Medical College; DO - NYITCOM
**Request Information:** *undergradadmissions.stevens.edu/register/inquiryform*
**Phone:** (201) 216-5194 | **E-mail:** *admissions@stevens.edu*
**International Students:** Not considered for BS/MD
**Preference to In-State Residents:** No, all students considered equally.
**Application Deadline:** November 1 (BS/MD)
**Min SAT/ACT:** 1400/32 (not superscored) | **GPA:** top 10% | **MCAT:** Yes

### COST OF ATTENDANCE

**Tuition & Fees:** ~$66,000 | **Addl Expenses:** $25,000 | **Total:** ~$91,000
**Scholarships:** The Presidential Achievement Scholarship, Global Impact, Martha Bayard Stevens Scholarship, A. James Clark Scholarship are based on academic excellence, standardized test scores, and/or extracurricular achievements. The Stevens Grant is available to those who demonstrate financial need. Students must submit the FAFSA and CSS Profile.

### ADDITIONAL INFORMATION

Apply to SIT and submit supplemental app to medical school partners. Students spend three years at Stevens completing a Bachelor of Science in Chemical Biology. Upon successful completion of the first year at NJMS, Stevens confers the bachelor's degree. The program is highly competitive with a limited number of seats available each year.

# STOCKTON UNIVERSITY
## BS/DO (7-YEARS)

**Stockton University BS/DO w/LECOM and Rowan-Virtua COM**
Campus Center, Suite 101 Vera King Farris Drive. Galloway, NJ 08205
**Affiliated Medical School:** Lake Erie College of Osteopathic Medicine and Rowan-Virtua School of Osteopathic Medicine
**Request Information:** *choose.stockton.edu/register/inquiryform*
**Phone:** (609) 652-4261 | **E-mail:** *admissions@stockton.edu*
**International Students:** Considered
**Preference to In-State Residents:** No
**Application Deadline:** November 30
**Min SAT/ACT:** 1310/27| **GPA:** top 10% | **MCAT:** Yes (No for LECOM)

### COST OF ATTENDANCE

**Tuition & Fees:** ~$17,000 (in-state), $25,000 (out-of-state)
**Addl Exp:** $25,000 | **Total:** $42,000 (in-state), $50,000 (out-of-state)
**Scholarships:** Approximately 200 privately funded scholarships awarded annually to qualified current Stockton students. Garden State Guarantee: A state program providing financial assistance to eligible New Jersey residents in their third and fourth years of study.

### ADDITIONAL INFORMATION

Students apply via the Common App or Stockton app. After submitting the application, eligible students receive access to the supplemental application through their Stockton portal. For LECOM, students must be accepted into the program before matriculating at Stockton.

## ADELPHI UNIVERSITY
## BS/MD & BS/DO (7-YEARS)

**Adelphi University BS/MD & BS/DO w/Rutgers NJMS**
One South Avenue, P.O. Box 701. Garden City, NY 11530
**Affiliated Medical Schools:**
Philadelphia College of Osteopathic Medicine (PCOM) – BS/DO
Lake Erie College of Osteopathic Medicine (LECOM) – BS/DO
**Request Information:** *adelphi.edu/admissions/contact/request-info*
**Phone:** (516) 877-3050 | **E-mail:** *admissions@adelphi.edu*
**International Students:** Eligible
**Preference to In-State Residents:** No
**Application Deadline:** Check each school.
**SAT/ACT:** Competitive | **GPA:** 3.5+ | **MCAT:** Yes (PCOM), No (LECOM)

### COST OF ATTENDANCE

**Tuition & Fees:** ~$52,000 | **Addl Expenses:** $25,000 | **Total**: $77,000
**Scholarships:** Automatically considered upon admission, with awards
ranging from $12,000 to $35,000 annually for full-time first-year
students. An additional $3,000 per year for students admitted into the
Honors College. $1,000 per year for achievements such as Eagle Scout,
Girl Scout Gold, or Explorer Awards.

### ADDITIONAL INFORMATION

Apply via the Common App or Adelphi app. Indicate interest in EAP or
Joint Degree program. Submit required documents.

---

## BROOKLYN COLLEGE
## BA/MD (8-YEARS)

**Brooklyn College BA/MD w/SUNY Downstate Medical Center**
222 West Quad Center, 2900 Bedford Avenue, Brooklyn, NY 11210
**Affiliated Medical Schools:** CUNY School of Medicine
**Request Information:** *brooklyn.edu/admissions-aid/take-the-next-step/
request-information*
**Phone:** (718) 951-5001 | **E-mail:** *adminqry@brooklyn.cuny.edu*
**International Students:** Not Considered
**Preference to In-State Residents:** Yes, but out-of-state considered
**Application Deadline:** CUNY December 1
**Ave. SAT/ACT:** Optional (check) | **GPA:** 3.5+ | **MCAT:** Yes

### COST OF ATTENDANCE

**Tuition & Fees:** ~$7,500 (in-state), ~$20,000 (out-of-state)
**Addl Exp:** $25,000 | **Total:** $32,500 (in-state), $45,000 (out-of-state)
**Scholarships:** Over 600 scholarships, awards, and prizes are available
annually, totaling more than $1 million in support. Presidential
Scholarships: Offered to students in the BA/MD program, covering
full tuition for undergraduate study. Approximately, 83% of students
receive financial aid averaging about $10,000.

### ADDITIONAL INFORMATION

Submit a general CUNY application, listing
Brooklyn College as a choice. Complete the
BA/MD program application through Brooklyn
College's Honors Academy.

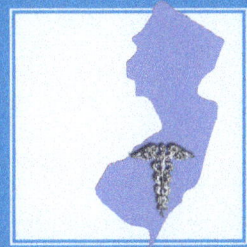

CONNECTICUT

MAINE

MASSACHUSETTS

NEW HAMPSHIRE

NEW JERSEY

NEW YORK

PENNSYLVANIA

RHODE ISLAND

VERMONT

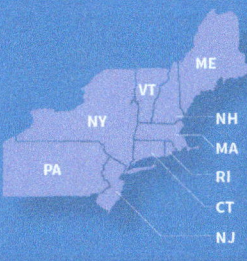

NORTHEAST

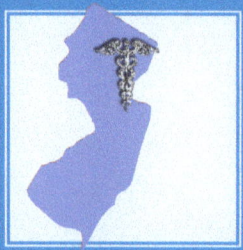

CONNECTICUT

MAINE

MASSACHUSETTS

NEW HAMPSHIRE

NEW JERSEY

NEW YORK

PENNSYLVANIA

RHODE ISLAND

VERMONT

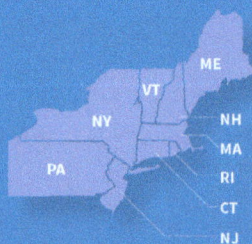

# CITY COLLEGE OF NEW YORK
## BS/MD (7-YEARS)

**CUNY BS/MD Sophie Davis Biomedical Education Program**
CUNY School of Medicine, Harris Hall, 160 Convent Avenue New York, NY 10031
**Affiliated Medical School:** CUNY School of Medicine
**Request Information:** *medicine.cuny.edu/request-information/*
**Phone:** (212) 650-7718 | **E-mail:** *admissions@med.cyny.edu*
**International Students:** Not Considered
**Preference to In-State Residents:** Yes, but out-of-state considered
**Application Deadline:** December 1
**Ave. SAT/ACT:** Optional (check) | **GPA:** 3.5+ | **MCAT:** No

## COST OF ATTENDANCE

**Tuition & Fees:** ~$7,500 (in-state), ~$20,000 (out-of-state)
**Addl Exp:** $25,000 | **Total:** $32,500 (in-state), $45,000 (out-of-state)
**Scholarships:** Steinfeld Pre-Med Fund Award: $5,000 for students with financial need. $4,834 for third-year undergrads w/notable academic achievement/research interest. $4,803 for deserving biomedical science undergrads. $1,563 to assist w/tuition and book costs...and more.

## ADDITIONAL INFORMATION

Submit both the general CUNY application (listing City College) and the supplemental CUNY School of Medicine application by Dec 1.

The CUNY Sophie Davis Biomedical Education Program admits high-achieving high school seniors, typically ≥95% GPA, SAT 1460–1560 or ACT 32–34, into a seamless 7-year BS/MD pathway with the CUNY School of Medicine in Manhattan, with an exceptionally low ~2.5% acceptance rate.

Students begin at The City College of New York following a tightly integrated biomedical sciences curriculum, including early clinical exposure, and must maintain ≥3.5 cumulative and ≥3.3 science GPA by junior year, with no MCAT required.

Admission is highly competitive and holistic, emphasizing academic excellence, community service in underserved areas, and passion for primary care. Three essays and five recommendations are required. The deadline is December 1 via CUNY, with interviews in winter and final decisions by April.

Advice for applicants: highlight commitment to urban/underserved medicine, showcase leadership and service, excel in STEM rigor, and ensure polished essays and recommendation letters that reflect sustained motivation and community orientation.

# HOFSTRA UNIVERSITY
# BS/MD (8-YEARS)

**Hofstra University BS-BA/MD 4+4 Program**
100 Hofstra University, Hempstead, NY 11549-1000
**Affiliated Medical School:** Donald and Barbara Zucker School of Medicine at Hofstra/Northwell
**4+4 FAQs:** *https://www.hofstra.edu/admission/4-plus-4.html*
**Phone:** (516) 463-5500
**International Students:** No
**Preference to In-State Residents:** No
**Application Deadline:** Nov 15, supplemental app deadline Jan 15
**SAT/ACT:** 1410+/32+ | **GPA:** 3.7+ | **MCAT:** Yes | **CASPer:** Yes

## COST OF ATTENDANCE

**Tuition & Fees:** ~$60,000 | **Addl Expenses:** $25,000 | **Total:** ~$85,000
**Financial Aid:** Hofstra University offers various financial aid options, including scholarships, grants, and loans. Approximately 64% of students receive financial aid, with an average aid package of $38,924.

## ADDITIONAL INFORMATION

Apply EA to Hofstra via the Common App. Indicate BS/MD. Qualified applicants receive a 4+4 supplement app in the Hofstra Portal. Decisions are returned by early March. Hofstra's BS-BA/MD program is our most competitive on campus. In a typical application season, about 2,000 students apply to fill a class of 10 to 15.

---

# NEW YORK INSTITUTE OF TECHNOLOGY
# BS/DO (8-YEARS)

**New York Institute of Technology**
NYC - 16 W. 61st Street, First Floor, New York, NY 10023
Long Island - Northern Blvd, P.O. Box 8000, Old Westbury, NY 11568
**Affiliated Medical School:** NYIT College of Osteopathic Medicine
**Request Information:** *https://apply.nyit.edu/register/inquire*
**Phone:** (800) 345-6948 | **E-Mail:** *admissions@nyit.edu*
**International Students:** No
**Preference to In-State Residents:** Yes, but all are considered
**Application Deadline:** November 15
**SAT/ACT:** 1400+/32+ | **GPA:** 3.7+ | **MCAT:** Yes

## COST OF ATTENDANCE

**Tuition & Fees:** ~$54,000 | **Addl Expenses:** $30,000 | **Total:** ~$84,000
**Scholarships:** NNYIT offers a range of financial aid options, including scholarships, grants, and work-study programs. Students are encouraged to complete the FAFSA to determine eligibility.

## ADDITIONAL INFORMATION

New York State residents benefit from in-state tuition rates at NYIT. Apply with the Common App or NYIT application. Indicate interest in BS/DO, qualified candidates will be invited for an interview.

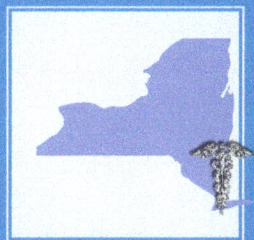

CONNECTICUT

MAINE

MASSACHUSETTS

NEW HAMPSHIRE

NEW JERSEY

NEW YORK

PENNSYLVANIA

RHODE ISLAND

VERMONT

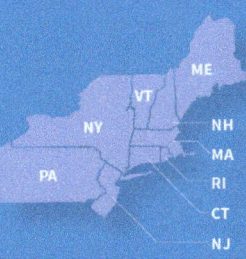

**NORTHEAST**

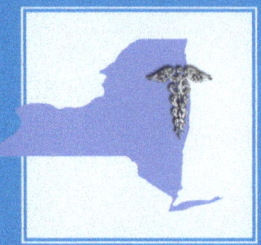

**CONNECTICUT**

**MAINE**

**MASSACHUSETTS**

**NEW HAMPSHIRE**

**NEW JERSEY**

**NEW YORK**

**PENNSYLVANIA**

**RHODE ISLAND**

**VERMONT**

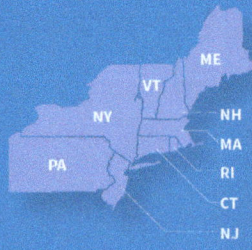

# RENSSELAER POLYTECHNIC INSTITUTE
# BS/MD (7-YEARS)

**Rensselaer Polytechnic Institute, Accel. Physician-Scientist Program**
Office of Admission, Troy, NY 12180-3590
**Affiliated Medical School:** Albany Medical College
**Request Information:** *https://www.rpi.edu/admissions*
**Phone:** (518) 276-6216 | **E-Mail:** *admissions@rpi.edu*
**International Students:** No
**Preference to In-State Residents:** No
**Application Deadline:** November 1 (supplement shortly thereafter)
**SAT/ACT:** 1360+/30+ | **GPA:** top 5% | **MCAT:** No | **CASPer:** No

## COST OF ATTENDANCE

**Tuition & Fees:** ~$67,000 | **Addl Exp:** ~$25,000 | **Total:** $92,000
**Financial Aid:** Apply for the Rensselaer Medal, a prestigious award valued at $40,000 per year, totaling $160,000 over four years. This scholarship is awarded to outstanding math and science students nominated by their high schools. Other scholarships are also available.

## ADDITIONAL INFORMATION

Rensselaer's prestigious Physician-Scientist Program invites exceptional high school seniors to apply. These students must be U.S. citizens or permanent residents and have completed rigorous STEM coursework. Applicants gain conditional admission to Albany Medical College alongside their B.S. in Biological Sciences in a streamlined seven-year trajectory.

Applicants apply via the Common App by November 1, indicating the Physician-Scientist major, and submit official SAT or ACT scores from a single testing date alongside a 500–750-word essay on their medical aspirations.

Admitted students spend three years at RPI, where they engage in intensive research and maintain high academic performance, followed by four years at Albany Medical College. Students skip both a second medical school application and the MCAT. The admission process is extremely selective (< 10% acceptance), featuring dual interviews and a holistic review of academic excellence, research interest, and service commitment.

Students should showcase real biomedical research or clinical exposure, articulate your passion effectively in essays, apply early, and prepare thoroughly for both RPI and AMC interview stages.

Albany Medical College will consider applicants to only one of its combined degree programs; dual applications are not permitted. High school seniors apply to RPI and indicate their interest in the BS/ MD.

# SIENA COLLEGE - BS/MD (8-YEARS)

**Siena College Science Humanities & Medicine Program w/AMC**
515 Loudon Road, Loudonville, NY 12211
**Affiliated Medical School:** Albany Medical College
**Request Information:** *https://www.siena.edu/programs/albany-medical-college-program/*
**Phone:** (518) 783-2423 | **E-Mail:** *admissions@siena.edu*
**International Students:** No
**Preference to In-State Residents:** No pref; out-of-state students eligible.
**Application Deadline:** Nov 1 (if selected, complete supplemental app)
**SAT/ACT:** 1380+/30+ | **GPA:** 3.5+ | **MCAT:** No

## COST OF ATTENDANCE

**Tuition & Fees:** ~$48,000 | **Addl Exp:** $25,000 | **Total:** $73,000
**Scholarships:** Siena offers merit scholarships ranging from $10,000 to $27,000 annually. All applicants are automatically considered. No separate application is required. Approximately 94% receive financial aid, with an average aid package of $38,559.

## ADDITIONAL INFORMATION

Siena College is a private Franciscan liberal arts college. The AMC BA/MD program emphasizes demonstrated service to the community. Each summer, Siena-AMC students embark on the Summer of Service, where they volunteer globally where there is demonstrated need. Students may stay in the U.S. or travel abroad to assist in orphanages/homes, medical clinics, and youth programs. Grants are provided for travel expenses. Albany Medical will consider applicants to only one of its combined degree programs. Dual applications are not permitted. High school seniors apply to Siena and indicate interest in BS/MD.

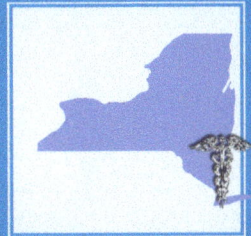

---

# ST. BONAVENTURE UNIVERSITY BS/MD AND BS/DO (7 & 8-YEARS)

**Saint Bonaventure University - BS/MD w/GWU, BSDO - 2 options**
3261 W State St, St Bonaventure, NY 14778
**Affiliated Medical School:**
BS/MD with GWU School of Medicine
BS/DO with NYITCOM Dual Degree Pathway and Duquesne University College of Osteopathic Medicine
**Request Information:** *https://www.sbu.edu/admission-aid/request-information*
**Phone:** (716) 375-2000 | **E-Mail:** *admissions@sbu.edu*
**International Students:** No (permanent residents okay)
**Preference to In-State Residents:** No
**Application Deadline:** November 30
**Min SAT/ACT:** 1390/28 | **GPA:** top 10% | **MCAT:** No

## COST OF ATTENDANCE

**Tuition & Fees:** ~$44,500 | **Addl Exp:** $25,000 | **Total:** $69,500
**Scholarships:** More than 95% of students receive financial assistance. Applying for scholarships and federal aid is recommended.

## ADDITIONAL INFORMATION

St. Bonaventure University is a private, Franciscan university. Upon successful completion of the SBU BS, students attend GWU Medical School. Requirements to transition into the MD program: GPA 3.60+ overall w/no C or lower in any science courses, and participation in medically-related experiences.

CONNECTICUT

MAINE

MASSACHUSETTS

NEW HAMPSHIRE

NEW JERSEY

NEW YORK

PENNSYLVANIA

RHODE ISLAND

VERMONT

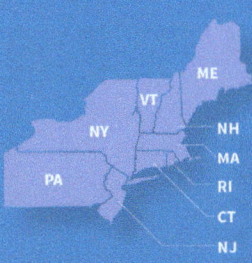

**NORTHEAST**

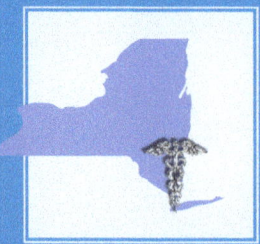

**CONNECTICUT**

**MAINE**

**MASSACHUSETTS**

**NEW HAMPSHIRE**

**NEW JERSEY**

**NEW YORK**

**PENNSYLVANIA**

**RHODE ISLAND**

**VERMONT**

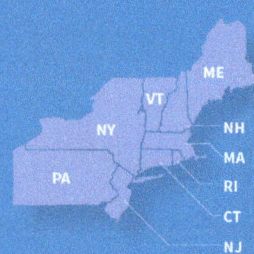

# STONY BROOK UNIVERSITY
# BA/MD SFM (8-YEARS)

**Stony Brook University Scholars for Medicine Program**
118 Administration Building, Stony Brook, NY 11794-1901
**Affiliated Medical School:** Renaissance School of Medicine at Stony Brook University
**Request Information:** *https://www.stonybrook.edu/undergraduate-admissions/contact/index.php*
**Phone:** (631) 632-6868 | **E-Mail:** *enroll@stonybrook.edu*
**International Students:** Not eligible
**Preference to In-State Residents:** Yes, but out-of-state applicants okay
**Application Deadline:** Nov 1 (EA), Jan 15 (RD) - EA Encouraged
**SAT/ACT:** 1540/35 | **GPA:** top 2% | **MCAT:** Yes

## COST OF ATTENDANCE

**Tuition & Fees:** ~$13,000 (in-state), ~$38,000 (out-of-state)
**Addl Exp:** $25,000 | **Total:** $38,000 (in-state), $63,000 (out-of-state)
**Scholarships:** Merit-Based Scholarships are swarded based on academic excellence. Special Talent scholarships are available for students with exceptional abilities in the arts, athletics, or leadership. "You Are Welcome Here" scholarship for international students, covering 50% of tuition.

## ADDITIONAL INFORMATION

Highly competitive admission is based on GPA, standardized test scores, strength of curriculum, honors/awards, leadership skills, extracurricular achievements, and unique individual talents. Open to high-achieving high school seniors admitted to Stony Brook's Honors College, WISE Program, or University Scholars Program

# SUNY OLD WESTBURY
# BS/DO (7-YEARS)

**SUNY Old Westbury NYITCOM Dual Degree Pathway**
Student Union Bldg, Suite 100. P.O. Box 210. Old Westbury, NY 11568
**Affiliated Medical School:** New York Institute of Technology College of Osteopathic Medicine
**Request Information:** *https://www.oldwestbury.edu/contact-admissions*
**Phone:** (516) 876-3200 | **E-Mail:** *enroll@oldwestbury.edu*
**International Students:** No
**Preference to In-State Residents:** Yes, but others considered.
**Application Deadline:** Nov 15 (EA), March 15 (RD) - EA Encouraged
**SAT/ACT:** 1270/28 | **GPA:** top 10% | **MCAT:** Yes

## COST OF ATTENDANCE

**Tuition & Fees:** ~$11,000 (in-state), ~$21,000 (out-of-state)
**Addl Exp:** $25,000 | **Total:** $36,000 (in-state), $46,000 (out-of-state)
**Scholarships:** Available to students who complete the University Scholarship Application. Excelsior scholarship are for eligible New York State residents, potentially covering full tuition.

## ADDITIONAL INFORMATION

Apply to SUNY Old Westbury in the SUNY App or the Common App. Indicate interest in the BS/DO program. Submit required documents, including transcripts, letters of rec, and personal essay. Deadlines may vary. It is advisable to check with SUNY Old Westbury's admissions office for current dates.

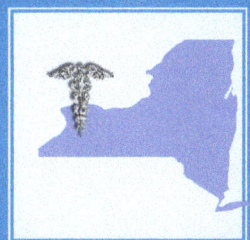

# UNION COLLEGE LEADERSHIP IN MEDICINE BS/MD (8-YEARS)

**Union College Leadership in Medicine Program**
Grant Hall, 807 Union Street, Schenectady, NY 12308
**Affiliated Medical School:** Albany Medical College
**Request Information:** *https://www.union.edu/admissions/contact-us*
**Phone:** (518) 388-6112 | **E-Mail:** *admissions@union.edu*
**International Students:** No
**Preference to In-State Residents:** Yes, but others considered.
**Application Deadline:** November 1
**Min SAT/ACT:** 1410/30 | **Min GPA:** top 5% | **MCAT:** No

## COST OF ATTENDANCE

**Tuition & Fees:** ~$69,000 | **Addl Exp:** ~$25,000 | **Total:** ~$94,000
**Scholarships:** Merit scholarships are awarded to top applicants based on academic credentials. Amounts range from $12,000 to $40,000 per year. Automatically renewed annually for up to four years.

## ADDITIONAL INFORMATION

This program is designed for high-achieving high school seniors committed to a career in medicine and healthcare leadership. Demonstrated clinical or volunteer service in medicine is required.

---

# UNIVERSITY OF ROCHESTER REMS BS/MD (8-YEARS)

**University of Rochester - Rochester Early Medical Scholars Program**
300 Wilson Boulevard, Rochester, NY 14627
**Affiliated Medical School:** University of Rochester School of Medicine and Dentistry
**Request Information:** *https://admissions.rochester.edu/contact/*
**Phone:** (585) 275-3221 | **E-Mail:** *admit@admissions.rochester.edu*
**International Students:** No
**Preference to In-State Residents:** No
**Application Deadline:** November 15
**Ave SAT/ACT:** 1500/33 | **Ave. GPA:** 3.95 | **MCAT:** No

## COST OF ATTENDANCE

**Tuition & Fees:** ~$72,000 | **Addl Exp:** ~$25,000 | **Total:** ~$97,000
**Scholarships:** Students pay an average net tuition cost of $38,156 for students with demonstrated financial need. Numerous scholarships available.

## ADDITIONAL INFORMATION

UR looks for a rigorous curriculum, shadowing, hospital volunteering, EMT experience, biomedical research, leadership roles, and community service. Students must also engage in non-medical activities, such as arts, athletics, or clubs. Apply through the Common App or Coalition App, indicating your interest in REMS. Finalists informed in January; interviews in February; decision in April. Clearly articulate your commitment to a medical career through experiences and essays.

**CONNECTICUT**

**MAINE**

**MASSACHUSETTS**

**NEW HAMPSHIRE**

**NEW JERSEY**

**NEW YORK**

**PENNSYLVANIA**

**RHODE ISLAND**

**VERMONT**

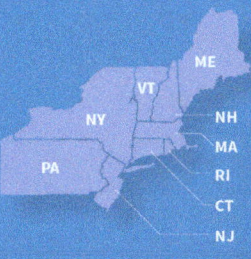

**NORTHEAST**

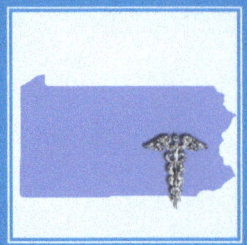

**CONNECTICUT**

**MAINE**

**MASSACHUSETTS**

**NEW HAMPSHIRE**

**NEW JERSEY**

**NEW YORK**

**PENNSYLVANIA**

**RHODE ISLAND**

**VERMONT**

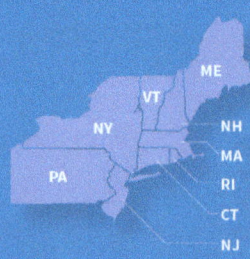

# DREXEL UNIVERSITY EARLY ASSURANCE PROGRAM BS/MD (8 YEARS)

**Drexel University EAP w/Drexel University College of Medicine**
3141 Chestnut Street, Philadelphia, PA 19104
**Affiliated Medical School:** Drexel University College of Medicine
**Request Information:** *https://drexel.edu/admissions/contact*
**Phone:** (215) 895-2400 | **E-Mail:** *enroll@drexel.edu* International
**Students:** Not Considered
**Preference to In-State Residents:** No
**Application Deadline:** November 1
**SAT/ACT:** 1420+/32+ | **GPA:** 3.5+ | **MCAT:** Yes

## COST OF ATTENDANCE

**Tuition & Fees:** ~$65,000 | **Addl Expenses:** $25,000 | **Total:** $90,000
**Scholarships:** Drexel offers merit scholarships and need-based aid.

## ADDITIONAL INFORMATION

HS seniors apply to Drexel for undergraduate admission through the Common App or Coalition App. Select BS/MD, complete supplemental essays in addition to the Drexel app. Submit the College of Medicine Supplemental Application through the Discover Drexel portal by November 1. Must major in Bio, Chem or acceptable major. Participate in designated clinical, research, and service activities with no disciplinary or academic violations.

# DUQUESNE UNIVERSITY BS/DO (7-YEARS)

**Duquesne University BS/DO Early Assurance Program**
600 Forbes Avenue, Pittsburgh, PA 15282
**Affiliated Medical School:** Duquesne College of Osteopathic Medicine
**Request Information:** *https://www.duq.edu/about/contact-us/index.php*
**Phone:** (412) 396-6000 | **E-Mail:** *admissions@duq.edu*
**International Students:** Yes, international students considered
**Preference to In-State Residents:** No pref, out-of-state considered
**Application Deadline:** Apply early
**SAT/ACT:** 1240+/26+ | **GPA:** 3.5+ | **MCAT:** Yes

## COST OF ATTENDANCE

**Tuition & Fees:** ~$46,000 | **Addl Expenses:** $25,000 | **Total:** $71,000
**Scholarships:** STEM Scholars Program: Designed for incoming students pursuing degrees in science, technology, engineering, or math. Application deadline: January 15. Rangos School of Health Sciences Empowering Inclusion No-Loan Tuition Scholarship: Covers 100% of tuition for five incoming first-year undergraduate students demonstrating academic excellence and a commitment to fostering inclusion. Application deadline: March 15.

## ADDITIONAL INFORMATION

Apply to Duquesne via the Common App or Duquesne's App Portal. Indicate interest in the Early Assurance Program during the application process.

# GANNON UNIVERSITY
## BS/DO (8-YEARS)

**Gannon University 4+4 Early Assurance Program w/LECOM & UMHS**
109 University Square, Erie, PA 16541
**Affiliated Medical School:** Lake Erie College of Osteopathic Medicine and the University of Medicine and Health Sciences
**Request Information:** *https://www.gannon.edu/admissions/request-information/*
**Phone:** (800) GANNON-U | **E-Mail:** *admissions@gannon.edu*
**International Students:** Yes, international students considered
**Preference to In-State Residents:** No pref, out-of-state considered
**Application Deadline:** Apply early
**SAT/ACT:** 1240+/26+ | **GPA:** 3.5+ | **MCAT:** No (Yes for UMHS)

### COST OF ATTENDANCE

**Tuition & Fees:** ~$45,000 | **Addl Expenses:** $25,000 | **Total:** ~$70,000
**Scholarships:** Academic, merit, and need-based scholarships are available.

### ADDITIONAL INFORMATION

Apply to Gannon University via the Common App or Gannon's App Portal. Indicate interest in the LECOM or UMHS EAP during the application process. Complete a separate application to LECOM or IMHS.

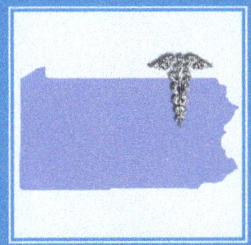

# PENNSYLVANIA STATE UNIVERSITY
## ACCELERATED MED - PPM BS/MD (7 YEARS)

**Penn State University BS/MD Premedical-Medical (PPM) Program**
230 Ritenour Building, Penn State University Park, PA 16802
**Affiliated Medical School:** Sidney Kimmel Medical College
**Additional Information:** *science.psu.edu/premed-med-bsmd*
**Phone:** (814) 865-5471 | **E-Mail:** *admissions@psu.edu*
**International Students:** Yes, international students considered
**Preference to In-State Residents:** No pref, out-of-state considered
**Application Deadline:** October 15
**SAT/ACT:** 1470+/32+ | **GPA:** 3.5+ | **MCAT:** Yes

### COST OF ATTENDANCE

**Tuition & Fees:** ~$22,000 (in-state), $40,000 (out-of-state)
**Addl Exp:** $25,000 | **Total:** $47,000 (in-state), $68,000 (out-of-state)
**Scholarships:** Students enrolled in Penn State's PMM Program are not eligible for certain undergraduate scholarships, including the Braddock Scholarship, McKinstry Scholarship, and awards from the Schreyer Honors College. This is due to the program's accelerated structure, which involves only three years of study at Penn State. However, once students transition to the Sidney Kimmel Medical College at Thomas Jefferson University for the medical portion of the program, they may be eligible for various scholarships and financial aid opportunities offered by SKMC

### ADDITIONAL INFORMATION

Approximately 25–30 students admitted annually. Complete the Penn State application via MyPennState or the Common Application. Indicate interest in the PMM program. Submit all required materials, including transcripts and test scores (if applicable), by the deadline. Initial screening by Penn State Admissions. Selected applicants are invited for interviews conducted jointly by Penn State and SKMC.

CONNECTICUT

MAINE

MASSACHUSETTS

NEW HAMPSHIRE

NEW JERSEY

NEW YORK

PENNSYLVANIA

RHODE ISLAND

VERMONT

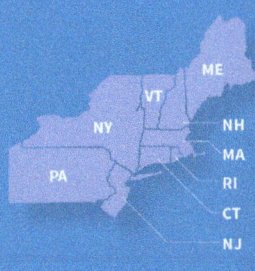

**NORTHEAST**

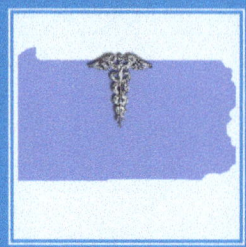

CONNECTICUT

MAINE

MASSACHUSETTS

NEW HAMPSHIRE

NEW JERSEY

NEW YORK

PENNSYLVANIA

RHODE ISLAND

VERMONT

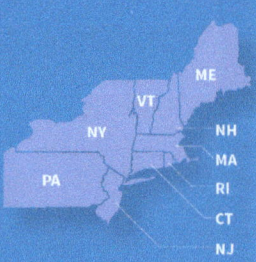

# UNIVERSITY OF PITTSBURGH
# BS/MD (8-YEARS)

**University of Pittsburgh GAP (Guaranteed Admission Program)**
4200 Fifth Avenue, Pittsburgh, PA 15260
**Affiliated Medical School:** University of Pittsburgh School of Medicine
**Request Information:** *https://admissions.pitt.edu/request-info/*
**Phone:** (412) 624-4141 | **E-Mail:** *admissions@medschool.pitt.edu*
**International Students:** No
**Preference to In-State Residents:** Yes, but out-of-state considered
**Application Deadline:** October 15 (Indicate GAP); GAP due Nov 1, Supplement may be due later - Check dates.
**SAT/ACT:** 1490+/34+ | **GPA:** ~3.8 | **MCAT:** No, if SAT/ACT was submitted.

## COST OF ATTENDANCE

**Tuition & Fees:** ~$22,000 (in-state), ~$42,000 (out-of-state)
**Addl Exp:** $25,000 | **Total:** ~$47,000 (in-state), $67,000 (out-of-state)
**Scholarships:** High-achieving GAP students often receive tuition scholarships, Honors funding, or department awards.

## ADDITIONAL INFORMATION

About 1,500 apply to GAP each year; ~400-600 candidates complete the supplemental med school application. Then, ~40-50 are interviewed in March and 5-15 students matriculate. The acceptance rate is between 5-10%. The rigorous multi-step selection includes university admission, GAP form, essays, and medical school interview. The program has ongoing mentorship and requires semester reviews, strong GPA (≥ 3.75+), extracurricular engagement, and academic excellence.

# BROWN UNIVERSITY PLME
# BS/MD (8-YEARS)

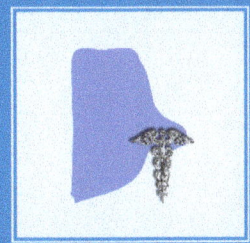

**Brown University BS/MD Program in Liberal Medical Education**
Providence, RI 02912
**Affiliated Medical School:** Brown's Warren Alpert Medical School
**Request Information:** *https://plme.med.brown.edu/about/*
information-prospective-students
**Phone:** (401) 863-1000 | **E-Mail:** *MedSchool_Admissions@brown.edu*
**International Students:** Yes
**In-State Residents:** No pref, out-of-state considered
**Application Deadline:** ED I: Nov 1, Video Portfolio: Nov 2, Decision mid-December; RD: Jan 3, Video Portfolio: Jan 4, Decisions March 28th.
**SAT/ACT:** 1530+/35+ | **GPA:** 3.8+ (unwt) | **MCAT:** No

## COST OF ATTENDANCE

**Tuition & Fees:** ~$74,000 (in-state) | **Addl Exp:** $25,000 | **Total:** $99,000
**Scholarships:** Brown is need-blind for U.S. citizens and meets 100% demonstrated need through grants, loans, and work-study. No separate PLME scholarship.

## ADDITIONAL INFORMATION

Brown's Program in Liberal Medical Education is the only Ivy League program enrolling ~60 students annually. Brown's PLME accepts a highly select cohort of high-achieving high school seniors. Only about 2–3% of applicants are selected for this elite 8-year combined B.A./Sc.B. + M.D. pathway linking Brown and its Warren Alpert Medical School.

Applicants apply via the same Common App as general undergraduate students. The due dates are - Early Decision (Nov 1) or Regular Decision (Jan 3). Students must complete three additional PLME-specific short essays and submitting at least one recommendation from a math or science teacher.

Ideal candidates present top-tier academic credentials (unweighted GPAs around 3.8+, SAT scores averaging 748 ERW / 779 Math or ACT ~34–35), strong extracurricular achievement in STEM, research, leadership, and demonstrate communication skills via optional video introductions.

Once admitted, PLME students are able to enroll in an open curriculum with unparalleled flexibility to explore non-science interests, assured medical school entry without MCATs, though other academic benchmarks remain. Students also have the option to defer medical matriculation for personal growth.

The program's difficulty lies in its low acceptance rate (~2%), holistic and rigorous selection, and high expectations for intellectual curiosity, academic excellence, and dedication to medicine. Applicants must aim for top test scores, deeply commit to service/research, craft polished personal essays, and apply early to strengthen candidacy.

CONNECTICUT

MAINE

MASSACHUSETTS

NEW HAMPSHIRE

NEW JERSEY

NEW YORK

PENNSYLVANIA

RHODE ISLAND

VERMONT

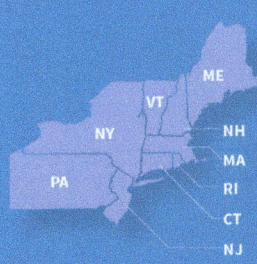

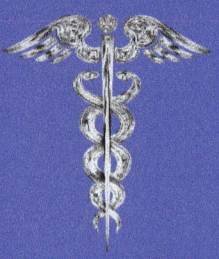

**ILLINOIS**

**INDIANA**

**IOWA**

**KANSAS**

**MICHIGAN**

**MINNESOTA**

**MISSOURI**

**NEBRASKA**

**NORTH DAKOTA**

**OHIO**

**SOUTH DAKOTA**

**WISCONSIN**

REGION TWO
# MIDWEST

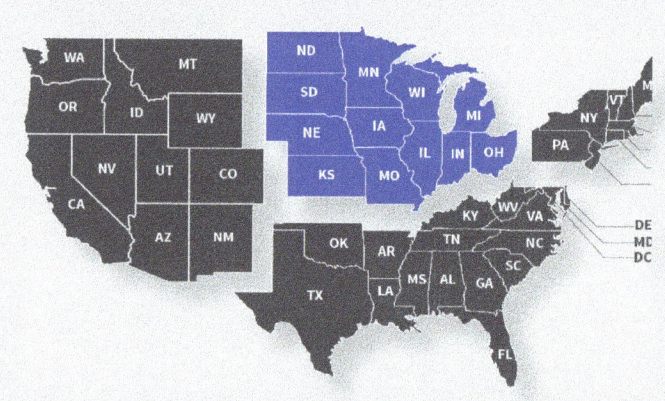

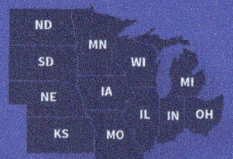

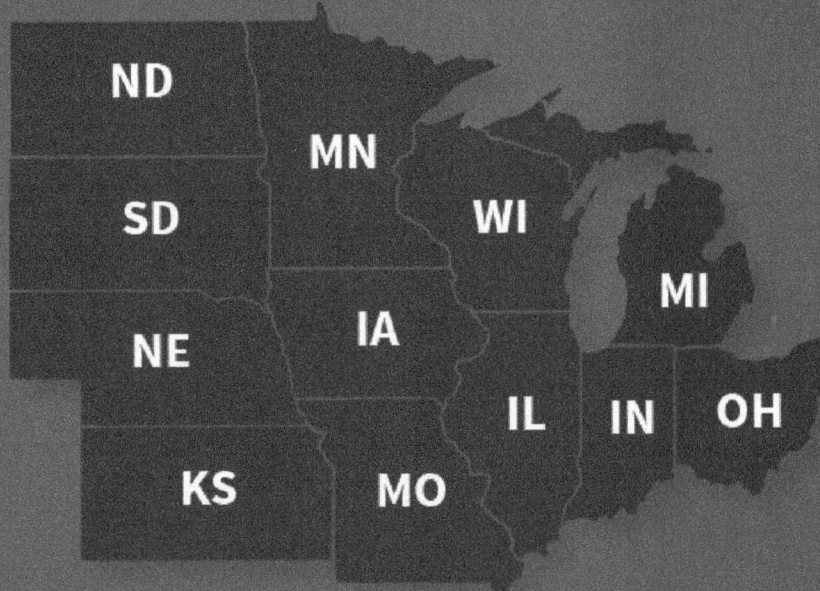

# 8 Programs | 12 States

1. IL – University of Illinois at Chicago GPPA - BS/MD
2. IN – University of Evansville - BS/MD
3. KS - Pittsburg State University - BS/MD and BS/DO
4. MO – Missouri Southern State Univ. "Yours to Lose" - BS/DO
5. MO – University of Missouri Kansas City - BS/MD
6. NE – Chadron State College (RHOP) - BS/MD and BS/DO
7. OH – John Carroll University - BS/DO
8. OH – University of Cincinnati - BS/MD

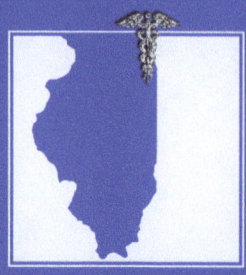

ILLINOIS

INDIANA

IOWA

KANSAS

MICHIGAN

MINNESOTA

MISSOURI

NEBRASKA

NORTH DAKOTA

OHIO

SOUTH DAKOTA

WISCONSIN

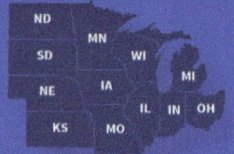

# UNIVERSITY OF ILLINOIS AT CHICAGO
## GPPA  BS/MD (8-YEARS)

**University of Illinois, Chicago Guaranteed Professional Program Admissions Medical Scholars Program**
828 Halsted Street, Burnham Hall, Chicago, IL 60607
**Affiliated Medical School:** University of Illinois College of Medicine
**Request Information:** *https://discover.uic.edu/*
**Phone:** (312) 413-2260 | **E-Mail:** *gppauic@uic.edu*
**International Students:** Yes, international students considered
**Preference to In-State Residents:** No pref, out-of-state considered
**Application Deadline:** November 1 for both UIC and GPPA
**SAT/ACT:** Not given. | **GPA:** 3.75+ | **MCAT:** Yes (target 513)

## COST OF ATTENDANCE

**Tuition & Fees:** ~$28,000 (in-state), ~$53,000 (out-of-state)
**Addl Exp:** $25,000 | **Total:** $53,000 (in-state), $78,000 (out-of-state)
**Scholarships:** New Aspire Grant (2025–26): Illinois families with incomes under $75k can attend UIC tuition-free.

## ADDITIONAL INFORMATION

UIC's GPPA Medical Scholars track provides a direct route to an MD degree. GPPA is in UIC's Honors College and is tailored for medicine. Accepted students earn provisional assurance into the University of Illinois Medical School (campuses in Chicago, Peoria, and Rockford) upon successful completion of their BS degree and fulfillment of program requirements. Apply in August. Complete the Common App and UIC's supplemental app with all materials (transcripts, GPPA/Honors supplement essays, letters) by the deadline. HS students only!

# UNIVERSITY OF EVANSVILLE
# BS/MD (8-YEARS)

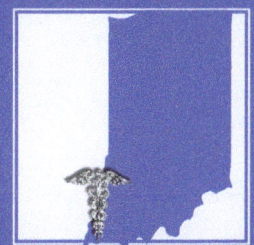

**University of Evansville BS/MD Program**
Room 324, Koch Center, 1800 Lincoln Ave, Evansville, IN 47722
**Affiliated Medical School:** Indiana University School of Medicine
**Request Information:** *https://www.evansville.edu/admission/
requestmore.cfm*
**Phone:** (812) 488-3250 | **E-Mail:** *fr25@evansville.edu*
**International Students:** No
**Preference to In-State Residents:** Yes, this program is for in-state only
**Application Deadline:** November 1 (Interview mid-Nov)
**SAT/ACT:** 1350+/29+ | **GPA:** 4.0+ | **MCAT:** Yes (must match/exceed
current class)

## COST OF ATTENDANCE

**Tuition & Fees:** ~$44,000 | **Addl Exp:** $20,000 | **Total:** $64,000
**Scholarships:** Participants in the program receive a $30,000 UE
scholarship per year during undergraduate studies evansville.edu,
significantly offsetting tuition costs.

## ADDITIONAL INFORMATION

If you are an Indiana resident applying this cycle, complete your
UE application by November 1 to enter the B/MD track. Plan for
interviews mid-November and commit by April 15 once accepted.
Approximately 8 students are admitted annually, with 2 alternates.
About 6-8 enroll each year.

Applicants must be an Indiana resident for 12 months. Guaranteed
provisional medical school admissions. Typically, an MCAT score
of 512 is required. Following undergraduate completion, students
submit the AMCAS application and interview at IU–Evansville.

ILLINOIS

INDIANA

IOWA

KANSAS

MICHIGAN

MINNESOTA

MISSOURI

NEBRASKA

NORTH DAKOTA

OHIO

SOUTH DAKOTA

WISCONSIN

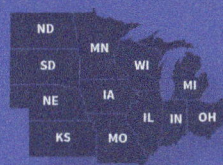

**MIDWEST**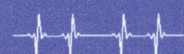

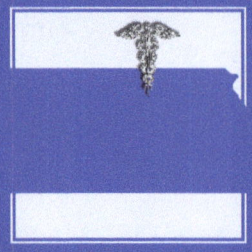

**ILLINOIS**

**INDIANA**

**IOWA**

**KANSAS**

**MICHIGAN**

**MINNESOTA**

**MISSOURI**

**NEBRASKA**

**NORTH DAKOTA**

**OHIO**

**SOUTH DAKOTA**

**WISCONSIN**

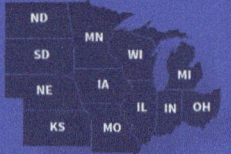

# PITTSBURG STATE UNIVERSITY
## BS/DO (7-YEARS - 3+4)

**Pittsburg State University BS/DO Accelerated Pre-Med Path**
1701 South Broadway Street, Pittsburg, KS 66762
**Affiliated Medical School:** Kansas City University College of Osteopathic Medicine
**Request Information:** *https://admit.pittstate.edu/register/request-for-information*
**Phone:** (620) 235-6541| **E-Mail:** *biology@pittstate.edu*
**International Students:** No, but possibly in some cases.
**Preference to In-State Residents:** No pref, out-of-state considered
**Application Deadline:** Apply to Pitt State and Amp-Up
**SAT/ACT:** 1300/26+ | **GPA:** 3.6+ | **MCAT:** No

## COST OF ATTENDANCE

**Tuition & Fees:** ~$9,000 (in-state), ~$12,000 (out-of-state)
**Addl Exp:** $20,000 | **Total:** $29,000 (in-state), $32,000 (out-of-state)
**Scholarships:** All students (including AMP-UP applicants) can apply via the PSU Online Scholarship Application, open until February 1 annually, for scholarships evaluating academic performance, leadership, and financial need.

## ADDITIONAL INFORMATION

Approximately 35 students (25 DO; 10 Dental) admitted annually. Amp-Up offers high-achieving, patient-care–focused students a secure and prestigious pathway into one of the nation's leading medical schools. After early review, qualifying students receive supplemental instructions in early December, followed by a January 15 application deadline.

Finalists are interviewed by Pitt Med in March, and admission is guaranteed for those who maintain performance targets through college. Students entering via AMP-UP are guaranteed an interview and reserved spots with 25 DO seats annually at KCU-Joplin, plus 10 reserved spots for dental school.

# MISSOURI SOUTHERN STATE UNIVERSITY "YOURS TO LOSE" - BS/DO (7-YEARS)

**Missouri Southern State University Early Acceptance)Program**
3950 E. Newman Road, Joplin, MO 64807
**Affiliated Medical School:** Kansas City University College of Osteopathic Medicine
**Request Information:** *https://mkeap.mssu.edu/*
**Phone:** (866) 818-6778 | **E-Mail:** *rhodes-v@mssu.edu*
**International Students:** Focus on domestic applicants
**Preference to In-State Residents:** Regional preferred; out of state okay
**Application Deadline:** November 1 (priority), December 1 (final)
**SAT/ACT:** 1310+/28+ | **GPA:** 3.7+ | **MCAT:** No

## COST OF ATTENDANCE

**Tuition & Fees:** Tuition for undergrad years is fully covered by MSSU for undergraduate years.

## ADDITIONAL INFORMATION

Every year, 25 DO seats and 10 dental seats are reserved for the cohort. Accelerated 3-year BS in Biomedical Sciences or Chemistry at MSSU. Guaranteed advancement to KCU after successful GPA performance (≥ 3.5 cumulative). Accelerated 3-year BS in Biomedical Sciences or Chemistry at MSSU. Guaranteed advancement to KCU after successful GPA performance (≥ 3.5 cumulative).

---

# UNIVERSITY OF MISSOURI KANSAS CITY BS/MD (6-YEARS)

**University of Missouri, Kansas City BA/MD Program**
Health Sciences Campus, 2411 Holmes Street, Kansas City, MO 64108
**Affiliated Medical School:** UMKC School of Medicine
**Request Information:** *https://futureroo.umkc.edu/*
**Phone:** (816) 235-1870 | E-Mail: *medicine@umkc.edu*
**International Students:** No
**Preference to In-State Residents:** Yes
**Application Deadline:** November 1 (general and supplemental)
**Ave. SAT/ACT:** 1420+/32+ | **Ave. GPA:** 3.9+ | **MCAT:** No

## COST OF ATTENDANCE

**Tuition & Fees:** ~$30,000 (in-state), ~$44,000 (regional), ~$60,000 (out-of-state)
**Addl Exp:** $20,000 | **Total:** ~$50,000 (in-state), ~$64,000 (regional), ~$80,000 (out-of-state)
**Scholarships:** About $10,000 per year is granted to 15 students. FAFSA required. Automatic merit scholarships: Based on ACT/SAT scores and high school GPA. Priority deadline: Jan 15.

## ADDITIONAL INFORMATION

Students bypass the competitive med school application provided they meet the program's progression benchmarks. High school students need a high GPA and standardized test scores. Students begin clinical work from Year 1 via "docent teams" under physician mentors. The accelerated six-year pace is intense; social life may be limited, though students bond deeply with their cohort and mentors.

ILLINOIS

INDIANA

IOWA

KANSAS

MICHIGAN

MINNESOTA

MISSOURI

NEBRASKA

NORTH DAKOTA

OHIO

SOUTH DAKOTA

WISCONSIN

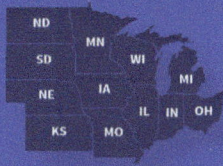

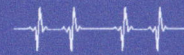

**MIDWEST**

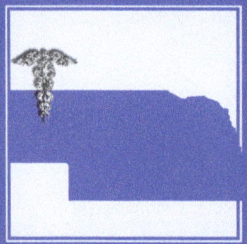

ILLINOIS

INDIANA

IOWA

KANSAS

MICHIGAN

MINNESOTA

MISSOURI

NEBRASKA

NORTH DAKOTA

OHIO

SOUTH DAKOTA

WISCONSIN

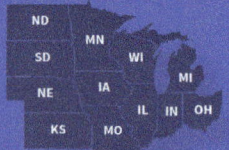

# CHADRON STATE COLLEGE (RHOP)
# BS/MD AND BS/DO (8-YEARS)

**Chadron State College BS/MD Rural Health Opportunities Program**
1000 Main Street, Chadron, NE 69337
**Affiliated Medical School:** University of Nebraska Medical Center
College of Medicine
**Request Information:** *https://info.csc.edu/*
**Phone:** 1-800-CHADRON | **E-Mail:** *hpoffice@csc.edu*
**International Students:** Yes (but RHOP is just for rural NE residents)
**Preference to In-State Residents:** RHOP is for rural Nebraska residents
**Application Deadline:** Apply early
**SAT/ACT:** 1240+/26+ | **GPA:** 3.5+ | **MCAT:** Yes

## COST OF ATTENDANCE

**Tuition & Fees:** Students in RHOP receive a full undergraduate tuition
waiver for CSC while completing their bachelor's degree, fall and spring
semesters only. Summer is excluded.
**Scholarships:** President Scholars: $7,000/year (GPA ≥ 3.95)
**Dean Scholars:** $2,000/year (GPA 3.50–3.94)
**Community Scholars:** $1,500/year (GPA 3.00–3.49)
State College Tuition Guarantee also may cover any tuition gaps
for Pell-eligible students, including non-residents once FAFSA is
submitted by April 1. Students must apply by March 1 for scholarship
consideration.

## ADDITIONAL INFORMATION

The Rural Health Opportunities Program is a selective high school–
entry track for rural Nebraska residents, offering conditional admission
into the University of Nebraska Medical Center's College of Medicine.
Applicants must apply to Chadron State College and submit the RHOP
application (with transcripts, test scores, three recommendations, and
a personal essay) by December 1.

This program targets students from non-urban Nebraska committed to
practicing in rural areas, accompanied by minimum ACT or SAT scores
(≥1 9 in all sections).

Successful candidates receive a full undergraduate tuition waiver
at Chadron State, priority registration, professional development
opportunities (including regular UNMC visits), and guaranteed med-

school entry upon maintaining ≥ 3 .5 cumulative and science
GPAs, earning at least C grades in science coursework, completing
shadowing requirements, and participating fully in RHOP activities.

Admission is competitive, with emphasis on academic potential, rural
community dedication, and readiness for rigorous health-profession
study. Advice for applicants: highlight strong ties to rural Nebraska,
demonstrate consistent academic success, show commitment through
service or leadership, and ensure a polished personal statement
emphasizing your long-term rural healthcare goals.

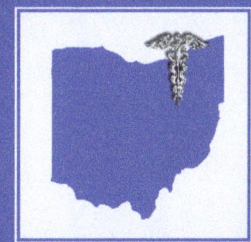

# JOHN CARROLL UNIVERSITY
## BS/DO (8-YEARS)

**John Carroll University OU-HCOM Early Assurance Program**
1 John Carroll Blvd, University Heights, OH 44118
**Affiliated Medical School:** Ohio University Heritage College of
Osteopathic Medicine with campuses in Athens, Cleveland, and Dublin
**Request Information:** *https://www.jcu.edu/request-info*
**Phone:** (216) 397-4248| **E-Mail:** *enrollment@jcu.edu*
**International Students:** No
**Preference to In-State Residents:** Yes, Ohio residents preferred.
**Application Deadline:** December 1. Virtual interviews in February
**SAT/ACT:** 1200+/25+ | **GPA:** 3.5+ | **MCAT:** No, but students must take a
mock MCAT.

## COST OF ATTENDANCE

**Tuition & Fees:** ~$52,000 | **Addl Exp:** ~$20,000 | **Total:** ~$72,000
**Scholarships:** Magis, Presidential, University, Ignatian Awards have
automatic consideration upon admission. Legacy, departmental, and
special-interest awards (e.g., Spanish Heritage, STEM-focused)
**Pre-Health-specific scholarships:** SANUM Scholars: $6,122/year for
declared pre-health (renewable) Kenneth & Joan Callahan Scholarship:
$4,400/year for pre-medical sophomores (renewable).

## ADDITIONAL INFORMATION

Heritage COM is a state-assisted public medical school, with strong
preference for Ohio residents. Students must maintain a 3.7+ GPA with
a 3.6+ at graduation from JCU. Students must maintain community
service, shadowing, leadership, and complete mock MCAT.

---

# UNIVERSITY OF CINCINNATI CONNECTIONS
## BS/MD (8-YEARS)

**University of Cincinnati Connections BS/MD Dual Admissions
Program** - Medical Sciences Building, Suite E-450, 231 Albert Sabin
Way, PO Box 670552, Cincinnati, OH 45267-0552
**Affiliated Medical School:** University of Cincinnati College of Medicine
**Request Information:** *https://med.uc.edu/connections-dual-
admissions?utm*
**Phone:** (513) 558-7314 | **E-Mail:** MDadmissions@uc.edu
**International Students:** No
**Preference to In-State Residents:** No pref, out-of-state considered
**Application Deadline:** December 1 with interviews in February
**Ave. SAT/ACT:** 1515+/32+ | **Ave. GPA:** 3.9+ | **MCAT:** Yes (507+)

## COST OF ATTENDANCE

**Tuition & Fees:** ~$15,000 (in-state), ~$31,000 (out-of-state)
**Addl Exp:** $20,000 | **Total:** $35,000 (in-state), $51,000 (out-of-state)
**Scholarships:** Students are automatically eligible for university-side
merit scholarships. Submit the undergraduate scholarship application
(via UC) to be considered for additional merit awards. Submit FAFSA
early to maximize eligibility for need-based and med school aid (up to
$6K/year).

## ADDITIONAL INFORMATION

The Connections program is hosted via the UC College of Medicine
site; includes program details, application steps,
and FAQs. The application opens September 1,
though it is due December 1. The supplemental
application is due by December 12 with interviews
in February and decisions delivered in March.
Students much choose to enroll by May 1.

ILLINOIS

INDIANA

IOWA

KANSAS

MICHIGAN

MINNESOTA

MISSOURI

NEBRASKA

NORTH DAKOTA

OHIO

SOUTH DAKOTA

WISCONSIN

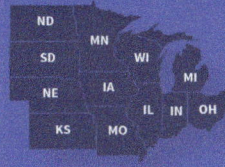

**MIDWEST**

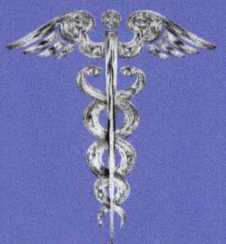

ALABAMA

ARKANSAS

DELAWARE

DISTRICT OF COLUMBIA

FLORIDA

GEORGIA

KENTUCKY

LOUISIANA

MARYLAND

MISSISSIPPI

NORTH CAROLINA

OKLAHOMA

SOUTH CAROLINA

TENNESSEE

TEXAS

VIRGINIA

WEST VIRGINIA

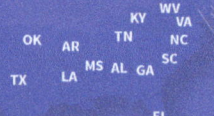

# REGION THREE
# SOUTH

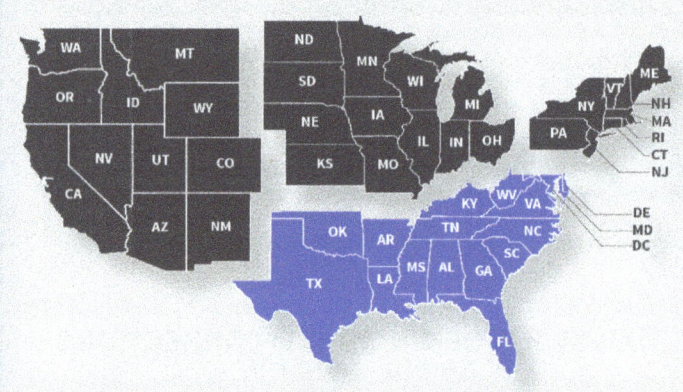

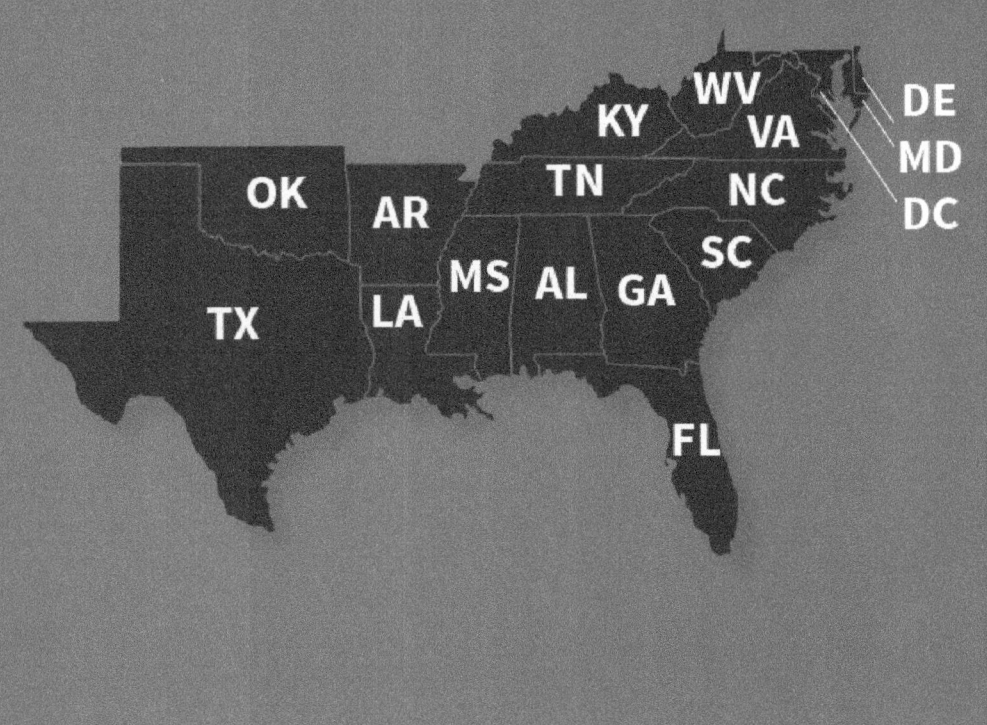

# 17 Programs | 17 States

1. *AL – University of Alabama – Birmingham EMSAP - BS/MD*
2. *AL – University of South Alabama - BS/MD*
3. *DC – The George Washington University - BS/MD*
4. *FL – Florida Southern College -BS/DO*
5. *FL – Florida International University - BS/MD*
6. *FL – Nova Southeastern University - BS/MD and BS/DO*
7. *FL – University of South Florida - BS.MD and BS/DO*
8. *GA – Augusta University - BS/MD*
9. *MD – Washington College - BS/DO*
10. *OK – University of Oklahoma - BS/MD*
11. *SC – University of South Carolina - BS/MD*
12. *TX – Texas Tech University - BS/MD*
13. *TX – University of Houston - BS/MD*
14. *TX – University of Texas at Dallas - BS/MD*
15. *TX – University of Texas Rio Grande Valley - BS/MD*
16. *VA – Virginia Commonwealth University - BS/MD*
17. *WV – West Virginia University - BS/MD*

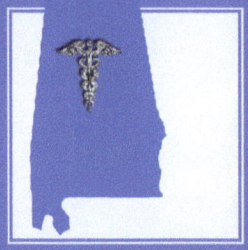

**ALABAMA**

**ARKANSAS**

**DELAWARE**

**DISTRICT OF COLUMBIA**

**FLORIDA**

**GEORGIA**

**KENTUCKY**

**LOUISIANA**

**MARYLAND**

**MISSISSIPPI**

**NORTH CAROLINA**

**OKLAHOMA**

**SOUTH CAROLINA**

**TENNESSEE**

**TEXAS**

**VIRGINIA**

**WEST VIRGINIA**

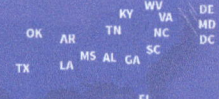

# UNIVERSITY OF ALABAMA, BIRMINGHAM EMSAP - BS/MD (8-YEARS)

**University of Alabama Early Medical School Acceptance Program**
1720 2nd Ave South, Birmingham, AL 35294
**Affiliated Medical School:** UAB Heersink School of Medicine
**Request Information:** *https://www.uab.edu/admissions/request-info*
**Phone:** (205) 934-8221 | **E-Mail:** *chooseuab@uab.edu*
**International Students:** No
**Preference to In-State Residents:** Out-of-state considered
**Application Deadline:** Apply by November.
**SAT/ACT:** 1360+/20+ | **GPA:** 3.5+ | **MCAT:** Yes

## COST OF ATTENDANCE

**Tuition & Fees:** ~$15,000 (in-state), ~$32,000 (out-of-state)
**Addl Exp:** $22,000 | **Total:** $37,000 (in-state), $54,000 (out-of-state)
**Scholarships:** Most EMSAP students receive UAB merit-based scholarships, which fully cover in-state tuition, even for out-of-state participants. Incoming students can complete the BSMART portal app (opens August 1) to access institutional and departmental awards.

## ADDITIONAL INFORMATION

EMSAP students are granted assured admission to the UAB School of Medicine upon meeting requirements. Students must maintain a 3.6 GPA complete required premed coursework (e.g., biology, chemistry, physics, etc.), attend EMSAP seminars, and reside on campus during the first two semesters and ensure contact with the program director.

# UNIVERSITY OF SOUTH ALABAMA COMEAP BS/MD (8-YEARS)

**University of South Alabama College of Medicine Early Acceptance Program** - 2500 Meisler Hall
390 Student Center Circle, Mobile, AL 36688-0002
**Affiliated Medical School:** Whiddon College of Medicine at the University of South Alabama
**Request Information:** *https://www.southalabama.edu/ departments/admissions/earlyacceptance/*
**Phone:** (251) 460-7834 | **E-Mail:** *recruitment@southalabama.edu*
**International Students:** No
**Preference to In-State Residents:** Out-of-state (MS and FL)
**Application Deadline:** Apply by December 16.
**SAT/ACT:** 1360+/30+ | **GPA:** 3.5+ | **MCAT:** Yes

## COST OF ATTENDANCE

**Tuition & Fees:** ~$15,000 (in-state), ~$25,000 (out-of-state)
**Addl Exp:** $22,000 | **Total:** $37,000 (in-state), $47,000 (out-of-state)
**Scholarships:** Merit-based freshmen scholarships (e.g. Board of Trustees, Valedictorian, Red & Blue Honors). Need-based awards like the Jaguar Dream, Retention, and Bridging the Gap Scholarships for Alabama residents or those in their final years.

## ADDITIONAL INFORMATION

COMEAP is an Early Acceptance Program jointly offered by the Honors College and the College of Medicine, awarding conditional admission to the M.D. program at the University of South Alabama's College of Medicine, contingent upon meeting academic milestones. Interviews are offered by invitation only in early February with interviews in March..

# THE GEORGE WASHINGTON UNIVERSITY BS/MD (7-YEARS)

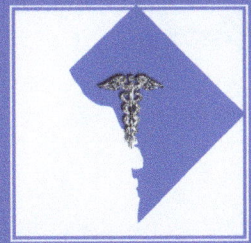

**George Washington University BS/MD**
800 21st St NW, Suite 100, Washington, DC 20052
**Affiliated Medical School:** George Washington University School of Medicine and Health Sciences Medicine
**Request Information:** *https://undergraduate.admissions.gwu.edu/contact-us*
**Phone:** (202) 994-6040 | **E-Mail:** *gwadm[at]gwu.edu*
**International Students:** No, Canada, yes.
**Preference to In-State Residents:** No
**Application Deadline:** Apply by November 15 to GW's Columbian College. When you apply, select BA/MD.
**SAT/ACT:** 1400+/32+ | **GPA:** 4.0 | **MCAT:** No

## COST OF ATTENDANCE

**Tuition & Fees:** ~$73,000 | **Addl Exp:** $25,000 | **Total:** $98,000
**Scholarships:** About 42% of students receive aid; of those with financial need, 97% are awarded assistance. Merit and need-based aid packages benefit qualifying students significantly.

## ADDITIONAL INFORMATION

Access the Dual BA/MD program page via GW SMHS "Combined & Joint Programs" section and click "7-Year BA/MD Program" to find info/application materials. Students must maintain GPA ≥ 3.6 overall, with no grade below C in any science course. Acceptance rate is extremely competitive, typically in the 2%–8% range, aligning with other top-tier dual-degree programs.

Students benefit from summer clinical exposure, mentoring from MD Admissions, and early. Students must maintain a track record of clinical or medically related experiences and service commitments. Embedded in Washington, DC, with rotations and clinical practice occurring at both main and regional campus sites like Sinai Hospital integration with medical faculty.

ALABAMA

ARKANSAS

DELAWARE

**DISTRICT OF COLUMBIA**

FLORIDA

GEORGIA

KENTUCKY

LOUISIANA

MARYLAND

MISSISSIPPI

NORTH CAROLINA

OKLAHOMA

SOUTH CAROLINA

TENNESSEE

TEXAS

VIRGINIA

WEST VIRGINIA

SOUTH

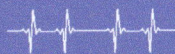

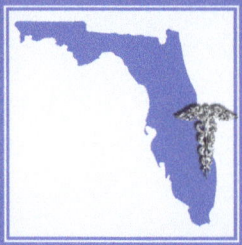

ALABAMA

ARKANSAS

DELAWARE

DISTRICT OF COLUMBIA

FLORIDA

GEORGIA

KENTUCKY

LOUISIANA

MARYLAND

MISSISSIPPI

NORTH CAROLINA

OKLAHOMA

SOUTH CAROLINA

TENNESSEE

TEXAS

VIRGINIA

WEST VIRGINIA

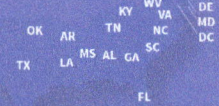

# NOVA SOUTHEASTERN UNIVERSITY
## BS/MD & BS/DO (6, 7, AND 8-YEARS)

**Nova Southeastern University - Dual Admission for Allopathic and Osteopathic Medicine** - different addresses for MD and DO
**Affiliated Medical Schools:** Dr. Kiran C. Patel College of Allopathic Medicine (MD) and Patel College of Osteopathic Medicine (DO)
**Request Information:** *https://nova.elluciancrmrecruit.com/Apply/ Account/Create*
**Phone:** (954) 262-1737 | **E-Mail:** *MDAdmissions@nova.edu*
**International Students:** No
**Preference to In-State Residents:** No preference for in-state
**Application Deadline:** February 1
**SAT/ACT:** 1520+/35+ | **GPA:** 3.5+ | **MCAT:** Yes (510+), not for 6-year students

## COST OF ATTENDANCE

**Tuition & Fees:** ~$44,000 | **Addl Exp:** $25,000 | **Total:** $69,000
**Scholarships:** At NSU, the full cost of attendance (including room, fees, etc.) reaches around $69,000/year. Still, with financial aid, the average net cost is about $29,600/year.

## ADDITIONAL INFORMATION

Admission is invitation-based at Shark Preview (admitted-student event). The 2+4 track awards a B.S. in Medical Science after the first year of med school; the 3+4 and 4+4 tracks allow any bachelor's major. The 2+4 track awards a B.S. in Medical Science after the first year of med school; the 3+4 and 4+4 tracks allow any bachelor's major. If admitted, you receive conditional acceptance into NSU's Doctor of Medicine (M.D.) or Doctor of Osteopathic Medicine (D.O.) program before starting college.

# UNIVERSITY OF SOUTH FLORIDA
## BS/MD (7-YEARS)

**University of South Florida BS/MD Pathway**
560 Channelside Drive, Tampa, FL 33602
**Affiliated Medical School:** University of South Florida Morsani College of Medicine
**Request Information:** *https://www.usf.edu/honors/programs/7-year-med.aspx*
**Phone:** (813) 396-9459 | **E-Mail:** *harbert@usf.edu*
**International Students:** No
**Preference to In-State Residents:** No preference
**Application Deadline:** November 15 (priority); March 15 (Final)
**SAT/ACT:** 1500+/34+ | **GPA:** 3.5+ | **MCAT:** Yes (516+)

## COST OF ATTENDANCE

**Tuition & Fees:** ~$8,000 (in-state), ~$20,000 (out-of-state)
**Addl Exp:** $25,000 | **Total:** $3,3000 (in-state), $45,000 (out-of-state)
**Scholarships:** All Honors students can obtain a $2,000 scholarship. The Genspiration Global Explorers Scholarship offers $10,000 for approved study abroad or domestic experiences. Honors and general USF scholarships are available through the Award Spring portal, including need and merit-based options (over $1 million annually).

## ADDITIONAL INFORMATION

No separate BS/MD application for this program. Students qualify by admission to USF Honors. Guaranteed conditional acceptance into USF Morsani upon maintaining a 3.7 BCPM and overall GPA after Year 1, then 3.8 GPAs by Year 3. Note that the 516 MCAT threshold is tough. Students must major in Biomedical Sciences. This program is reserved for top academic achievers since the course requirements demands sustained excellence.

# AUGUSTA UNIVERSITY
## BS/MD & BS/DMD  (8-YEARS)

**Augusta University Medical Scholars Program**
Benet House, 2500 Walton Way, Augusta, GA 30904
**Affiliated Medical School:** The Medical College of Georgia
**Request Information:** *https://www.augusta.edu/admissions/ professionalscholars.php*
**Phone:** (706) 737-1632 | **E-Mail:** *admissions@augusta.edu*
**International Students:** No
**Preference to In-State Residents:** Preference for GA residents.
**Application Deadline:** October 31, supplement due December 16
**SAT/ACT:** 1450+/32+ | **GPA:** 3.7+ | **MCAT:** Yes

## COST OF ATTENDANCE

**Tuition & Fees:** ~$22,000 (in-state), ~$25,000 (out-of-state)
**Addl Exp:** $23,000 | **Total:** $45,000 (in-state), $48,000 (out-of-state)
**Scholarships:** Institutional scholarship deadline is February 1 for program and general awards.

## ADDITIONAL INFORMATION

The Augusta University BS/MD Medical Scholars Program offers exceptional high school students a streamlined, conditional pathway to the Medical College of Georgia, one of the oldest and most prestigious public medical schools in the Southeast. Students benefit from early assurance, access to clinical and research opportunities, and close mentorship throughout their undergraduate years. However, this path is highly competitive, with a rigorous screening process requiring a minimum 3.7 GPA and a 1450+ SAT or 32+ ACT, followed by a supplemental application, interviews, and academic review.

Applicants must also navigate the challenge of maintaining a strong college GPA and achieving a competitive MCAT score, making the program both an opportunity and a significant academic commitment. In-state Georgia residents receive preference, and only U.S. citizens or permanent residents may apply, making it a selective but rewarding option for students committed to a career in medicine.

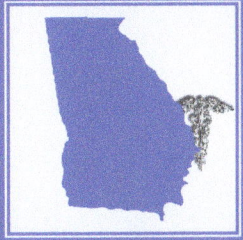

ALABAMA

ARKANSAS

DELAWARE

DISTRICT OF COLUMBIA

FLORIDA

GEORGIA

KENTUCKY

LOUISIANA

MARYLAND

MISSISSIPPI

NORTH CAROLINA

OKLAHOMA

SOUTH CAROLINA

TENNESSEE

TEXAS

VIRGINIA

WEST VIRGINIA

SOUTH

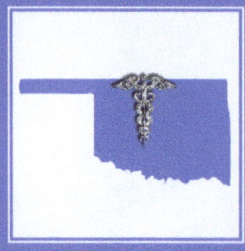

ALABAMA

ARKANSAS

DELAWARE

DISTRICT OF COLUMBIA

FLORIDA

GEORGIA

KENTUCKY

LOUISIANA

MARYLAND

MISSISSIPPI

NORTH CAROLINA

OKLAHOMA

SOUTH CAROLINA

TENNESSEE

TEXAS

VIRGINIA

WEST VIRGINIA

# UNIVERSITY OF OKLAHOMA
# MHSP BA/MD (8-YEARS)

**University of Oklahoma Medical Humanities Scholars Program**
Boren Hall, 1300 Asp Avenue, Norman, OK 73019-0385
**Affiliated Medical School:** University of Oklahoma College of Medicine
**Request Information:** *https://hello.ou.edu/portal/mailing-list*
**Phone:** (405) 325-5291 | **E-Mail:** *honors@ou.edu*
**International Students:** No
**Preference to In-State Residents:** Out-of-state considered
**Application Deadline:** December 1, though apps are accepted until January 15; interview in March
**SAT/ACT:** 1450+/32+ | **GPA:** 4.0 | **MCAT:** Yes (509+)

## COST OF ATTENDANCE

**Tuition & Fees:** ~$22,000 (in-state), ~$29,000 (out-of-state)
**Addl Exp:** $20,000 | **Total:** $42,000 (in-state), $49,000 (out-of-state)
**Scholarships:** MHSP offers up to $2,000 reimbursement for MCAT prep courses/materials. Open to all MHSP students in good standing. Check the current deadlines.

Vision Scholarship is available for up to $5,000 total ($2,500 per semester/year 1–2) for incoming freshmen with financial need and GPA ≥ 3.4. Other awards (e.g. travel, research, study abroad, leadership) ranging from $500–$1,500, all requiring Honors College enrollment and 3.4+ GPA.

## ADDITIONAL INFORMATION

MHSP is a selective BA/MD pathway in the OU Honors College. Students must have strong extracurriculars: clinical shadowing, community service, arts/humanities. They earn a BA in Medical Humanities. Students must maintain a 3.7+ GPA and earn a 509 MCAT score by junior year.

Once students begin at the Health Sciences Center, MHSP students can apply for college-specific scholarships such as the Physicians Manpower/Oklahoma Rural Medical Scholarship, Tulsa County Medical Society Foundation, and others; some scholarships offering multi-year support.

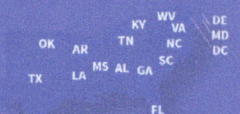

# UNIVERSITY OF SOUTH CAROLINA
# BS/MD (7-YEARS)

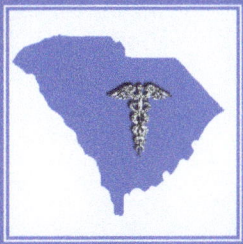

**USC & South Carolina Honors College BARSC w/Accel. Pre-Med**
Harper College 120, USC, Columbia, SC 29208
**Affiliated Medical School:** USC School of Medicine
**Request Information:** *https://sc.edu/study/colleges_schools/ honors_college/about/contact/*
**Phone:** (803) 777-8102 | **E-Mail:** *admhonor@mailbox.sc.edu*
**International Students:** No
**Preference to In-State Residents:** In-state pref, out-of-state okay
**Application Deadline:** November 15 (BARSC-MD app closes Feb 7)
**SAT/ACT:** 1450+/33+ | **GPA:** top 3% | **MCAT:** No

## COST OF ATTENDANCE

**Tuition & Fees:** ~$31,000 (in-state), ~$55,000 (out-of-state)
**Addl Exp:** $22,000 | Total: $53,000 (in-state), $77,000 (out-of-state)
**Scholarships:** Incoming Honors students are automatically considered for university-wide scholarships, and can additionally apply (via a spring departmental application) for awards like David W. Robinson ($1,000), Belser Full-Tuition, Aitchison $1,000, Gray-Mims $2,000, and others ($1k–full-tuition).

High-achieving students may receive national-level merit scholarships (Stamps, Carolina, McNair, Horseshoe, etc.), which can include full or substantial tuition, room & board, and enrichment funding. Honors students (including those in the accelerated track) can apply annually for awards ($1,000 each) like Kepper, Guerin, McAnulty, Timko, etc., typically requiring GPA ≥ 3.5 and good standing.

## ADDITIONAL INFORMATION

The BARSC Accelerated program, offered through the Honors College, is a 7-year track that admits high-achieving freshman applicants (top ~3%, high SAT/ACT) to earn a Bachelor of Arts with Science (BARSC) and seamlessly transition to USC School of Medicine–Columbia without taking the MCAT. This program combines 3 years undergraduate coursework (including honors thesis/research) with 4 years of medical school.

ALABAMA

ARKANSAS

DELAWARE

DISTRICT OF COLUMBIA

FLORIDA

GEORGIA

KENTUCKY

LOUISIANA

MARYLAND

MISSISSIPPI

NORTH CAROLINA

OKLAHOMA

SOUTH CAROLINA

TENNESSEE

TEXAS

VIRGINIA

WEST VIRGINIA

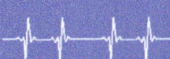

# SOUTH

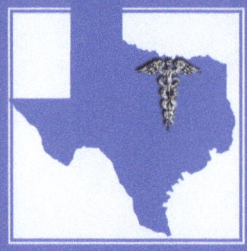

**ALABAMA**

**ARKANSAS**

**DELAWARE**

**DISTRICT OF COLUMBIA**

**FLORIDA**

**GEORGIA**

**KENTUCKY**

**LOUISIANA**

**MARYLAND**

**MISSISSIPPI**

**NORTH CAROLINA**

**OKLAHOMA**

**SOUTH CAROLINA**

**TENNESSEE**

**TEXAS**

**VIRGINIA**

**WEST VIRGINIA**

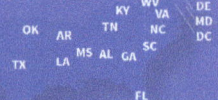

# TEXAS TECH UNIVERSITY
## UMSI BS/MD (8-YEARS)

**Texas Tech University Undergraduate to Medical School Initiative**
Honors College & Pre-Professional Advising, 147 Drane Hall, Box 41038, Texas Tech University, Lubbock, TX 79409-1038
**Affiliated Medical School:** Texas Tech University Health Sciences Center School of Medicine
**Phone:** (806)742-2189 | **E-Mail:** *pphc@ttu.edu*
**International Students:** No
**Preference to In-State Residents:** Only Texas residents considered.
**Application Deadline:** Apply to TTU and Honors College by Dec 1
**SAT/ACT:** 1360+/30+ | **GPA:** top10% | **MCAT:** No

### COST OF ATTENDANCE

**Tuition & Fees:** ~$15,000 (in-state) | **Addl Exp:** $22,000 | **Total:** $37,000
**Scholarships:** Students are automatically considered when applying to Honors College by Dec 1. Awards vary. Multiple awards for juniors/seniors in pre-med tracks.

### ADDITIONAL INFORMATION

Maintain a 3.7 GPA to assure medical school slot. Complete the required coursework, activities, and events in the Honors College. Students admitted to UMSI must maintain 100 hours of volunteer and/or shadowing activity per academic year. By waiving the MCAT requirement and guaranteeing medical school admission, UMSI gives students the opportunity to have a varied undergraduate education, which could include internships or study abroad.

# UNIVERSITY OF HOUSTON
## HONORSMED BS/MD (8-YEARS)

**University of Houston – HonorsMed BS/MD Honors College Pathway**
4434 University Drive, Houston, TX 77204
**Affiliated Medical School:** Fertitta Family College of Medicine at University of Houston
**Request Information:** https://www.uh.edu/honors/programs-minors/curricular-programs/honors-med/
**Phone:** (713) 743-9010| E-Mail: honors@uh.edu
**International Students:** No
**Preference to In-State Residents:** No pref, out-of-state considered
**Application Deadline:** November 1
**SAT/ACT:** 1400+/30+ | **GPA:** 3.5+ | **MCAT:** Yes (500+)

### COST OF ATTENDANCE

**Tuition & Fees:** ~$12,000 (in-state), ~$29,000 (out-of-state)
**Addl Exp:** $25,000 | **Total**: $37,000 (in-state), $54,000 (out-of-state)
**Scholarships:** Merit- and need-based awards available to students who attend an Honors Open House. Annual Honors awards re-open each July for returning students. SURF–UH: $4,000 summer research fellowship for undergrad STEM students.

### ADDITIONAL INFORMATION

Applicants must be accepted to UH + Honors College and complete HonorsMed application. Matriculation into the College of Medicine is contingent upon students maintaining a 3.5 cumulative GPA and scoring a minimum of 500 on the MCAT. Selected students will be invited to interview with the Fertitta Family College of Medicine in the spring, and up to six students will be chosen for the program after interviews.

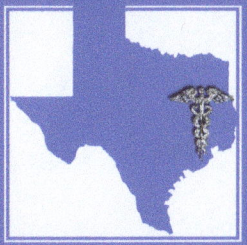

# UNIVERSITY OF TEXAS AT DALLAS
## PACT BS/MD (8-YEARS)

**University of Texas at Dallas Partnership in Advancing Clinical Transition**
800 W. Campbell Rd, Richardson, TX 75080
**Affiliated Medical School:** UT Southwestern Medical School, Dallas
**Request Information:** *https://enroll.utdallas.edu/apply/request-info/*
**Phone:** (972) 883-2700 | **E-Mail:** *hpac@utdallas.edu*
**International Students:** No
**Preference to In-State Residents:** Out-of-state considered
**Application Deadline:** December 1; Interviews in Feb/March
**SAT/ACT:** 1400+/32+ | **GPA:** 3.8+ | **MCAT:** No

### COST OF ATTENDANCE

**Tuition & Fees:** ~$32,000 (in-state), ~$84,000 (out-of-state)
**Addl Exp:** $25,000 | **Total:** $57,000 (in-state), $109,000 (out-of-state)
**Scholarships:** Both universities offer strong financial support for high-achieving students, UT Dallas through prestigious merit awards, through a combination of merit-based and need-based grants.

### ADDITIONAL INFORMATION

UT PACT is an early assurance BS/MD program that students apply to while in high school. Students accepted into the program are guaranteed conditional admission to the UT Southwestern Medical School. CASPer or similar pre-screening: Required (via PPHC). Conditional medical-school acceptance granted after interviews.

# UNIVERSITY OF TEXAS RIO GRANDE VALLEY
## BS/MD (8-YEARS)

**University of Texas Rio Grande Valley Vaqueros MD Early Assurance Program** - Student Services Building, 1201 W University Dr, Edinburg, TX 78539
**Affiliated Medical School:** UTRGV School of Medicine
**Request Information:** *https://www.utrgv.edu/admissions/info/request/index.htm*
**Phone:** (956) 882-4026 | **E-Mail:** *VaquerosMD@utrgv.edu*
**International Students:** No
**Preference to In-State Residents:** Only Texas residents may apply.
**Application Deadline:** March 1
**SAT/ACT:** 1450+/32+ | **GPA:** 3.8+ | **MCAT:** Yes (60th percentile)

### COST OF ATTENDANCE

**Tuition & Fees:** ~$18,000 (in-state) | **Addl Exp:** $25,000 | **Total:** ~$43,000
**Scholarships:** The UTRGV Tuition Advantage Grant covers tuition/fees for students with family income ≤ $125K and unmet need, via FAFSA/TASFA. Prestigious merit program for exceptional undergrads.

### ADDITIONAL INFORMATION

High school applicants to UTRGV and Honors College from thirteen South Texas counties, or via online/boarding school with residency in the region. Must apply as freshmen, rank in top 5%, SAT ≥ 90th percentile, GPA ≥ 3.8 overall and ≥ 3.75 in science, letters, interviews, video personal statement. During undergrad: complete Honors College requirements, TMDSAS application, MCAT ≥ 60th percentile, GPA ≥ 3.2 overall and 3.5 science.

ALABAMA

ARKANSAS

DELAWARE

DISTRICT OF COLUMBIA

FLORIDA

GEORGIA

KENTUCKY

LOUISIANA

MARYLAND

MISSISSIPPI

NORTH CAROLINA

OKLAHOMA

SOUTH CAROLINA

TENNESSEE

TEXAS

VIRGINIA

WEST VIRGINIA

**SOUTH**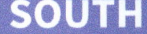

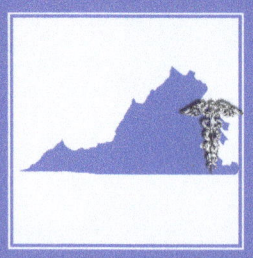

**ALABAMA**

**ARKANSAS**

**DELAWARE**

**DISTRICT OF COLUMBIA**

**FLORIDA**

**GEORGIA**

**KENTUCKY**

**LOUISIANA**

**MARYLAND**

**MISSISSIPPI**

**NORTH CAROLINA**

**OKLAHOMA**

**SOUTH CAROLINA**

**TENNESSEE**

**TEXAS**

**VIRGINIA**

**WEST VIRGINIA**

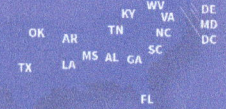

# VIRGINIA COMMONWEALTH UNIVERSITY GMED - BS/MD (8-YEARS)

**Virginia Commonwealth University Guaranteed Admission to Med**
701 W. Grace St, Box 843010, Richmond, VA 23284-3010
**Affiliated Medical School:** VCU School of Medicine
**Request Information:** *https://admissions.vcu.edu/connect/request-information/*
**Phone:** (804) 828-1803 | **E-Mail:** *honors@vcu.edu*
**International Students:** No
**Preference to In-State Residents:** No pref, out-of-state considered
**Application Deadline:** November 1
**Ave. SAT/ACT:** 1560+/36+ | **Ave. GPA:** 4.0 | **MCAT:** Yes (503+)

## COST OF ATTENDANCE

**Tuition & Fees:** ~$15,000 (in-state), ~$38,000 (out-of-state)
**Addl Exp:** $24,000 | **Total:** $39,000 (in-state), $62,000 (out-of-state)
**Scholarships:** Scholarships cover tuition/fees up to $16,000/year, plus room & board, total value of $114,356 over four years and up to $16,000/year in tuition/fees for a total of $64,000. Additionally, out-of-state students may qualify for at least $10,000/year merit awards. Honors College Scholarships are available to incoming and current Honors students, awards typically range from $500 to $3,000/year, renewable with GPA ≥3.5.

## ADDITIONAL INFORMATION

The VCU Guaranteed Admission to Medicine program is an accelerated, early-admission track designed for exceptional high school students who are admitted to both VCU and its Honors College. Successful applicants, typically with GPAs near 3.9 and SAT scores in the 1500+ range (or ACT 33+), receive conditional acceptance to the VCU School of Medicine under the agreement that they sustain strong academic performance (usually a GPA of 3.5 or higher) and submit a qualifying MCAT score (typically 503+) by the summer before medical matriculation.

GMED ensures that students who maintain program requirements bypass the traditional med school admissions process, offering a seamless BS-to-MD pathway enriched with honors-level advising, mentorship, and a clear route to a medical career.

# WEST VIRGINIA UNIVERSITY
## BS/MD (8-YEARS)

**West Virginia University MAP & Early Assurance Pathways**
Office of Admissions, 1 Waterfront Place, Morgantown, WV 26506
**Affiliated Medical School:** WVU School of Medicine
**Request Information:** *https://medicine.hsc.wvu.edu/md-admissions/programs/wvu-mountaineer-accelerated-pathway-map-to-md/*
**Phone:** (304) 293-5355 | **E-Mail:** *medadmissions@hsc.wvu.edu*
**International Students:** No
**Preference to In-State Residents:** West Virginia residents only
**Application Deadline:** Apply early fall.
**SAT/ACT:** 1360+/30+ | **GPA:** 3.8+ | **MCAT:** Yes

## COST OF ATTENDANCE

**Tuition & Fees:** ~$12,000 (in-state) | **Addl Exp:** $25,000 |
**Total:** ~$37,000
**Scholarships:** Medical tuition supported with $10K+/year scholarship.

## ADDITIONAL INFORMATION

Student must enroll in a Health Sciences major (e.g., Biomedical Lab Diagnostics, Immunology, Exercise Physiology). Upon enrollment at WVU Health Sciences undergraduate major, if requirements are met, students receive a guaranteed med-school interview; actual MD admission not guaranteed.

Medical tuition is supported with $10K+/year scholarship. This program provides guaranteed interview; not guaranteed admission. MAP limited to WV residents/dependents; Pre-Med track open to any WVU student.

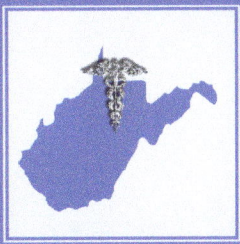

ALABAMA

ARKANSAS

DELAWARE

DISTRICT OF COLUMBIA

FLORIDA

GEORGIA

KENTUCKY

LOUISIANA

MARYLAND

MISSISSIPPI

NORTH CAROLINA

OKLAHOMA

SOUTH CAROLINA

TENNESSEE

TEXAS

VIRGINIA

WEST VIRGINIA

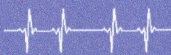

**SOUTH**

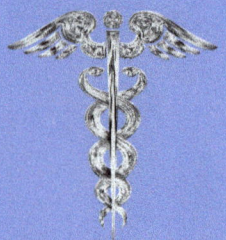

# REGION FOUR
# WEST

**ALASKA**

**ARIZONA**

**CALIFORNIA**

**COLORADO**

**HAWAII**

**IDAHO**

**MONTANA**

**NEVADA**

**NEW MEXICO**

**OREGON**

**UTAH**

**WASHINGTON**

**WYOMING**

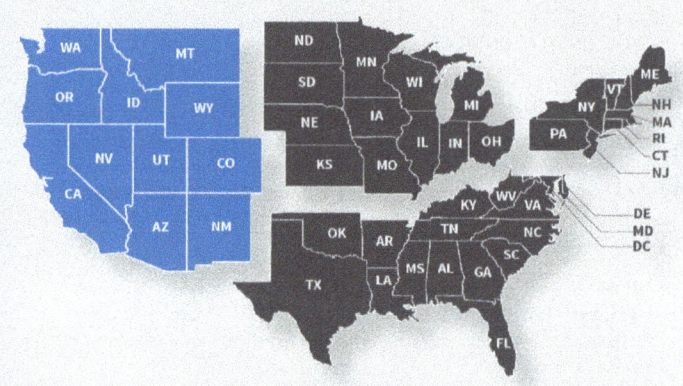

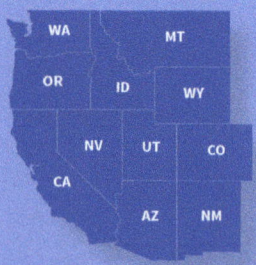

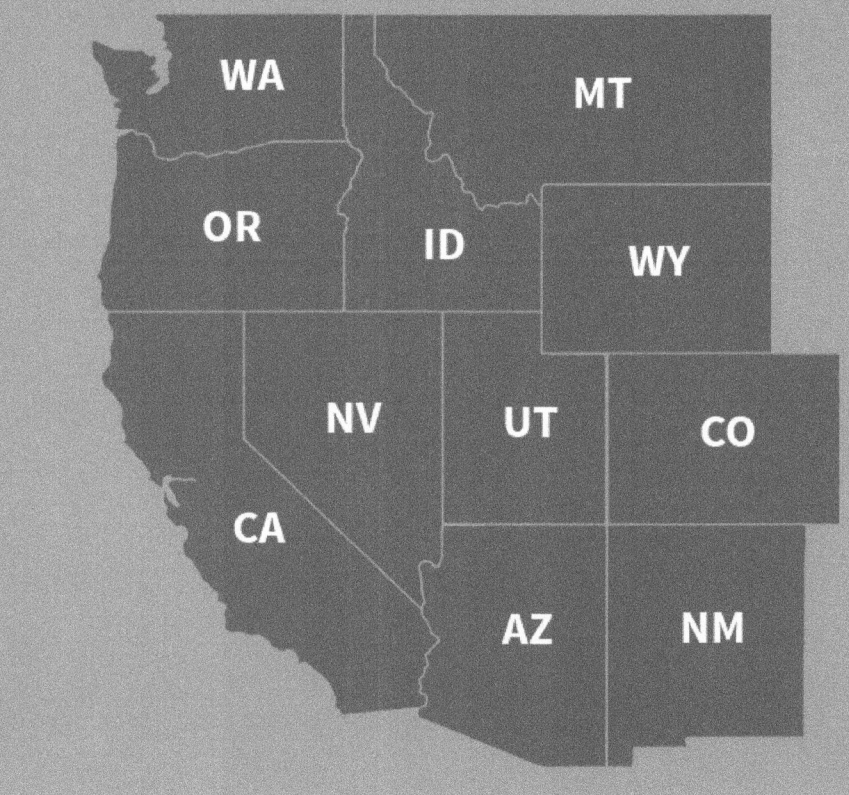

# 5 Programs | 13 States

1. CA - California Northstate University - BS/MD
2. CA - University of California Merced, UCSF - BS/MD
3. CO – University of Colorado at Denver - BA/MD
4. NM – University of New Mexico - BA/MD
5. NV – University of Nevada - BS/MD

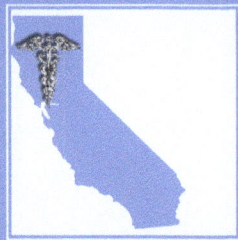

ALASKA

ARIZONA

CALIFORNIA

COLORADO

HAWAII

IDAHO

MONTANA

NEVADA

NEW MEXICO

OREGON

UTAH

WASHINGTON

WYOMING

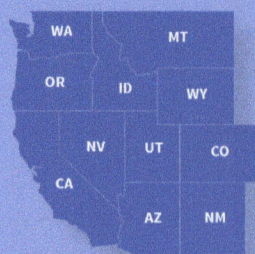

# CALIFORNIA NORTHSTATE UNIVERSITY BS/MD (8-YEARS)

**California Northstate University – BS/MD Program**
2910 Prospect Park Drive, Rancho Cordova, CA 95670
**Affiliated Medical School:** California Northstate University College of Medicine
**Phone:** (916) 686-7674 | **E-Mail:** *COMadmissions@cnsu.edu*
**International Students:** Yes, international students considered
**Preference to In-State Residents:** No pref, out-of-state considered
**Application Deadline:** November 15
**SAT/ACT:** Optional, but check if changed | **GPA:** 3.5+ | **MCAT:** Yes

## COST OF ATTENDANCE

**Tuition & Fees:** ~$57,000, **Addl Exp:** $28,000 | **Total:** ~$85,000
**Scholarships:** CNUCHS awards three levels of merit scholarships: president's, dean's, and scholastic. Also, the Duruisseau President Academic & Diversity Scholarship covers tuition, fees, and health insurance (retention requirement: cumulative GPA ≥ 3.0). There are also College & COM Grants based funding available across colleges.

## ADDITIONAL INFORMATION

California Northstate offers a combined BS/MD pathway through its College of Medicine, accepting students directly from HS. Apply by November 15 under Early Action. SAT/ACT scores are optional for those w/25+ transferable college credits. A 3.5+ GPA w/a 510+ MCAT score before medical school.

# UNIVERSITY OF CALIFORNIA, MERCED SJV PRIME+ BS/MD (8-YEARS)

**UC Merced San Joaquin Valley (SJV) PRIME+ BS/MD**
5200 North Lake Road, Merced, CA 95343
**Affiliated Medical School:** UCSF School of Medicine
**Request Information:** *https://admissions.ucmerced.edu/information/request*
**Phone:** (209) 228-7178 | **E-Mail:** *primeplus@ucmerced.edu*
**International Students:** No
**Preference to In-State Residents:** CA residents, pref to those in SJV
**Application Deadline:** November 30, supplement by December 3
**SAT/ACT:** N/A | **GPA:** 3.6+ | **MCAT:** No

## COST OF ATTENDANCE

**Tuition & Fees:** ~$18,000 | **Addl Exp:** $29,000 | **Total:** $47,000
**Scholarships:** Students automatically qualify for Pell, Cal Grants, UC scholarships. In addition, SJV PRIME+ students often receive priority need- and merit-based aid due to the program's focus on health equity and Central Valley representation.

## ADDITIONAL INFORMATION

The SJV PRIME+ BS/MD is an eight-year, early-admission partnership between UC Merced and the UCSF School of Medicine (training in Fresno and Merced). HS seniors from SJV counties apply via the UC application, choosing a major in Bio, Chem, Bioengineering, or Public Health, and submit a supplemental application by Dec 3. A minimum UC GPA of 3.6 and demonstration of strong ties to SJV. No MCAT is required, as admission to UCSF Med is conditional upon meeting BA/BS milestones. Preference is given to SJV residents.

# UNIVERSITY OF COLORADO AT DENVER
# BA/MD (8-YEARS)

**University of Colorado Denver – BA/BS-MD Program**
1200 Larimer Street, North Classroom Building, Suite 3002
Denver, CO 80204
**Affiliated Medical School:** University of Colorado School of
Medicine at Anschutz Medical Campus
**Request Information:** *https://application.admissions.ucdenver.edu/
register/UGRDRequestInformation*
**Phone:** (303) 315-7536 | **E-Mail:** *BABSMD@ucdenver.edu*
**International Students:** No
**Preference to In-State Residents:** Colorado residents only.
**Application Deadline:** Mid-Oct w/BS/MD supplement by Oct 31.
Interviews are held in early December.
**SAT/ACT:** 1200+/27+ | **GPA:** 3.5+ | **MCAT:** Yes

## COST OF ATTENDANCE

**Tuition & Fees:** ~$15,000 (in-state) | **Addl Exp:** $22,000 |
**Total:** $37,000
**Scholarships:** New full-time undergraduates with a strong GPA are
automatically considered. Scholarships range based on GPA:
GPA 3.0–3.29: $5,000/year
GPA 3.3–3.69: $7,500/year
GPA ≥ 3.7: $10,000/year

Through CU Denver's Scholarship Universe, students (including
international) can access over $30 million in institutional, private,
state, and national scholarships. This includes both merit- and need-
based awards.

## ADDITIONAL INFORMATION

Accepted students are guaranteed a reserved slot at CU med school,
contingent on meeting requirements during undergrad. The process
includes a holistic review; top 10 academically and community
service. Students must intend to practice medicine in Colorado.

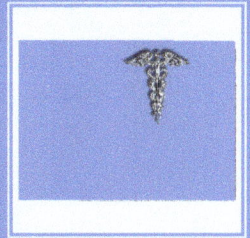

ALASKA

ARIZONA

CALIFORNIA

COLORADO

HAWAII

IDAHO

MONTANA

NEVADA

NEW MEXICO

OREGON

UTAH

WASHINGTON

WYOMING

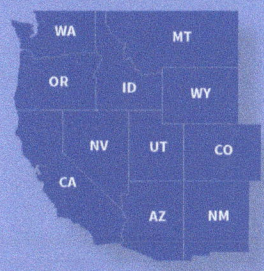

SOUTH

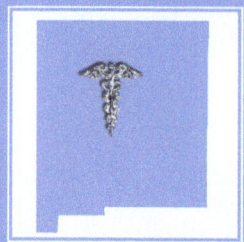

**ALASKA**

**ARIZONA**

**CALIFORNIA**

**COLORADO**

**HAWAII**

**IDAHO**

**MONTANA**

**NEVADA**

**NEW MEXICO**

**OREGON**

**UTAH**

**WASHINGTON**

**WYOMING**

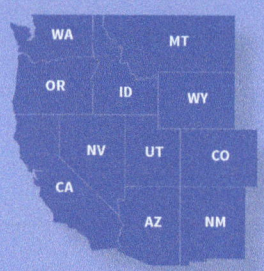

# UNIVERSITY OF NEW MEXICO
# BA/MD  (8-YEARS)

**University of New Mexico – Combined BA/MD Program**
Health Sciences & Services Building, Suite 102
2500 Marble Avenue NE, Albuquerque, NM 87106
**Affiliated Medical School:** University of New Mexico School of Medicine
**Request Information:** *https://admissions.unm.edu/connect-with-us/index.html*
**Phone:** (505) 925-4500 |
**E-Mail:** *HSC-CombinedBAMD@salud.unm.edu*
**International Students:** No
**Preference to In-State Residents:** NM high school or tribal/living on Navajo Nation; commitment to rural/underserved NM practice.
**Application Deadline:** Apply between August to the first Thursday in November with both the UNM application and the BA/MD supplemental application.
**SAT/ACT:** 1100+/22+ | **GPA:** 3.5+ | **MCAT:** Yes

## COST OF ATTENDANCE

**Tuition & Fees:** $0 (full ride scholarship for students in this program)

## ADDITIONAL INFORMATION

New Mexico high school seniors or tribal students only. This program is limited to 28 spots/year; includes full-ride scholarship and conditional med-school acceptance. BA/MD students are required to complete the Kaplan MCAT preparatory course during their third year of undergraduate school.

Students must sit for the MCAT by August 1 of their fourth undergraduate year, with a score meeting or exceeding the UNM School of Medicine's minimum threshold (usually around 494). Failing to achieve the required MCAT score by this deadline may result in release from the program.

# UNIVERSITY OF NEVADA, RENO
## BS/MD (7-YEARS)

**University of Nevada, Reno – BS/MD Program**
Office of Admissions & Student Affairs, School of Medicine
Reno, NV 89557-0071
**Affiliated Medical School:** University of Nevada, Reno School of Medicine
**Phone:** (775) 784-6063 | **E-Mail:** *asa@unr.edu*
**International Students:** No
**Preference to In-State Residents:** Nevada residents only.
**Application Deadline:** November 15
**Ave. SAT/ACT:** 1430+/32+ | **Ave. GPA:** 3.8+ | **MCAT:** Yes (509+)

## COST OF ATTENDANCE

**Tuition & Fees:** ~$13,000 | **Addl Exp:** $22,000 | **Total:** $35,000
**Scholarships:**
*Presidential Scholarship* - $8,000/year (renewable up to 4 years) - Requires GPA 3.7–4.0 ACT 31–36 (or SAT 1390–1600).
*Nevada Scholars Scholarship* - $3,000 for the first year; Awards are ba sed on a GPA between 3.2–3.99 and ACT 22–36 (or SAT 1100–1600).
*Pack Pride, Alphie, Luna or Wolfie Scholarship:* Awards range from $2,000 down to $500 based on GPA and test scores.
*National Merit Scholarship* - Up to $16,000/year for recognized National Merit Finalists who list UNR as their first choice by May 1
*ASUN Student Government Scholarships* - Annual $1,000–$1,500 awards for leadership, public service, diversity, and more. Applications are due early February via MyNevada.

## ADDITIONAL INFORMATION

The University of Nevada, Reno offers a competitive and fast-track 7-year BS/MD pathway, initially admitting freshmen high school students. Only Nevada residents can apply for this rigorous Bachelor of Science in Biological Sciences curriculum at UNR.

High school seniors apply directly for provisional BS/MD. Students start their undergraduate education at the University of Nevada, Reno. After three years, they transition to medical school. Approximately twelve students are accepted each year.

Applicants typically rank in the top 10% of their class with a minimum unweighted GPA of 3.7 and standardized test scores of SAT 1270+ (CR ≥ 600) or ACT 29+ (English ≥ 26). Throughout their first three college years, BS/MD students must maintain a strong academic record (minimum 3.5 cumulative and science GPA), complete required science coursework, and engage in clinical experiences and extracurriculars.

Upon meeting these benchmarks and their MCAT requirement, these students advance directly into the UNR School of Medicine, avoiding the traditional medical school application process. Acceptance is highly selective, usually limited to around a dozen students per cycle, with emphasis on academic excellence, maturity, and dedication to medicine, all aimed at retaining top Nevada talent in-state.

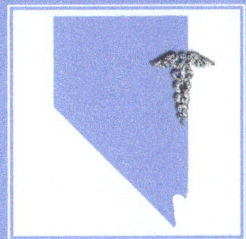

ALASKA
ARIZONA
CALIFORNIA
COLORADO
HAWAII
IDAHO
MONTANA
NEVADA
NEW MEXICO
OREGON
UTAH
WASHINGTON
WYOMING

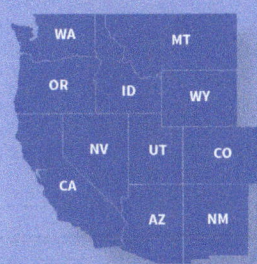

**SOUTH**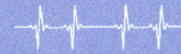

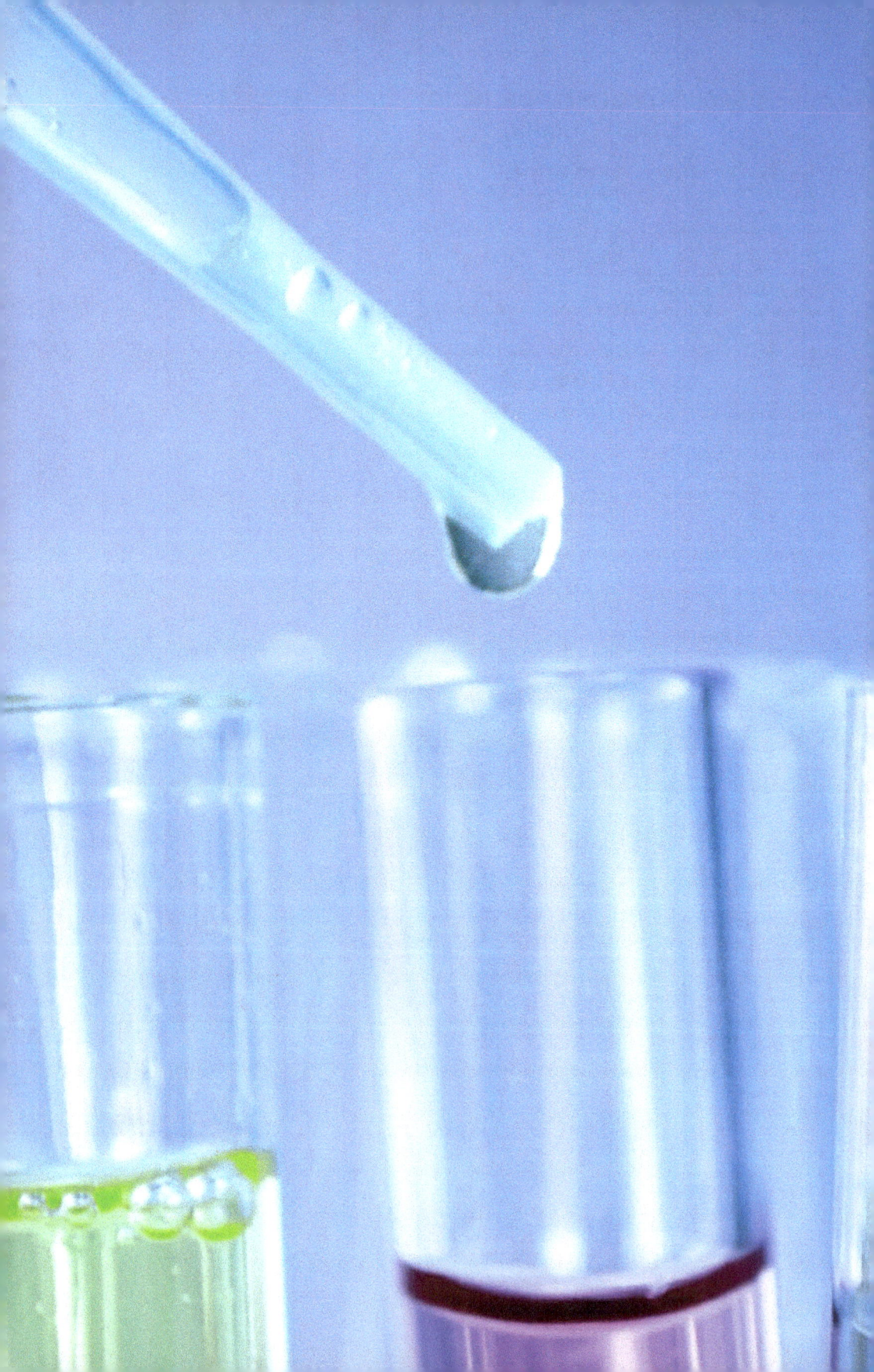

# PART 7

# LISTS OF COLLEGE PROGRAMS

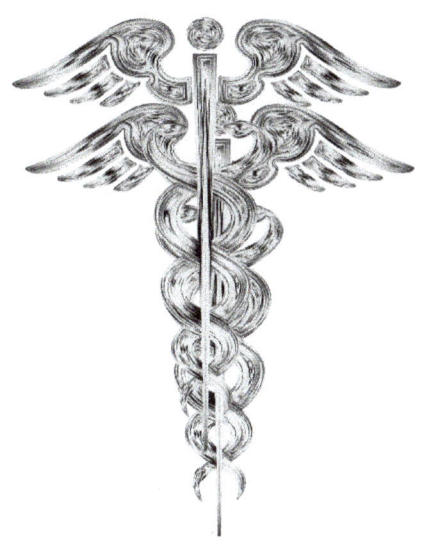

# LISTS AND GUIDES

## LIST OF B/MD, B/DO, EAP, AND DIRECT MED BY STATE/CITY

| UNIVERSITY/PROGRAM | CITY | STATE |
|---|---|---|
| University of Alabama at Birmingham | Birmingham | AL |
| University of South Alabama | Mobile | AL |
| California Northstate University | Rancho Cordova | CA |
| UC Merced's SJV PRIM | Merced | CA |
| University of Colorado, Denver | Denver | CO |
| University of Connecticut | Storrs | CT |
| George Washington University | Washington | DC |
| Howard University | Washington | DC |
| University of Delaware | Newark | DE |
| Florida Atlantic University | Boca Raton | FL |
| Florida International University | Miami | FL |
| Florida Southern College | Lakeland | FL |
| University of Miami | Coral Gables | FL |
| University of South Florida | Tampa | FL |
| Nova Southeastern University | Ft. Lauderdale | FL |
| Spelman College | Atlanta | GA |
| Augusta University | Augusta | GA |
| Mercer University | Macon | GA |
| St. George's University | Saint George's | Grenada |
| Loyola University Chicago | Chicago | IL |
| University of Illinois Chicago | Chicago | IL |
| Grambling State University | Grambling | LA |
| Tufts University Early Assurance | Medford | MA |
| Wayne State University Med-Direct Program | Detroit | MI |
| University of Missouri, Kansas City | Kansas City | MO |
| St. Louis University Medical Scholar Program | St. Louis | MO |
| Caldwell University w/ St. George's University | Caldwell | NJ |
| Montclair University | Montclair | NJ |
| Rutgers University | Newark | NJ |
| New Jersey Inst. of Tech. w/ St. George's | Newark | NJ |

| UNIVERSITY/PROGRAM | CITY | STATE |
|---|---|---|
| Monmouth University | West Long Branch | NJ |
| University of New Mexico | Albuquerque | NM |
| University of Nevada | Reno | NV |
| Albany College of Pharmacy & Health Sciences | Albany | NY |
| University at Albany - SUNY | Albany | NY |
| Brooklyn College BA/MD | Brooklyn | NY |
| Adelphi University | Garden City | NY |
| Hofstra University BS-BA/MD | Hempstead | NY |
| Siena College with Albany Medical College | Loudonville | NY |
| CUNY/CCNY Sophie Davis | New York | NY |
| Yeshiva University | New York | NY |
| Purchase College | Purchase | NY |
| Rochester University REMS | Rochester | NY |
| Rochester Institute of Technology | Rochester | NY |
| Union College Leadership in Medicine w/Albany Medical | Schenectady | NY |
| Saint Bonaventure Univeristy - GWU Medical School | St Bonaventure | NY |
| Stony Brook University BA/MD Scholars Program | Stony Brook | NY |
| Rensselaer Polytechnic Institute | Troy | NY |
| SUNY Polytechnic Institute | Utica | NY |
| Case Western Reserve University | Cleveland | OH |
| University of Toledo | Toledo | OH |
| University of Oklahoma | Norman | OK |
| Lehigh University | Bethlehem | PA |
| Drexel University | Philadelphia | PA |
| Temple University Health Scholars | Philadelphia | PA |
| University of the Sciences with Cooper Medical | Philadelphia | PA |
| Duquesne University | Pittsburgh | PA |
| University of Pittsburgh, Guaranteed Admissions | Pittsburgh | PA |
| Rosemont College Dual Degree | Rosemont | PA |
| Penn State University Accelerated Med | University Park | PA |
| Washington and Jefferson College | Washington | PA |

| UNIVERSITY/PROGRAM | CITY | STATE |
|---|---|---|
| West Chester University | West Chester | PA |
| Brown College PLME | Providence | RI |
| Fisk University | Nashville | TN |
| Texas JAMP | Austin | TX |
| Texas Tech University | Lubbock | TX |
| Baylor University | Waco | TX |
| Hampton University | Hampton | VA |
| Virginia Commonwealth University | Richmond | VA |
| Marshall University | Huntington | WV |

## BS/MD STATE RESIDENCY REQUIRED LIST

| UNIVERSITY/PROGRAM | | |
|---|---|---|
| Chadron State College | Texas JAMP | University of Louisville |
| Indiana State University | Texas Tech University | University of Minnesota |
| Marshall University | Univ. of Colorado, Denver | University of Nevada |
| Mercer University | University of Evansville | University of New Mexico |
| Montclair University | University of Illinois Chicago | |

## MEDICAL SCHOOLS BY MCAT SCORE AVERAGES

| MEDICAL SCHOOL | AVE. MCAT | AVE. GPA |
|---|---|---|
| New York University | 523 | 3.98 |
| University of Pennsylvania | 522 | 3.94 |
| Columbia University | 522 | 3.90 |
| Johns Hopkins University | 521 | 3.92 |
| Yale University | 521 | 3.92 |
| University of Chicago | 521 | 3.91 |
| Mayo Clinic | 521 | 3.94 |
| Harvard University | 520 | 3.90 |
| Northwestern University | 520 | 3.93 |
| Washington University in St. Louis | 520 | 3.88 |
| Icahn SOM at Mt. Sinai | 519 | 3.81 |
| Duke University | 519 | 3.90 |
| University of California San Francisco | 519 | 3.87 |
| University of South Florida | 519 | 3.95 |
| Weill Cornell | 519 | 3.90 |
| Stanford University | 518 | 3.89 |
| Vanderbilt University | 518 | 3.88 |
| Case Western Reserve | 518 | 3.87 |
| Baylor College of Med. | 518 | 3.91 |
| University of Texas SOM at San Antonio | 518 | 3.88 |
| Hofstra University | 518 | 3.86 |
| Keck School of Medicine of the University of Southern California | 517 | 3.85 |
| Emory University | 517 | 3.8 |
| University of Colorado | 517 | 3.7 |
| Boston University | 517 | 3.7 |
| University of Rochester | 517 | 3.6 |
| UCLA | 517 | 3.8 |
| UCSD | 517 | 3.8 |
| UCI | 517 | 3.89 |
| University of Virginia | 517 | 3.85 |

| MEDICAL SCHOOL | AVE. MCAT | AVE. GPA |
|---|---|---|
| Rowan University | 511 | 3.7 |
| Drexel University College of Medicine | 511 | 3.7 |
| Penn State University | 511 | 3.75 |
| Medical University of S. Carolina | 511 | 3.86 |
| University of South Carolina | 511 | 3.75 |
| University of Tennessee | 511 | 3.83 |
| Texas Christian University, Anne Burnett Marion School of Medicine | 511 | 3.7 |
| University of Texas Medical Branch | 511 | 3.80 |
| University of Washington | 511 | 3.7 |
| Florida International University Herbert Wertheim College of Medicine | 510 | 3.82 |
| Loyola University | 510 | 3.6 |
| Oakland University | 510 | 3.87 |
| University of Nevada Las Vegas | 510 | 3.65 |
| University of Buffalo | 510 | 3.7 |
| University of Oklahoma | 510 | 3.8 |
| East Tennessee State | 510 | 3.78 |
| West Virginia University | 510 | 3.76 |
| Med. Col. of Wisconsin | 510 | 3,78 |
| SUNY Upstate | 510 | 3.64 |
| Louisiana State Univ. | 509 | 3.76 |
| University of Alabama | 509 | 3.83 |
| Loma Linda University | 509 | 3.84 |
| University of California Davis | 509 | 3.58 |
| Chicago Medical School at Rosalind Franklin University of Medicine & Science | 511 | 3.7 |
| Rush University | 509 | 3.67 |
| University of Kansas | 509 | 3.84 |
| Tulane University | 509 | 3.61 |
| University of Missouri | 509 | 3.83 |

| MEDICAL SCHOOL | AVE. MCAT | AVE. GPA |
|---|---|---|
| Stony Brook University | 516 | 3.93 |
| University of Arizona - Phoenix | 516 | 3.8 |
| Florida Atlantic Univ. | 516 | 3.8 |
| Albert Einstein College of Medicine | 516 | 3.8 |
| NYU Long Island SOM | 516 | 3.94 |
| Brown University | 516 | 3.83 |
| Emory University | 516 | 3.81 |
| UT Southwestern | 516 | 3.89 |
| University of Michigan | 515 | 3.84 |
| Kaiser Permanente Bernard J. Tyson School of Medicine | 515 | 3.84 |
| University of Miami | 515 | 3.83 |
| University of Iowa | 515 | 3.81 |
| University of Nebraska | 515 | 3.75 |
| Rutgers New Jersey | 515 | 3.7 |
| New York Medical College | 515 | 3.6 |
| Northeast Ohio Medical | 515 | 3.74 |
| University of Pittsburgh | 515 | 3.83 |
| University of Central Florida | 514 | 3.89 |
| Tufts University | 514 | 3.8 |
| Wayne State University | 514 | 3.8 |
| Dartmouth University | 514 | 3.8 |
| Rutgers Robert Wood Johnson | 514 | 3.7 |
| Hackensack Meridian | 514 | 3.8 |
| The Ohio State University | 514 | 3.8 |
| Thomas Jefferson University | 514 | 3.8 |
| University of Texas Austin | 514 | 3.8 |
| University of Utah | 514 | 3.87 |
| University of Connecticut | 513 | 3.76 |
| Georgetown University | 513 | 3.76 |
| Carle Illinois COM | 513 | 3.73 |
| University of Maryland | 513 | 3.76 |
| Western Michigan University | 513 | 3.81 |
| Saint Louis University | 513 | 3.89 |

| MEDICAL SCHOOL | AVE. MCAT | AVE. GPA |
|---|---|---|
| University of Nevada Reno | 509 | 3.68 |
| University of Toledo | 509 | 3.77 |
| Oregon Health & Science | 509 | 3.69 |
| Texas Tech University | 509 | 3.85 |
| Texas Tech University - Lubbock | 509 | 3.85 |
| Washington State University | 509 | 3.65 |
| Wright State University | 509 | 3.68 |
| University of South Dakota | 509 | 3.79 |
| University of South Alabama | 508 | 3.85 |
| University of Arizona | 508 | 3.74 |
| University of California, Riverside | 508 | 3.6 |
| Southern Illinois University | 508 | 3.7 |
| University of Louisville | 508 | 3.73 |
| Central Michigan University College of Medicine | 507 | 3.6 |
| East Carolina University | 508 | 3.63 |
| University of South Carolina Columbia | 508 | 3.78 |
| University of Texas, Rio Grande Valley | 508 | 3.87 |
| University of Arkansas | 507 | 3.85 |
| Howard University | 507 | 3.61 |
| Florida State University | 507 | 3.68 |
| LSU Shreveport | 507 | 3.77 |
| Michigan State University | 507 | 3.7 |
| University of North Dakota | 507 | 3.8 |
| University of Kentucky | 506 | 3.82 |
| University of Houston | 506 | 3.59 |
| University of Mississippi | 505 | 3.53 |
| University of New Mexico | 505 | 3.76 |
| University of Puerto Rico | 505 | 3.81 |
| Charles R. Drew University of Medicine & Science | 505 | 3.5 |
| Morehouse University | 504 | 3.64 |
| Marshall University | 504 | 3.8 |

| MEDICAL SCHOOL | AVE. MCAT | AVE. GPA |
|---|---|---|
| Creighton University | 513 | 3.87 |
| SUNY Downstate | 513 | 3.73 |
| Temple University | 513 | 3.76 |
| Eastern Virginia University | 513 | 3.6 |
| California Northstate University College of Medicine | 510 | 3.7 |
| George Washington University School of Medicine and Health Science | 512 | 3.72 |
| Nova Southeastern University | 512 | 3.75 |
| Augusta University | 512 | 3.8 |
| University of Hawaii | 512 | 3.77 |
| University of Massachusetts | 512 | 3.87 |
| University of North Carolina | 512 | 3.79 |
| Albany Medical College | 512 | 3.78 |
| Texas A&M University | 512 | 3.86 |
| UT McGovern at Houston | 512 | 3.85 |
| Virginia Commonwealth | 512 | 3.79 |
| Virginia Tech | 512 | 3.65 |
| University of Vermont | 512 | 3.7 |
| Geisinger Commonwealth | 512 | 3.82 |
| University of Minnesota – Twin Cities | 511 | 3.77 |
| University of Minnesota– Duluth | 511 | 3.77 |
| California University of Science & Medicine | 510 | 3.7 |
| Frank H. Netter School of Medicine at Quinnipiac University | 511 | 3.7 |
| University of Illinois | 511 | 3.7 |
| Indiana University | 511 | 3.8 |
| Uniformed Services Univ. | 511 | 3.7 |
| Wake Forest University | 511 | 3.83 |

| MEDICAL SCHOOL | AVE. MCAT | AVE. GPA |
|---|---|---|
| Mercer University | 503 | 3.72 |
| Meharry Medical College | 503 | 3.46 |
| University Central Del Caribe | 501 | 3.8 |
| Ponce School of Medicine | 499 | 3.5 |
| San Juan Bautista SOM | 499 | 3.57 |
| University of Missouri (UMKC) | 495 | 3.94 |
| Western University | 508 | 3.66 |
| Midwestern University Chicago | 508 | 3.65 |
| Des Moines University | 507 | 3.71 |
| Rowan University | 507 | 3.6 |
| Western University Pacific NW | 507 | 3.62 |
| University of North Texas | 507 | 3.81 |
| Touro University, Nevada | 507 | 3.54 |
| Michigan State University | 507 | 3.6 |
| Touro University – CA | 506 | 3.58 |
| Rocky Vista University | 506 | 3.61 |
| Nova Southeastern University | 506 | 3.6 |
| New York Inst. of Technology | 506 | 3.62 |
| Sam Houston State University | 506 | 3.65 |
| Midwestern Univ. – AZ | 505 | 3.65 |
| Kansas City University | 505 | 3.62 |
| William Carey University | 505 | 3.53 |
| Campbell University | 505 | 3.61 |
| Philadelphia College | 505 | 3.5 |
| California Health Science Univ. | 504 | 3.54 |
| U. of the Incarnate Word | 504 | 3.6 |
| Liberty University | 504 | 3.6 |
| Idaho College | 504 | 3.56 |

## BS/DDS AND BS/DMD PROGRAMS

| INSTITUTION | DEGREE TRACK | DURATION |
|---|---|---|
| Boston University | BA/BS-DMD | 8 years |
| Case Western Reserve | BA/BS-DMD | 8 years |
| Howard University | BS/DDS, BS/DMD | 6–8 years |
| Marquette University | BS/DDS | 7 years |
| NYU | BA-DDS | 7 years |
| Nova Southeastern University | BS/DMD or BA/DMD | 6–8 years |
| Rutgers University | BS/DMD | 7 years |
| Temple University | BA/DMD | 7 years |
| University of Colorado Denver | BS/BA-DDS | 8 years |
| University of Connecticut | BS/DMD | 8 years |
| University of Detroit Mercy | BS/DDS | 7 years |
| University of Louisville | BS/DMD | 8 years |
| University of Pittsburgh | BS/DMD | 8 years |
| University of the Pacific | BS/DDS or BS/DMD | 5–7 years |
| Virginia Commonwealth U. | BS/DDS | 8 years |

## D.O. SCHOOLS LIST

**Note: COM is College of Osteopathic Medicine & SOM is School of Osteopathic Medicine**

| UNIVERSITY/PROGRAM | |
|---|---|
| **Alabama**<br>Alabama COM – Dothan<br>Edward Via COM – Auburn | **Mississippi**<br>William Carey University COM– Hattiesburg |
| **Arizona**<br>A.T. Still University – SOM – Mesa<br>Midwestern University – Arizona COM – Glendale | **Missouri**<br>Kansas City University COM – Kansas City & Joplin |
| **Arkansas**<br>Arkansas COM – Fort Smith<br>New York Institute of Technology COM at Arkansas State University – Jonesboro | **Montana**<br>Rocky Vista University – Montana COM – Billings<br>Touro COM – Great Falls |
| **California**<br>California Health Sciences University COM Touro University California COM – Vallejo Western University of Health Sciences COM of the Pacific – Pomona | **Nevada**<br>Touro University Nevada COM – Henderson |
| **Colorado**<br>Rocky Vista University COM – Parker | **New Jersey**<br>Rowan University SOM – Stratford & Sewell |
| **Florida**<br>Burrell COM - Melbourne<br>Lake Erie COM – Bradenton<br>Nova Southeastern University Dr. Kiran C. Patel COM – Fort Lauderdale & Clearwater Orlando COM – Winter Garden | **New Mexico**<br>Burrell COM - Las Cruces |
| | **New York**<br>New York Institute of Technology COM – Old Westbury<br>Touro COM – Harlem & Middletown |
| **Georgia**<br>Philadelphia COM – Suwanee & South Georgia | **North Carolina**<br>Campbell University Jerry M. Wallace SOM – Buies Creek |
| **Idaho**<br>Idaho COM – Meridian | **Ohio**<br>Ohio University Heritage COM – Athens, Cleveland & Dublin |
| **Illinois**<br>Illinois COM (opening 2026)<br>Midwestern University Chicago COM – Downers Grove | **Oklahoma**<br>Oklahoma State University Center for Health Sciences COM – Tulsa & Cherokee Nation |
| **Indiana**<br>Marian University COM – Indianapolis | **Pennsylvania**<br>Lake Erie COM – Elmira & Seton Hill<br>Philadelphia COM – Philadelphia |
| **Iowa**<br>Des Moines University COM – Des Moines | **South Carolina**<br>Edward Via COM – Spartanburg |

| UNIVERSITY/PROGRAM | |
|---|---|
| **Kansas** <br> Kansas Health Science University – Kansas COM – Wichita | **Tennessee** <br> Baptist Health Sciences University COM – Memphis Lincoln Memorial University DeBusk COM – Harrogate & Knoxville |
| **Kentucky** <br> University of Pikeville – Kentucky COM – Pikeville | **Texas** <br> Sam Houston State University COM – Conroe <br> University of the Incarnate Word SOM – San Antonio <br> University of North Texas Health Science Center Texas COM – Fort Worth |
| **Louisiana** <br> Edward Via COM – Monroe | **Utah** <br> Noorda COM – Provo <br> Rocky Vista University COM – Ivins |
| **Maine** <br> University of New England COM – Biddeford | **Virginia** <br> Liberty University COM – Lynchburg <br> Edward Via COM (Virginia Tech) – Blacksburg |
| **Maryland** <br> Meritus SOM – Hagerstown | **Washington** <br> Pacific Northwest University of Health Sciences COM – Yakima |
| **Michigan** <br> Michigan State University COM – East Lansing, Detroit & Clinton Township | **West Virginia** <br> West Virginia SOM – Lewisburg |

## DENTAL SCHOOLS LIST

| DENTAL SCHOOLS | |
|---|---|
| **Alabama** | |
| Univ. of AL at Birmingham School of Dentistry | |
| **Arizona** | |
| A.T. Still Univ., AZ School of Dentistry & Oral Health | Midwestern Univ. College of Dental Medicine-AZ |
| **Arkansas** | |
| Lyon College School of Dental Medicine | |
| **California** | UCLA School of Dentistry |
| CA Northstate College of Dental Medicine | UCSF School of Dentistry |
| Herman Ostrow School of Dentistry of USC | Univ. of the Pacific Arthur A. Dugoni School of Dentistry |
| Loma Linda Univ. School of Dentistry | Western U. of Health Sci. College of Dental Medicine |
| **Colorado** | |
| Univ. of CO School of Dental Medicine | |
| **Connecticut** | |
| Univ. of CT School of Dental Medicine | |
| **District of Columbia** | |
| Howard Univ. College of Dentistry | |
| **Florida** | Nova Southeastern Univ. College of Dental Medicine |
| LECOM School of Dental Medicine | Univ. of Florida College of Dentistry |
| **Georgia** | |
| Dental College of GA at Augusta Univ | |
| **Illinois** | Southern Illinois Univ. School of Dental Medicine |
| Midwestern Univ. College of Dental Medicine-IL | Univ. of Illinois College of Dentistry |
| **Indiana** | |
| Indiana Univ. School of Dentistry | |
| **Iowa** | |
| Univ. of Iowa College of Dentistry | |
| **Kentucky** | |
| Univ. of Kentucky College of Dentistry | Univ. of Louisville School of Dentistry |
| **Louisiana** | |
| LSU School of Dentistry | |
| **Maine** | |
| Univ. of New England College of Dental Medicine | |
| **Maryland** | |
| Univ. of Maryland School of Dentistry | |

# LISTS AND GUIDES

| DENTAL SCHOOLS | |
|---|---|
| **Massachusetts** | Harvard School of Dental Medicine |
| Boston Univ. School of Dental Medicine | Tufts Univ. School of Dental Medicine |
| **Michigan** | |
| Univ. of Detroit Mercy School of Dentistry | Univ. of Michigan School of Dentistry |
| **Minnesota** | |
| Univ. of Minnesota School of Dentistry | |
| **Mississippi** | |
| Univ. of MS Medical Center School of Dentistry | |
| **Missouri** | Kansas City Univ. College of Dental Medicine |
| A.T. Still Univ. MO School of Dentistry & Oral Health | UMKC School of Dentistry |
| **Nebraska** | |
| Creighton Univ. School of Dentistry | Univ. of Nebraska Medical Ctr College of Dentistry |
| **Nevada** | |
| Roseman Univ. of Health Science College of Dental Medicine | Univ. of Nevada, Las Vegas School of Dental Medicine |
| **New Jersey** | |
| Rutgers School of Dental Medicine | |
| **New York** | Stony Brook Univ. School of Dental Medicine |
| Columbia Univ. College of Dental Medicine | Touro College of Dental Medicine at NYMC |
| NYU College of Dentistry | Univ. at Buffalo School of Dental Medicine |
| **North Carolina** | |
| East Carolina Univ. School of Dental Medicine | UNC Chapel Hill School of Dentistry |
| **Ohio** | |
| Case Western Reserve School of Dental Medicine | The Ohio State Univ. College of Dentistry |
| **Oklahoma** | |
| Univ. of Oklahoma College of Dentistry | |
| **Oregon** | |
| OR Health & Science Univ. School of Dentistry | |
| **Pennsylvania** | UPenn School of Dental Medicine |
| Temple Univ. School of Dentistry | Univ. of Pittsburgh School of Dental Medicine |
| **Puerto Rico** | |
| Univ. of Puerto Rico School of Dental Medicine | |
| **South Carolina** | |
| Univ. of S. Carolina College of Dental Medicine | |
| **Tennessee** | UT Health Sci. Ctr at San Antonio School of Dentistry |
| | Texas Tech School of Dental Medicine, Univ. Health |
| Lincoln Memorial Univ. College of Dental Medicine | Science Center, El Paso |

| DENTAL SCHOOLS | |
|---|---|
| **Texas** | |
| Texas A&M Univ. School of Dentistry<br>UT Health Sci. Ctr at Houston School of Dentistry | UT Health Sci. Ctr at San Antonio School of Dentistry<br>Texas Tech School of Dental Medicine, Univ. Health<br>Sci. Ctr El Paso |
| **Utah** | |
| Roseman Univ. of Health Science College of<br>Dental Medicine | Univ. of Utah School of Dentistry |
| **Virginia** | |
| Univ. of Washington School of Dentistry | |
| **Washington** | |
| Univ. of WA School of Dentistry | |
| **West Virginia** | |
| West Virginia U. School of Dentistry | |
| **Wisconsin** | |
| Marquette Univ. School of Dentistry | |

# PHARMD SCHOOLS LIST

| PHARMD SCHOOLS | |
|---|---|
| **Alabama** | |
| Auburn University Harrison College of Pharmacy<br>Samford University McWhorter School of Pharmacy | |
| **Alaska** | |
| University of Alaska Anchorage/Idaho State University Doctor of Pharmacy Program | |
| **Arizona** | |
| Midwestern University College of Pharmacy–Glendale<br>University of Arizona R. Ken Coit College of Pharmacy | |
| **Arkansas** | |
| Harding University College of Pharmacy<br>University of Arkansas for Medical Sciences College of Pharmacy | |
| **California** | |
| American University of Health Sciences<br>California Health Sciences University<br>California Northstate University<br>Chapman University<br>Keck Graduate Institute<br>Loma Linda University | Marshall B. Ketchum University<br>Touro University California<br>UC Irvine; UC San Diego<br>UC San Francisco<br>University of the Pacific<br>USC Alfred E. Mann School<br>West Coast University<br>Western University of Health Sciences |
| **Colorado** | |
| Regis University<br>University of Colorado Skaggs School of Pharmacy | |

## PHARMD SCHOOLS

### Connecticut

University of Connecticut
University of Saint Joseph

### District of Columbia

Howard University College of Pharmacy

### Florida

Florida A&M University
LECOM Bradenton
Larkin University

Palm Beach Atlantic University
University of Florida
University of South Florida
Nova Southeastern University

### Georgia

Mercer University
PCOM Georgia

South University
University of Georgia

### Hawaii

University of Hawaii at Hilo

### Idaho

Idaho State University College of Pharmacy

### Illinois

Chicago State University
Midwestern University Chicago
Roosevelt University

Rosalind Franklin University
SIU Edwardsville
University of Illinois at Chicago

### Indiana

Butler University

Manchester University
Purdue University

### Iowa

Drake University

University of Iowa

### Kansas

University of Kansas School of Pharmacy

### Kentucky

Sullivan University

University of Kentucky

### Louisiana

University of Louisiana at Monroe

Xavier University of Louisiana

### Maine

Husson University

University of New England

### Maryland

Notre Dame of Maryland University

University of Maryland Eastern Shore
University of Maryland Baltimore

### Massachusetts

MCPHS Boston
MCPHS Worcester

Northeastern University
Western New England University

| PHARMD SCHOOLS | |
|---|---|
| **Michigan** | |
| Ferris State University | University of Michigan<br>Wayne State University |
| **Minnesota** | |
| University of Minnesota College of Pharmacy | |
| **Mississippi** | |
| University of Mississippi | William Carey University |
| **Missouri** | |
| University of Health Sciences and Pharmacy in St. Louis | University of Missouri–Kansas City |
| **Montana** | |
| University of Montana Skaggs School of Pharmacy | |
| **Nebraska** | |
| Creighton University | University of Nebraska Medical Center |
| **Nevada** | |
| Roseman University of Health Sciences | |
| **New Hampshire** | |
| MCPHS Manchester | |
| **New Jersey** | |
| Fairleigh Dickinson University | Rutgers University |
| **New Mexico** | |
| University of New Mexico College of Pharmacy | |
| **New York** | Long Island University<br>St. John Fisher University |
| Albany College of Pharmacy<br>Binghamton University<br>D'Youville University | St. John's University<br>Touro College of Pharmacy<br>University at Buffalo |
| **North Carolina** | |
| Campbell University<br>Wingate University | High Point University<br>UNC Chapel Hill |
| **North Dakota** | |
| North Dakota State University | |
| **Ohio** | Ohio State University |
| Cedarville University<br>NEOMED<br>Ohio Northern University | University of Cincinnati<br>University of Findlay<br>University of Toledo |
| **Oklahoma** | |
| Southwestern Oklahoma State University | University of Oklahoma |

# LISTS AND GUIDES

| PHARMD SCHOOLS | |
|---|---|
| **Oregon** | |
| Oregon State University | Pacific University |
| **Pennsylvania** | |
| | Temple University |
| Duquesne University | Thomas Jefferson University |
| LECOM Erie | University of Pittsburgh |
| Saint Joseph's University | Wilkes University |
| **Puerto Rico** | |
| University of Puerto Rico School of Pharmacy | |
| **Rhode Island** | |
| University of Rhode Island | |
| **South Carolina** | |
| Medical University of South Carolina | South Carolina College of Pharmacy |
| Presbyterian College | University of South Carolina |
| **South Dakota** | |
| South Dakota State University | |
| **Tennessee** | Lipscomb University |
| | South College |
| Belmont University | Union University |
| East Tennessee State University | University of Tennessee |
| **Texas** | University of Houston |
| | UNT Health Science Center |
| Texas A&M University | UT Austin; UT El Paso |
| Texas Southern University | UT Tyler |
| Texas Tech University | University of the Incarnate Word |
| **Utah** | |
| University of Utah College of Pharmacy | |
| **Virginia** | |
| Appalachian College of Pharmacy | Shenandoah University |
| Hampton University | Virginia Commonwealth University |
| **Washington** | |
| University of Washington | Washington State University |
| **West Virginia** | University of Charleston |
| Marshall University | West Virginia University |
| **Wisconsin** | Medical College of Wisconsin |
| Concordia University Wisconsin | University of Wisconsin–Madison |
| **Wyoming** | |
| University of Wyoming School of Pharmacy | |

# VET SCHOOLS LIST

## US & INTERNATIONAL VETERINARY MEDICAL SCHOOLS

### ALABAMA

Auburn University
College of Veterinary Medicine

Tuskegee University
College of Veterinary Medicine

### ARIZONA

Midwestern University College of Veterinary Medicine

University of Arizona
College of Veterinary Medicine

### CALIFORNIA

University of California, Davis
School of Veterinary Medicine

Western University of Health Sciences
College of Veterinary Medicine

### COLORADO

Colorado State University
College of Veterinary Medicine and Biomedical Sciences Fort

### FLORIDA

University of Florida
College of Veterinary Medicine,

### GEORGIA

University of Georgia
College of Veterinary Medicine

### ILLINOIS

University of Illinois
College of Veterinary Medicine

### INDIANA

Purdue University
College of Veterinary Medicine

### IOWA

Iowa State University
College of Veterinary Medicine

### KANSAS

Kansas State University College of Veterinary Medicine

### LOUISIANA

Louisiana State University
School of Veterinary Medicine

### MASSACHUSETTS

Tufts University
School of Veterinary Medicine

### MICHIGAN

Michigan State University
College of Veterinary Medicine

### MINNESOTA

University of Minnesota College of Veterinary Medicine

### MISSISSIPPI

Mississippi State University
College of Veterinary Medicine

### MISSOURI

University of Missouri-Columbia College of Veterinary Medicine

### NEW JERSEY

Rowan University
Shreiber School of Veterinary Medicine

### NEW YORK

College of Veterinary Medicine
Long Island University

### NEW YORK

Cornell University
College of Veterinary Medicine

### NORTH CAROLINA

North Carolina State University
College of Veterinary Medicine

### OHIO

The Ohio State University
College of Veterinary Medicine

### OKLAHOMA

Oklahoma State University
College of Veterinary Medicine

### OREGON

Oregon State University College of Veterinary Medicine

### PENNSYLVANIA

University of Pennsylvania
School of Veterinary Medicine

### TENNESSEE

University of Tennessee
College of Veterinary Medicine

Lincoln Memorial University
College of Veterinary Medicine

### TEXAS

Texas A&M University
College of Veterinary Medicine & Biomedical Sciences

### TEXAS

Texas Tech University
School of Veterinary Medicine & Biomedical Sciences

### UTAH

Utah State University
College of Veterinary Medicine

### VIRGINIA

Virginia-Maryland College of Veterinary Medicine
Virginia Tech

### WASHINGTON

Washington State University
College of Veterinary Medicine

### WISCONSIN

University of Wisconsin-Madison
School of Veterinary Medicine

## AUSTRALIA

**MELBOURNE**
University of Melbourne
Melbourne Veterinary School

**QUEENSLAND**
University of Queensland
School of Veterinary Science

**SYDNEY**
The University of Sydney
School of Veterinary Science

**WESTERN AUSTRALIA**
Murdoch University College of
Veterinary Medicine, Murdoch

## CANADA

**ALBERTA**
University of Calgary
Faculty of Veterinary Medicine

**ONTARIO**
University of Guelph Ontario
Veterinary College Guelph,

**PRINCE EDWARD ISLAND**
University of Prince Edward Island
Atlantic Veterinary College

**QUEBEC**
Université de Montréal
Faculté de Médecine Vétérinaire

**SASKATCHEWAN**
University of Saskatchewan
Western College of Veterinary
Medicine

## FRANCE

**LYON**
VetAgro Sup
l'École Nationale des Services
Vétérinaires à Lyon

## IRELAND

**DUBLIN**
University College, Dublin
School of Veterinary Medicine

## KOREA

**SEOUL**
Seoul National University
College of Veterinary Medicine

## MEXICO

**COYOACAN**
Universidad Nacional
Autonoma de México
Facultad de Medicina
Veterinaria y Zootecnia

## NEW ZEALAND

**PALMERSTON NORTH**
Massey University
School of Veterinary Science

## PUERTO RICO

Universidad Ana G. Mendez
School of Veterinary Medicine

## SCOTLAND

**EDINBURGH**
The University of Edinburgh
Royal Dick School of Veterinary
Studies

**GLASGOW**
University of Glasgow
School of Biodiversity, One
Health and Veterinary Medicine

## THE NETHERLANDS

**UTRECHT**
Utrecht University
School of Veterinary Medicine

## UNITED KINGDOM

**BRISTOL**
University of Bristol
Bristol Veterinary School

**LEICESTERSHIRE**
University of Nottingham
School of Veterinary Medicine
and Science

**LIVERPOOL**
University of Liverpool School
of Veterinary Science

**LONDON**
University of London
The Royal Veterinary College

## WEST INDIES

**ST.KITT**
Ross University
School of Veterinary Medicine
Basseterre

**WEST INDIES**
St. George's University School
of Veterinary Medicine

## BS/MD TIMELINE

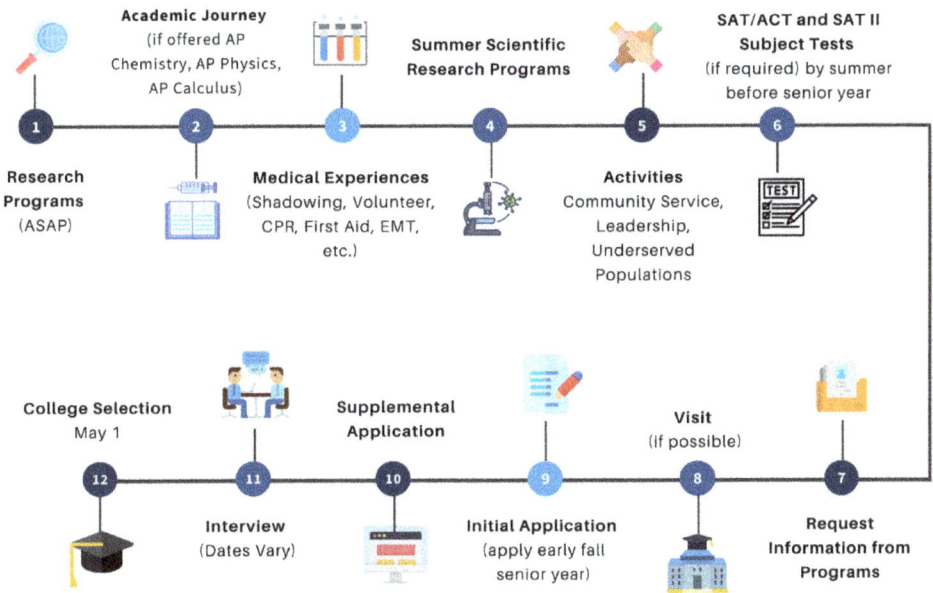

| BS/MD PROGRAMS | INITIAL APPLICATION DATES | BS/MD SUPPLEMENTAL APPLICATION DATES | INTERVIEW DATES |
|---|---|---|---|
|  |  |  |  |
|  |  |  |  |
|  |  |  |  |
|  |  |  |  |
|  |  |  |  |
|  |  |  |  |
|  |  |  |  |
|  |  |  |  |
|  |  |  |  |
|  |  |  |  |
|  |  |  |  |

# INDEX

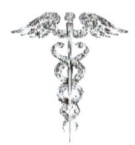

## A

Accreditation Council for Occupational Therapy Education (ACOTE) — 22

Accreditation Council for Pharmacy Education (ACPE) — 21

Accreditation Review Commission on Education for the Physician Assistant (ARC-PA) — 22

Adelphi University — 295, 301, 341

Albany Medical College — 304, 305, 307, 341, 345

Albert Schweitzer — 42

Allopathic Medicine — 20, 165

AMCAS — 10, 11, 17, 21, 174, 211, 217, 218, 219, 225, 253, 288, 315

American Academy of Physician Assistants (AAPA) — 22

American Association of Colleges of Nursing (AACN) — 22

American Association of Colleges of Podiatry Medicine (AACPM) — 21

American Association of Medical Colleges (AAMC) — 21, 235

American Association of Nurse Practitioners (AANP) — 22

American Chiropractic Association (ACA) — 22

American Dental Association (ADA) — 21

American Dental Education Association (ADEA) — 21

American Medical College Application Service — 11, 217

American Occupational Therapy Association — 22

American Osteopathic Association (AOA) — 21

American Pharmacists Association (APhA) — 21

American Physical Therapy Association (APTA) — 22,

American Psychological Association (APA) — 21, 69

American Veterinary Medical Association (AVMA) — 21

Amherst College — 97, 229

Application Process — 43, 156, 172, 173, 174, 178, 201, 267, 279, 280, 287, 308, 309, 337

AP Tests — 39, 40, 280

Association of American Veterinary Medical Colleges (AAVMC) — 21

Association of Chiropractic Colleges (ACC) — 22

Association of Optometrists (AOP) — 21

Association of Schools and Colleges of Optometry (ASCO) — 21

Athletic Trainer — 23,

Auburn University — 78

Audiologist — 23

Augusta University — 321, 325, 340, 345

# B

Baylor University — 113, 342

Benjamin Franklin — 32, 192

Biology, Chemistry, Physics, and Math (BCPM) — 11, 218

Boston College — 96, 229

Boston University — 96, 283, 343, 346

Brooklyn College — 104, 295, 301, 341

Brown University — 111

Bureau of Labor Statistics — 19, 21, 22

Bureau of Osteopathic Specialists — 21

# C

Caldwell University — 340

California Northstate University — 333, 334, 340, 345, 351

Capstone Diploma — 40

Cardiovascular Technologist — 23

Carnegie Mellon — 48, 61, 110

Case Western Reserve University — 186, 203, 206, 254, 341, 341

CASPer — 113

Cedars Sinai — 48–51

Certifying Board Services (CBS) — 21

Chadron State College — 313, 342

Chiropractor — 20

City College of New York — 104, 295, 302

Clark Scholars Program — 48, 115

Clemson University — 112

Clinical Experience — 51, 202

Clinical Laboratory Technician — 23

Clinical Laboratory Technologist — 23

Coalition Application — 225, 243, 244, 361

Coca Cola Scholarship — 274

Cognitive Science — 84

College Credit — 84, 97

Columbia University — 104

Commission on Accreditation in Physical Therapy Education (CAPTE) — 22, 23

Common Application — 243

Community College — 34, 122, 148, 179

Community Involvement — 241

Contests — 59, 69

Cornell University — 48, 105, 283, 355

COSMOS — 48, 80

Cost of Attendance — 296, 297, 298, 299, 300, 301, 302, 303, 304, 305, 306, 307, 308, 309, 310, 311, 314, 315, 316, 317, 318, 319, 322, 323, 324, 325, 326, 327, 328, 329, 330, 331, 334, 335, 336, 337

Council on Academic Accreditation in Audiology and Speech Language Pathology — 22

Council on Chiropractic Education — 22

Council on Podiatric Medical Education (CPME) — 21

COVID-19 — 6, 25, 26, 29

CUNY School of Medicine — 172, 180, 184, 185, 301, 302

# D

Debt Burden — 269, 277

Dental Assistant — 23

Department of Veterans Affairs — 270

Diagnostic Medical Sonographer — 23

Dietician (RD, RDN) — 23

Direct Med Program — 17, 126, 127, 140, 141, 201, 203, 209, 211

Dispensing Optician — 23

Drexel University — 110, 295, 308, 341, 343

Duke University — 108, 229

Duquesne University — 295, 305, 308, 341, 341, 354

## E

Early Action (EA) — 227

Early Assurance Program — 175, 255, 308, 309, 319, 329, 340

Early Decision (ED) — 227

Early Medical School Acceptance Program — 322

Elements — 1

Emergency Medical Technician — 23

Emory University — 89, 229

Euclid of Alexandria — 1, 14

Exercise Physiologists — 1, 14

## F

Fisk University — 342

Florida International University — 88, 321, 340, 343

Florida Southern College — 321, 340

## G

Gannon University — 110, 295, 309

Gates Millennium Scholarship — 274

Genetics Counselors — 23

Georgetown University — 87

George Washington University — 199, 321, 323, 340, 345

Georgia Institute of Technology — 89

Gettysburg College — 110

Grambling State University — 340

Guaranteed Professional Programs Admissions — 11

## H

Hackathons — 61, 62, 110

Hampton University — 342, 354

Harvard University — 97

Harvey Mudd — 81, 229

Haverford College — 110

Health Information Technician — 23, 23

Hippocrates — 130, 134, 212

Hispanic Scholarship Fund — 275

Hofstra University — 105, 202, 295, 303, 305, 341, 343

Home Health Aide — 23

Honors Program in Medical Education — 11

Howard University — 340, 344, 346, 352

## I

Illinois Institute of Technology — 91

Indiana State University — 342

Indiana University — 93

Indiana University School of Medicine — 315

Indian Health Service — 270

Internships — 58, 78, 79, 80, 85, 86, 87, 88, 90, 91, 92, 93, 94, 95, 96, 99, 100, 101, 102, 103, 104, 108, 109, 110, 111, 112, 113, 115, 116, 117, 119, 163

Interviews — 2, 2, 3, 59, 74, 140, 152, 157, 168, 201, 224, 249, 257, 263, 289, 302, 304, 307, 309, 315, 319, 322, 325, 328, 329

## J

John Carroll University — 313, 319

John Jay College — 105

# K

Khan Academy — 37, 122, 132
Kinesiologist — 23

# L

Lake Erie College of Osteopathic
        Medicine — 11, 203, 297, 300,
        301, 309
Lehigh University — 110, 341
Letters of Recommendation — 132, 135,
        136, 140, 149, 207, 211, 215, 224,
        239, 255, 287, 288
LinkedIn — 248
Loyola University Chicago — 340, 343

# M

Marshall University — 342, 344, 354
Massachusetts College of Pharmacy and
        Health Sciences — 295, 297
Massachusetts Institute of Technology
        — 97
Massage Therapist — 23
Medical Assistant — 23
Medical College Admissions Test — 219
Medical College of Georgia — 325
Medical Records Assistant — 23
Medical Scholars Program — 11, 17,
        202, 203, 307, 314, 325
Medical Transcriptionist — 23
Meharry Medical College — 345
Mercer University — 340, 342, 345, 352
Michigan Math and Science Scholars —
        48
Michigan State University — 48, 99, 203,
        344, 348, 355
Midwife — 23
Minority Introduction to Engineering

and Science — 11, 48, 97
Missouri Southern State Univ. — 313
Monmouth University — 341
Montclair University — 340, 342
Morsani College of Medicine — 324
MRI Technologist — 23

# N

National Institutes of Health — 87, 270
Networking — 62, 78, 79, 81, 85, 86, 87,
        88, 89, 90, 91, 92, 94, 95, 96, 99,
        100, 101, 102, 103, 105, 108, 109,
        110, 112, 114, 116, 117, 119
Neuroplasticity — 91
Neuropsychology — 96
New Jersey Institute of Technology —
        102, 295, 298
New York Institute of Technology — 203,
        206, 295, 303, 306, 347
New York University — 106
Northwestern University — 91, 254, 343
Nova Southeastern University — 185,
        203, 321, 324, 340, 345, 346, 347,
        352
Nuclear Medicine Technologists — 23
Nurse Anesthetist — 22
Nurse Practitioner (NP) — 22
Nursing — 22, 23, 44, 359
Nursing Assistant (CNA) — 23
Nutritionist — 23

# O

Occupational Therapy — 22, 23
Occupational Therapy Assistant — 23
Optometry — 21, 297
Orderly — 23, 365
Organic Chemistry — 28, 217, 218, 286
Orthotists — 23, 365

Osteopathic Medicine — 7, 11, 21, 165, 167, 203, 206, 217, 236, 297, 299, 300, 301, 303, 305, 306, 308, 309, 316, 317, 319, 324, 347

# P

Paramedics — 23
Pennsylvania State University — 111
Personal Statement — 29, 136, 140, 144, 145, 149, 224, 233, 243, 252, 272, 318, 329
Pharmacy — 21, 23, 107, 213, 214, 215, 217, 295, 297, 341, 341, 351, 352, 353, 354
Pharmacy Technician — 23
Philadelphia College of Osteopathic Medicine — 203, 301
Phlebotomist — 23
Physical Therapist (PT) — 20
Physical Therapy Assistant — 23
Physician's Assistant — 14, 20
Pittsburg State University — 313, 316
Podiatry — 21
Portal — 279, 280
Post-Bacc programs — 218
President's Volunteer Service Award — 45
Princeton University — 66, 102
Program in Liberal Medical Education (PLME) — 172, 202, 206, 253, 342
Prosthetists — 23
Psychiatric Aide — 23
Psychiatric Disorders — 104
Psychiatry — 23
Psychology — 16, 21, 65, 69, 83, 84, 89, 92, 104, 105, 108, 114, 273
Public Service Loan Forgiveness (PSLF) — 270
Purchase College — 106, 341

Purdue University — 93

# Q

Questbridge Scholarship — 276

# R

Radiation Therapists — 23
Radiologic Technologist — 23
Recreational Therapist — 23
Registered Nurse — 23
Regular Decision — 11, 227, 228, 229, 268, 311
Rensselaer Polytechnic Institute — 295, 304, 341, 341, 366
Research Apprenticeship in Biological Sciences — 48
Research in the Biological Sciences (RIBS) — 92
Research Science Institute — 48, 98
Respiratory Therapist — 23
Resume — 118
Rice University — 114, 229, 254
RISE — 48, 96, 136
Rochester Institute of Technology — 106, 341
Rochester Institute of Technology (RIT) — 307, 341
Rosemont College — 341
ROTC — 276
Rowan University — 203, 295, 299, 343, 345, 347, 355
Rutgers University — 202, 295, 299, 300, 340, 340, 346, 353

# S

Saint Louis University — 344
Scholarships — 63, 66, 70, 78, 270, 274, 276

Shadowing — 10, 51, 168, 184, 213, 233, 287

Sidney Kimmel Medical College — 309

Siena College — 295, 305, 341

Social Media — 87, 277

Southern Methodist University — 115

Speech Pathologist — 20, 22

Spelman College — 340

Stamps Scholarship — 99

Stanford Institutes of Medicine Summer Research Program (SIMR) — 8

St. Bonaventure University — 295, 305

Stevens Institute of Technology — 295, 300

St. George's University — 340, 356

Stockton University — 295, 300

Stony Brook University — 107, 202, 203, 255, 295, 306, 341, 344

Summer Academy for Math & Science (SAMS) — 110

Summer Programs — 82, 83, 85, 93, 95, 104, 115, 118

Summer Science Program — 48, 85, 93, 103, 108

SUNY Old Westbury — 295, 306

SUNY Polytechnic Institute — 310, 341

SUNY Upstate Medical University — 255

Super-Score — 181

T

Temple University — 111, 341, 345, 346, 354

Test Prep — 38, 39, 152, 155, 233

Texas A&M — 113, 114

Texas JAMP — 342

Texas Tech University — 321, 328, 342, 344, 354, 355

Touro College of Osteopathic Medicine — 203

Tufts University — 98, 175, 229, 255, 283, 340, 340, 340, 344, 355

Tulane University — 229

U

Ultrasound Technician — 23

Uniformed Services University — 270

Union College — 295, 307, 341, 341

University of Alabama — 321, 322, 340, 343

University of Arizona — 79

University of California, Berkeley — 83

University of California, Davis — 84

University of California, Merced — 333

University of California, San Diego — 84

University of California, San Francisco — 343

University of California, Santa Barbara — 84

University of Chicago — 48, 92, 343

University of Cincinnati — 313, 319, 353

University of Colorado — 85, 333, 335, 340, 343, 346, 351

University of Connecticut — 180, 202, 203, 295, 296, 340, 344, 346, 352

University of Delaware — 340

University of Evansville — 313, 315, 342

University of Florida — 88

University of Houston — 115, 321, 328, 344

University of Illinois — 62, 92

University of Illinois, Chicago — 314, 340, 342

University of Louisville — 342, 344, 346

University of Maryland — 65, 95, 96

University of Miami — 88, 283, 340, 340, 344

University of Michigan — 62, 99

University of Minnesota — 265, 342, 345, 353, 355

University of Missouri, Kansas City — 11, 317, 340, 340

University of Nebraska — 101, 318, 344, 353

University of Nevada — 102, 333, 337, 341, 342, 343, 344

University of New Mexico — 333, 336, 341, 341, 342, 342, 344, 353

University of North Carolina — 108

University of Notre Dame — 93

University of Oklahoma — 109, 321, 326, 341, 341, 343, 353

University of Pittsburgh — 111, 202, 203, 255, 295, 310, 341, 341, 344, 346, 354

University of Rochester — 13, 107, 202, 206, 255, 265, 295, 307, 343

University of South Alabama — 321, 322, 340, 340, 344

University of South Carolina — 112, 321, 343, 344, 354

University of Southern California — 84

University of South Florida — 181, 321, 324, 340, 340, 343, 352

University of Texas at Austin — 115

University of Texas at Dallas — 321, 329

University of Texas Rio Grande Valley — 321, 329

University of the Sciences — 341, 341

University of Toledo — 341, 344, 353

University of Washington — 118

University of Wisconsin — 119

U.S. Census Bureau — 2, 19, 292, 292

# V

Veterinary Assistant — 23

Veterinary Medicine — 21, 213, 215, 355, 356

Veterinary Technologist — 23

Virginia Commonwealth University — 117, 321, 330, 342, 342, 354

Virginia Tech — 116, 117

Volunteer Service Award — 45

# W

Waitlist — 228

Warren Alpert Medical School — 311

Washington and Jefferson College — 341

Washington College — 321

Washington University — 87, 100

Washington University in St. Louis — 100, 343

Wayne State University — 202, 340, 340, 344, 353

Wellesley College — 98

West Chester University — 342, 342

West Virginia University — 321, 331, 343, 354

William & Mary — 229

Williams College — 229

Women's Technology Program — 48, 98

# Y

Yeshiva University — 341

# Z

Zucker School of Medicine at Hofstra/ Northwell — 303